[illegible]

A HISTORY OF
JEWISH GYNAECOLOGICAL TEXTS
IN THE MIDDLE AGES

BRILL'S SERIES IN JEWISH STUDIES

GENERAL EDITOR

DAVID S. KATZ (Tel Aviv)

ADVISORY EDITORS

STUART COHEN (Bar-Ilan)

ANTHONY T. GRAFTON (Princeton)

YOSEF KAPLAN (Jerusalem)

FERGUS MILLAR (Oxford)

VOL. XX

A HISTORY OF JEWISH GYNAECOLOGICAL TEXTS IN THE MIDDLE AGES

BY

RON BARKAI

BRILL
LEIDEN · BOSTON · KÖLN
1998

This book is printed on acid-free paper.

RG
85
.B369
1998

Library of Congress Cataloging-in-Publication Data

Barkai, Ron.
A history of Jewish gynaecological texts in the middle ages / by Ron Barkai.
p. cm. — (Brill's series in Jewish studies, ISSN 0926–2261 ; vol. 20)
Includes bibliographical references and index.
ISBN 9004109951 (cloth : alk. paper)
1. Gynecology—Early works to 1800. 2. Medicine, Medieval. 3. Jews—Medicine—History—Sources. I. Title. II. Series.
RG85.B369 1998
618.1'009'02—dc21 97–52122
CIP

Die Deutsche Bibliothek – CIP-Einheitsaufnahme

Barqây, Rôn:
A history of jewish gynaecological texts in the middle ages / by Ron Barkai. – Leiden ; New York ; Köln : Brill, 1998
(Brill's series in Jewish studies ; Vol. 20)
ISBN 90-04-10995–1

ISSN 0926-2261
ISBN 90 04 10995 1

© Copyright 1998 by Koninklijke Brill NV, Leiden, The Netherlands

All rights reserved. No part of this publication may be reproduced, translated, stored in a retrieval system, or transmitted in any form or by any means, electronic, mechanical, photocopying, recording or otherwise, without prior written permission from the publisher.

Authorization to photocopy items for internal or personal use is granted by Brill provided that the appropriate fees are paid directly to The Copyright Clearance Center, 222 Rosewood Drive, Suite 910 Danvers MA 01923, USA. Fees are subject to change.

PRINTED IN THE NETHERLANDS

Para mi consuelo

For my daughters Adva and Moran

CONTENTS

PART TWO: JEWISH GYNAECOLOGICAL TEXTS

ACKNOWLEDGEMENTS

This volume could not have seen the light of day without the help and encouragement of a number of institutions, friends and colleagues. No amount of words can adequately express my gratitude.

The book was completed during the 1994-1995 academic year, while on sabbatical in Salamanca, Spain. Thanks to this sabbatical, awarded to me by the Ministry of Science and Higher education of the Government of Spain in cooperation with the University of Salamanca, I was able to devote part of the year to completing the required research. I was privileged to receive the assistance and support of colleagues and friends, who also strove to make my stay in this ancient university town truly agreeable. Special thanks to Prof. Carlos Carrete Parrondo, of the Department of Aramaic and Hebrew Studies, who made every effort to guarantee that the sabbatical would be both effective and enjoyable; to Prof. Felipe Maíllo Salgado, of the Department of Arabic Studies, whose vast knowledge and sincere friendship strongly influenced me; and to Prof. Martine Torrens-Frandji, who was always ready to respond to my every request.

Historical research of this sort is highly dependent on the assistance of curators and librarians, whose intense love for ancient manuscripts and wealth of information, transmitted with such humility, permit the historian to reveal the legacies bequeathed by time. Among the many who helped me, I would like to make special mention of my friend, Michel Garel, Chief Curator of Hebrew Manuscripts, the National Library, Paris, who made inordinate efforts in assisting me while I conducted my research in this Library, and who relayed information crucial to the project even from afar. I would also like to extend special, heartfelt thanks to the personnel of the Department of Oriental Manuscripts, the Bodleian Library, Oxford, as well to the dedicated, gracious staff of the Institute of Hebrew Manuscripts, the National Library, Jerusalem.

But most of all, I owe a lasting debt to Prof. Monica H. Green of the Department of History, Duke University, Durham, North Carolina. Prof. Green's unique personality combines an extraordinary knowledge about medieval Latin gynaecology with exceptional analytic skills, ample curiosity about subjects touching upon her work and, not least, a passion for generous, collegial sharing of ideas. My many conversations with her, our intensive exchange of letters, in which she has not only critically commented upon my ideas but also offered to let me peruse her yet unpublished work, enabled me to correct erroneous assumptions I had previously held as well as immeasurably improve the form and the content of the present volume. As the reader will soon note, I am indebted to her for the identification of important medieval gynaecological texts translated from Latin into Hebrew.

I would also like to express my thanks to my friend Dr. Ilana Bat-El, who reviewed the preliminary English version of this work, and to Nina Reshef, who edited the final text and prepared it for publication. I am sincerely grateful to them both.

ABBREVIATIONS AND SIGLA

LSM 3	*Liber de sinthomatibus mulierum*, version 3
DPM B	*De passionibus mulierum*, version B
P	Parma manuscript
P. M.	Pessarium Muscionis
[...]	lacuna in the manuscript
[ ]	text reconstructed according to another manuscript
{ }	reconstructed according to the latin text

PART ONE

JEWISH MEDICINE AND HEBREW GYNAECOLOGY

INTRODUCTION

The history of medicine has come to occupy an important place in the *general histories* of ancient, medieval and modern societies in the last few decades. The history of medicine is no longer the preserve of a few scholars having a special interest in the area. This branch of the history of science has gradually been incorporated as an important part of mainstream contemporary historiography, along with social and intellectual history, the history of institutions, gender history and the "history of mentalities".

Unfortunately, this process has almost no parallel in Jewish historiography or Judaic studies. The studies and monumental bibliographical work of Moritz Steinschneider, published in the second half of the nineteenth century, have provided important methodological starting points as well as a substantive basis for further comprehensive research.[1] Some valuable works on Biblical and Talmudic medicine were also published at the end of the nineteenth and the beginning of the twentieth centuries.[2] But since then, very little research of any importance has appeared in this field.[3] The crux

---

[1] M. Steinschneider, "Jüdische Aertze", *Zeitschrift für hebraeische Bibliographie*, 17 (1914), pp. 63-96; 121-167; 18 (1915), pp. 25-57. For his works on the History of medicine, see F.H.Garrison, "Bibliographie der Arbeiten Moritz Stenschneider zur Geschichte der Medizin und Naturwissenschaften", *Archiv für Geschichte der Medizin*, 25 (1932), pp. 249-278. M. Steinschneider, *Die hebraeischen Übersetzungen des Mittelalters und die Juden als Dolmetscher*, Berlin, 1893, reprinted at Gratz, 1956, especially pp. 650-843.

[2] Hithertho, the classical work on Jewish ancient medicine has been J. Preuss, *Biblische talmudische Medizin, Beiträge zur Geschichte der Heilkunde und der Kulture überhaupt*, 1st. ed. 1911, latest ed. New York, 1971; translated into English by F. Rosner, New York and London, 1978.

[3] Most of the studies on medieval Jewish medicine have focused on the works of Maimonides, see R. Y. Ebied, *Bibliography of Medieval Arabic and Jewish Medicine and Allied Sciences*, London, 1971, pp. 110-116. Other important Jewish authors such as Nathan ben Joel Falaquera, Joshua ha-Lorki, Ilyâs ibn Ibrâhîm and the Qashlaries, have been almost completely neglected. The works of Joseph Shatzmiller are of importance for medieval Jewish social history, especially his *Jews, Medicine, and Medieval Society*, Berkeley, Los Angeles and London, 1994; cf. his bibliography, *ibid.*, pp. 229-230.

of the problem remains the lack of critical editions of the important medical texts written in Jewish languages (such as Hebrew, Judeo-Arabic, Judeo-Spanish and Yiddish) or their translations into one of the common European tongues. This kind of work may enable scholars unfamiliar with Jewish languages to study Jewish medicine and to evaluate its place in the general history of science.

In my book *Les infortunes de Dinah, ou la gynécologie juive au moyen âge*,[4] I tried to examine the methods used by Jewish medieval authors in their attempts to assimilate foreign concepts of female physiology, anatomy and pathology. As an illustration of this procedure, I included a critical edition of *Sefer ha-toledet* (Book on Generation). The treatise was derived from a work written in the second century by the Greek physician Soranus of Ephesus.[5] The Latin version, from which the Hebrew adaptation was made, was written by Muscio, perhaps in the sixth century.[6] While preparing the book, I was surprised to discover that no less than fifteen gynaecological treatises in Hebrew, of which at least 22 manuscripts survive, had circulated among the medieval Jewish communities (see Table I). Some of these texts are Hebrew translations, others are original Hebrew compositions. Some are short in length, including only prescriptions; others are more comprehensive and provide a detailed description of female anatomy, aetiology and pathology, together with a variety of treatments.

It seems apparent that, on the basis of the large treasury of specialized medical literature, ample justification exists for the attempt to analyze the practical application of these works, the routes by which foreign medical ideas were absorbed by Jewish society, and the various medical trends adopted by Jewish physicians in the

---

[4] Paris, 1991.

[5] For an excellent critical edition and French translation, see: *Soranos d'Éphèse: maladies des femmes*, texte établi, traduit et commenté par P. Burguière, D. Gourevitch et Y. Malinas, Paris 1988 (I), 1990 (II). For an English translation, see: O. Temkin, *Soranus' Gynecology*, Baltimore, 1956 (reprint, 1991). On Soranus, his medicine and writings, see: A. E. Hanson and M. H. Green, "Soranus of Ephesus: Methodicorum princeps", in: W. Hasse and H. Temporini (eds.), *Rise and Decline of the Roman World*, Part II, Principate, vol. 37.2, Berlin and New York, 1994, pp. 968-1073.

[6] V. Rose, *Sorani Gynaeciorum vetus translatio latina*, Leipzig, 1882; R. Radicchi, *La Gynaecia di Muscione: manuale per le ostetriche e le mamme del VI sec. d. C.*, Traduzione italiana e note con testo latino tratto dai codici e ampio glossario, Pisa, 1970. On this Latin translation, see: Hanson and Green, "Soranus of Ephesus", pp. 1046-1047.

Middle Ages. The study of these texts may also contribute to the understanding of some aspects of the lives of medieval women. First and foremost, the large quantity of treatises and their available manuscripts is clear evidence that Jewish physicians had great interest in women's medicine as a specialized branch. In this respect they were undoubtedly closer to Latin medical culture than to the Arabic model. Second, some of these writings reveal the respective roles ascribed to the male physician and to the female midwife in the treatment of women's suffering. Last but not least, the two genuinely Hebrew treatises dealing with both male and female diseases and physical disorders (especially sterility) convey important information on the conceptions of sex differences held by their medieval authors.[7]

This history is confined geographically to the European Jewish communities, especially those of Spain, Southern France and Italy, in other words, Mediterranean Europe. This constraint was imposed by the nature of our sources, since almost all of the treatises originated in this region. This phenomenon is not surprising, given that the communities of this region represented the core of Jewish intellectual activities during the high and late Middle Ages. Furthermore, temporal limits have been imposed by the literature itself: from the first appearance of Hebrew gynaecological texts in the 12th century to the end of Middle Ages.

---

[7] On this subject see: J. Cadden, *Meanings of Sex Difference in the Middle Ages Medicine*, Science and Culture, Cambridge, 1993.

Table I: Jewish Medieval Gynaecological Texts

Title	Original Language	Number of Existing Mss.
Sefer ha-herayon ve-ha-reḥem le-abuqrat (Hippocrates' Book on Pregnancy and the Womb) [Hebrew]	Arabic	1
Sefer yeṣirat ha-'ubar ve-hanhagat ha-harot ve-hanoladim (Book on the Creation of the Foetus and the Treatment of Pregnant Women and Babies) [Hebrew]	Arabic	2 (fragments)
Sefer ha-em el Galenus (Galen's Book on the Womb) [Hebrew]	Latin	2
Sefer ha-seter (Book on the Hidden [Places]) [Hebrew]	Latin	1 (fragment)
Sefer Dinah (Dinah's Book) [Judeo-Arabic]	Latin	1
Sefer ha-toledet (Book on Generation) [Hebrew]	Latin	3
Sitrei nashim (?) (Secrets of Women) [Hebrew]	Latin? ["Trotula" text? or *Secreta mulierum*, pseudo-Albertus Magnus?]	none
Zikhron ha-ḥolayim ha-hovim bi-khlei ha-herayon (A Record of the Diseases Occuring in the Genital Members) [Hebrew]	Hebrew	1

Terufut le-herayon (Medicaments for Pregnancy) [Hebrew]	Hebrew	1
Ha-ma'mar ba-tolada niqra sod ha-'ibur (The Treatise on Procreation Called the Secret of Conception) [Hebrew]	Hebrew	1
Merkaḥat mo'il le-herayon (A Useful Composition for Pregnancy) [Hebrew]	Hebrew	1
Sha'ar be-sibat 'aqarut ha-nashim (Chapter on the Cause of Women's Sterility) [Hebrew]	Hebrew	2
Trufot le-'ishah she-tikanes le-herayon (Medicaments for the Woman to Help her get Pregnant) [Hebrew]	Hebrew	1
Sha'ar ha-nashim (Women's Chapter) [Hebrew]	Hebrew	1
Liqutei Rabbenu Mosheh be-'inyanei veset ve-herayon (Maimonides' Compilation on Menstruation and Pregnancy) [Hebrew]	Arabic	2
Mi-qoshiyei ha-ledah (On Birth Difficulties) [Hebrew]	Hebrew	2

CHAPTER ONE

THE RISE OF HEBREW MEDICAL LITERATURE

The creation of the corpus of medieval Jewish texts on gynaecology and obstetrics was directly related to the process of secularisation of the Holy tongue and the formation of "Jewish science", written essentially in Hebrew. Involved in this process, which began with secular poetry in the tenth century and continued in other domains in the High Middle Ages, were political, cultural and sociological factors. However, the amazing history of the revival of Hebrew culture in the Middle Ages has yet to be fully investigated and related. In the present chapter, I will try to trace the causes and the paths of its evolution, especially in medicine.

A. The Preeminence of the Arabic Language

During the early Middle Ages, the Arabic language dominated the scientific literature written by Jews in the Orient as well as in the Occident.[1] However, two important exceptions must be mentioned:The first is *Sefer refu'ot* (Book on Remedies), attributed to Asaph ha-Rofé (Asaph the Physician), surnamed in some manuscripts as ha-Yarḥoni (the Astrologer). To our knowledge, it is the earliest medical treatise written in Hebrew, probably dating from the seventh or the eighth centuries.[2] *Sefer refu'ot* is composed of four

---

[1] For an analysis of the process by which Arabic replaced Aramaic as a written language of the Jewish repertoire and the division of functions of Hebrew and Arabic see: R. Drory, "'Words beautifully put', Hebrew versus Arabic in tenth-century Jewish Literature", in J. Blau and S. C. Reif (eds.), *Genizah Research after Ninety Years: The Case of Judeo-Arabic*, Cambridge, 1992, pp. 53-66.

[2] On this treatise see S. Muntner, *Introduction to the Book of Asaph the Physician - the Oldest Existing Text of a Medical Book Written in Hebrew*, Jerusalem, 1957 (Hebrew); Muntner also published the text "Asaph the Physician - 'Sefer harefuoth'", *Koroth*, 4 (1966), pp. 11-40; 4 (1967), pp. 170-207, 389-443; 4 (1968),

parts: A legend on the transmission of the entire knowledge of medicine from God to mankind; a general survey on medicine; a lexicon of *Materia medica*; and finally, a list of medical aphorisms. Unfortunately, we do not have any direct evidence about the presumed author, nor of where the book was written; however, from the number of its manuscripts that circulated during the Middle Ages, we can learn that the treatise attained great popularity within the Jewish communities. Of lesser importance is the second Hebrew medical text, which was written by Shabbetai ben Abraham ben Joel Donnolo (913-985), who lived in Brindisi, Italy.[3]

The Jews who lived in Muslim territories, especially in Spain, were integrated into the ruling society and assimilated Arabic culture into their own. That meant, first of all, that Middle-Arabic was adopted as a spoken language and that Arabic, written in Hebrew letters (Judeo-Arabic), was employed in the composition of their literary works.[4] Thus, the assimilation of Arabic culture in general, and the Arabic language in particular, inferred the acceptance of the literary forms and modes of expression peculiar to this culture. Furthermore, the Jews took part in the scientific activities and debates which preoccupied their Muslim colleagues. By and large, the scientific works of these learned Jews were by no means different from those composed by Muslims. For example, the North African Isaac ben Solomon ha-Yisraeli (more familiar under his Arabic name: Isḥâq al-Isrâ'ilî, 850-932?), a prominent physician, wrote his medical treatises in Arabic.[5] The only traces of his religious identity may be found in his ethical conception of the practice of medicine.[6]

---

pp. 531-572) (Hebrew); note that his edition is based only on a part of the known manuscripts.

[3] S. Muntner, *The Medical Writings of Rabbi Shabtai Donnolo*, Jerusalem, 1949 (Hebrew); see also G. Nebbia, *Donnolo, medico e sapiente ebreo di Oria in provincia di Brindisi,* Verona, 1963; S. Muntner, "Donnolo et la contribution des juifs aux premières oeuvres de la médecine salernitaine", *Revue d'histoire de la médecine hébraïque*, 32 (1956), pp. 155-161.

[4] R. Drory, *The Emergence of Jewish-Arabic Literary Contacts in the Beginning of the Tenth Century*, Tel Aviv, 1988 (Hebrew; English version in preparation).

[5] On ha-Yisraeli's medical and philosophical works see F. Sezgin, *Geschichte des arabischen Schrifttums*, Band III, Leiden, 1970, pp. 295-297; A. Alteman and S. Stern, *Isaac Israeli. A Neoplatonic Philosopher of the Early Tenth Century. His Works, Translated with Comments and an Outline of his Philosophy*, Oxford, 1958.

[6] A. Bar Sela and H. E. Hoff, "Isaac Israeli's Fifty Admonitions to the Physicians", *Journal of the History of Medicine and Allied Sciences*, 17 (1962), pp. 245-257; S. Jarcho, "Guide for Physicians (Musar Harofim) by Isaac Judaeus (880?-

Even more significant is the case of Maimonides, who was not only an eminent physician and the author of various important medical works, but also a Rabbi of great authority in religious matters. Maimonides employed two entirely different languages: For his scientific and philosophical works he adopted the Arabic language, thus following the accepted view of Arabic as the most appropriate idiom for the expression of ideas in these realms. In his religious works, on the other hand, Maimonides remained deeply attached to the traditional vocabulary and lexicon of post-Biblical Jewish literature. This dichotomous attitude is well illustrated in his pharmaceutical glossary *Kitâb sharḥ 'asmâ' al-'uqâr* (Book on the Explication of the Names of Drugs).[7] In this work, Maimonides provides the Arabic terms and their synonyms in Castilian, Persian, Greek and Syriac, but not one is given in Hebrew. Yet, as I. Löw has indicated, 170 plants' names are mentioned in the Bible, and no less than 320 were employed in the *Mishnah.*[8] Maimonides was undoubtedly familiar with these Hebrew terms since he used many of them in his monumental work *Mishneh Torah*, written in Hebrew. Moreover, he was perfectly familiar with their Arabic synonyms, which he employed in his commentary to the *Mishnah*, written in Arabic. In trying to explain this peculiar phenomenon, Max Meyerhof wrote: "Si malgré cela il n'a pas employé un seul nom synonym de drogues en hébreu c'est, je suppose, parce qu'il a écrit son glossaire surtout à l'usage de ses élèves non-juifs, comme du reste tous ses autres livres médicaux qui, eux aussi, ne contiennent pas de termes en hébreu".[9]

This explanation is hardly convincing for two major reasons: in the first place, by their very nature, these medieval glossaries attempted to furnish as many synonyms as possible. Thus the Egyptian disciples of Maimonides did not have the slightest knowledge of the Castilian language yet he eagerly cited synonyms in this idiom. Second, at least two other authors, Kohen al-'Attâr and al-'Idrîsî, both mentioned by Meyerhof, employed Hebrew synonyms in their Ara-

---

932?), Translated from the Hebrew with Introduction", *Bulletin of the History of Medicine*, 15 (1944), pp. 180-188.

[7] The Arabic text has been published according to the only known manuscript in M. Meyerhof: *L'explication des noms de drogues - un glossaire de matière médicale composé par Maïmonide*, Cairo, 1940. It was translated into Hebrew by S. Muntner (Jerusalem, 1969). A second edition was included in *Maimonides' Medical Writings*, Jerusalem, 1987, vol. IV.

[8] I. Löw, *Die Flora der Juden*, Vienna, 1934, p. 75

[9] Meyerhof, *L'explication des noms de drogues*, p. LXVI.

bic glossaries.[10] It therefore seems that Maimonides, similar to many other Jewish erudites, availed himself of the two languages according to their functions: Hebrew, the sacred language, was employed essentially for religious issues whereas Arabic, the more expressive and prevalent language, was used as a daily instrument of communication and for the expression of worldly ideas.

The norms for the use of Hebrew and Arabic were actually established in the 10th century, in Al-Andalus, at the "Extreme Occident" of the Muslim territories.[11] Ḥasdai ibn Shaprut (c.910-975) played a decisive role in this process as the *Nagid* ("President") of the Jewish community. He served as personal physician to the Caliph ʻAbd al-Raḥmân III and as a senior member of his court. Due to his many talents and proficiency in languages (including Latin and Romance), Ḥasdai undertook important diplomatic missions for his sovereign and, at the same time, participated in the scientific activities patronized by the Caliph himself.[12] In cooperation with Nicholas, a Christian monk, he completed the Arabic translation of Dioscorides' *Materia medica,* a project initiated by Stephanos b. Basileios and Ḥunain ibn Isḥâq.[13]

Ḥasdai strongly encouraged Jewish participation in scientific writing, but in Arabic of course. Concurrently, he nonetheless supported the "Renaissance" of the Hebrew language as a symbol of Jewish cultural identity. Thus, while under Arabic influence, the Jews of Al-Andalus wrote Hebrew grammatical treatises, and more importantly, composed poetry, both secular and religious, in Hebrew.[14]

---

[10] *Ibid.*

[11] I am referring, of course, to the West; regarding the East, see Drory, "'Words beautifully put", pp. 53-58.

[12] For a description of his broad reach and exceptional career, see E. Ashtor, *The Jews of Moslem Spain,* translated from the Hebrew by A. Klein and J. Machlowitz Klein, Philadelphia, 1973, vol. I, pp. 155-227.

[13] On the transmission of Dioscorides' treatise to Arabic medicine, see C. E. Dubler y E. Terés, *La versión árabe de la "Materia Médica" de Dioscórides.* Estudio de la transcripción de los nombres griegos al árabe y comparación de las versiones griega, árabe y castellana, Tetuán y Barcelona, 1952-1957. The information regarding the participation of Ḥasdai ibn Shaprut in the translation is provided by the Cordoban Ibn Juljul, in particular; see J. Vernét, *La cultura hispanoárabe en Oriente y Occidente*, Barcelona, 1978, pp. 69-72.

[14] See A. Schippers, *Arabic Tradition and Hebrew Innovation: Arabic Themes in Hebrew Andalusian Poetry*, Amsterdam, 1988, pp. 54-57; T. Rosen-Moqued, "La

This was indeed a two-fold revolution: For the first time, secular poems were written in the Holy Language; and, whilst thematically and structurally the new Hebrew poetry followed Arabic models, the language itself was almost purely Biblical. Hebrew poetry in Al-Andalus reached its "golden age" in the eleventh and twelfth centuries, with writers such as Samuel ha-Nagid, Solomon ibn Gabirol and Yehudah ha-Levi symbolizing, each within the confines of his own style, the integration of the Jewish élite into the surrounding society. Samuel ha-Nagid composed his war-poems and poetry in other genres while serving his Muslim master in Granada as a military commander and administrator; Solomon ibn Gabirol integrated the neoplatonic philosophical trends of the time within his poetry; and, perhaps most significantly, Yehudah ha-Levi intermittently employed Hebrew, Arabic, and Romance in his *kharjas* (the last part of the *muwashshaha*, a poetical genre which was conceived in Muslim Spain).[15]

Put succinctly, the Arabic language in its two forms, the literary and the Judeo-Arabic, was well established as the formal means of expression for scientific purposes amongst the Jews in Al-Andalus. In order to better understand the attachment of the Spanish Jewish élite to the Arabic language, it is worthwhile reading the following evaluation by Moses ibn 'Ezra, written in the middle of the twelfth century: "They [the Arabs] have translated into Arabic all the sciences, ancient as well as modern, which they have appropriated and accomplished with explanations and clarifications. No nation has composed or translated such a quantity in the domain of science as has been translated and written by this nation. They were able to do so thanks to the richness of their language and the excellence of its rhetoric".[16]

This estimation, incorporated in the Spanish Jewish poet's theoretical treatise on Hebrew Poetry (the treatise itself was written in Arabic), was undoubtedly shared by most Jewish scholars of his time and the following generations. In fact, even when Hebrew became the dominant written language of the Jews in the Latin West, Jews of Christian Spain continued to use medical works written in Arabic

poésie juive espagnole", in R. Barkaï (ed.), *Chrétiens, musulmans et juifs dans l'Espagne médiévale, De la convergence à l'expulsion*, Paris, 1994, pp. 103-133.

[15] Schippers, *Arabic Tradition and Hebrew Innovation*, pp. 60-74.

[16] Mosheh ibn 'Ezra, *Kitâb al-muḥâdarah wa-l-mudhâkarah*, edición y traducción por M. Abumalham, Madrid, 1986, vol. II, p. 42.

and to write a portion of their medical treatises in this language. Research conducted in recent years has shown that the Arabic medical manuscripts written in Christian Spain circulated within the Jewish communities almost exclusively. They were written for Jews and used by Jewish masters and students of medicine until the end of the fifteenth century,[17] that is to say, more than three centuries after the Jews were obliged to leave Al-Andalus and to abandon Arabic culture.[18]

Not less significant is the fact that eminent Jewish physicians of Christian Spain preferred to write their important medical works in the Arabic language. The most remarkable of these medical treatises is the *Kitâb al-ṭibb al-qastâlî al-malûkî*, written in the beginning of the fourteenth century, probably by a member of the famous family of Jewish physicians, the Banû Shushan of Toledo. Since the Arabic manuscript has never been published, historians of medieval medicine have yet to evaluate its importance. In the last few years, however, two Spanish historians, in the process of preparing a critical edition of the manuscript, were able to conclude in a preliminary study of the text that: "It is a highly elaborated intellectual product, an expression of mature Galenism, based on direct knowledge of Galen's medical *corpus* and the extensive repertoire of medical works of Arabic Galenism. Due to its formal structure, its subject matter, and its didactic character, it is indeed a singular piece of

---

[17] These are the conclusions of the excellent study by P. Sj. van Koningsveld: "As far as one can tell from the materials preserved, the Arabic medical and scientific manuscripts of Christian Spain almost exclusively circulated in Jewish circles... Our information about the scribes, students and owners of the medical and scientific manuscripts is in fact quiet detailed. Several manuscripts copied for Jewish owners, were written by Muslim scribes living as war captives in Christian Spain... Other manuscripts were written by Jewish scribes... Not only were many manuscripts directly copied for Jewish owners they also remained in Jewish ownership during following generations, as we can gauge from the owner's entries...", *Festschrift H. R. Singer*, (forthcoming). This article is in fact a complement to a previous one, in which the author provides a list and analysis of the existing manuscripts, see note 18. Cf. L. García Ballester and C. Vázquez de Benito, "Los médicos judíos castellanos del siglo XIV y el galenismo árabe: El kitab al-tibb al-qastali al-maluki (Libro de medicina castellana regia) (c. 1312)", *Asclepio: Archivo iberoamericano de historia de la medicina y antropología médica*, 1 (1990), esp. pp. 121-122.

[18] P. Sj. van Koningsveld, "Andalusian-Arabic Manuscripts from Christian Spain: A Comparative Intercultural Approach", *Israel Oriental Studies*, 12 (1992), pp. 75-110; García Ballester y Vázquez de Benito, "Los médicos judíos castellanos del siglo XIV y el galenismo árabe", pp. 119-147.

medical literature of the Late Middle Ages, whether Latin, Arabic, or Jewish. Its content reveals valuable information about the transmission and elaboration of medical learning within the Jewish community, and on the so-called "open" system of medical teaching. The work is the result of a penetrating intelligence by a practising Jewish physician who worked among Christians, and who took part in the medical-scientific polemics of his time. These debates originated in the Christian-Castilian circles in which he lived, but also took place within the rationalist circles of the Castilian Jewish community... Beyond its intellectual concerns, the eminently practical aim of the treatise conveys first-hand material enabling us to reconstruct the unknown world of medicine practiced daily in the Late Middle Ages..."[19]

This tradition of writing medical treatises in Arabic among Spanish Jews was continued by the eminent physician Joshua ha-Lorki, who served Pope Benedict XIII as his personal physician. (In 1412, ha-Lorki was baptized under the name Hieronymus de Sancta Fide.[20]) While still a respectable member of the Jewish community, he was asked by its dignitaries to write an up-to-date book on medicine for the benefit of Jewish physicians. It is instructive that Joshua ha-Lorki, because of his esteem for the Arabic language, preferred to write the treatise in this idiom rather than in Hebrew. The work was later translated into Hebrew by Joseph Benvenisti ben Lavi de la Caballeria under the title *Guerem ha-ma'alot* (The Staircase). Many manuscripts of the Hebrew translation circulated in various Jewish communities but, unfortunately, the original Arabic text has been lost.

The chain of medical works written in Arabic by Jews of Spanish origin is closed by a treatise on the Black Death, *Kitâb majannat al-ta'ûn wa-al-wabâ'*,[21] written by Eliya ben Abraham shortly after the expulsion in 1492, and dedicated to the Ottoman Sultan Selim I. The Spanish origin of the author is attested to by his Arabic appellation in the manuscript - 'Ilyâs ibn 'Ibrâhîm al-Yahûdî al-'Ishbânî [*sic*].

---

[19] García Ballester and Vázquez de Benito, "Los médicos judíos castellanos del siglo XIV y el galenismo árabe", p. 120.

[20] I. F. Baer, *A History of the Jews in Christian Spain*, translated by L. Schoffman, Philadelphia, 1961, vol. II, p. 139-150.

[21] Chester Beatty Collection, Dublin, ms. 3676,6, ff. 185r-216r. For a preliminary study of the work, its form and content, see R. Barkai, "Between East and West: A Jewish Doctor from Spain", *Mediterranean Historical Review*, 10 (1995), pp. 42-64. I am currently working on the critical edition of the treatise.

While stressing the fact that Arabic continued to play a considerable role in the scholarly efforts of the Jewish physicians living in Christian Spain, we should keep in mind that it had a limited impact on medieval Jewish medicine in general. In other parts of Latin Europe, Hebrew completely dominated medical writings. Even in Spain, as is clearly expressed by the translator of *Guerem ha-ma'alot*, most fifteenth-century Jewish physicians preferred Hebrew texts. Yet we should recall that Jewish physicians in the medieval West also used Latin and vernacular treatises in their study of medicine, especially when trained by non-Jewish masters.

B. The Passage from Arabic to Hebrew

Due to their special legal status, the lives of medieval Jews were by far more tenuous than those of their Muslim or Christian neighbours. Independent of the level of their integration in the ruling society, political or religious fluctuations in the regime had an immediate impact on their situation and, in extreme cases, they were even obliged to convert or to leave their homeland. Such events profoundly influenced not only the social and economic structure of entire Jewish communities, they also had broad cultural implications, as seen in the transformations that took place as a result of the extensive Jewish immigration from Al-Andalus.

The political events that troubled Muslim Spain from the end of the eleventh to the middle of the twelfth century were crucial in determining the fate of the Jews living in the area as well as of the medieval Hebrew culture. The conquest of Al-Andalus by two successive Berber dynasties, the Almoravides (1090) and the Almohades (1145), provoked a radical change in the country's political regime and cultural climate. These traditionalist Muslim regimes put an end to the relative tolerance and open-mindedness which had characterized Al-Andalus up to the time of the invasions. They placed constraints on the relative freedom to study unorthodox branches of science, and reinforced the power of their rigid religious leadership. In consequence, what may be deemed "the free and hedonistic spirit" of Al-Andalus gradually disappeared, to be replaced by an uncompromising orthodoxy.[22]

[22] R. Arié, *Historia de España (III), España musulmana (siglos VIII-XV)*, Barcelona, 1982, pp. 31-36.

These extreme measures, initiated by the Almoravides, were carried even further by the Almohades, who forced the two resident minorities, the Christians and the Jews, to embrace Islam. In response, most members of these communities fled from Al-Andalus to Christian Spain. Many Jewish families even chose to abandon the Iberian Peninsula which for generations they had considered a genuine *patria*, and immigrated to southern France, Italy or to the Orient. In a short time, the once-prolific coexistence of Muslims, Christians and Jews in Muslim Spain came to an unhappy end. In tandem, a new confluence of the three monotheistic cultures, which would last until 1492, began to emerge in Christian Spain.

The Jews who settled in Christian lands were quickly integrated and, like their co-religionists already residing there, played important roles in the economic and cultural life of these countries. After a generation, Arabic was replaced by the vernacular languages of Christian Spain and southern France as a means of communication with non-Jewish neighbors and even within the community itself. However, although Jews mastered the "Christian languages", and some members of the educated class knew Latin, they did not employ these languages in writing their scientific works. Hebrew thus became the "common" written idiom, a kind of "international language" for the Jewish communities of the Western Diaspora. Hebrew had an additional advantage of course: It could be used also by the Oriental Jewish communities. This "second Renaissance" of Hebrew culture in the Middle Ages coincided perfectly with the revival of philosophy and science in the Latin West, a development more generally defined as the "twelfth century Renaissance" by Charles Haskins.

As far as we can learn from the existing sources, this new era of Jewish science did not begin with Hebrew medical writings but, rather, in fields such as astronomy, astrology, cosmology, geometry and mathematics. Two eminent Jewish scholars, Abraham bar Ḥiyya (the second half of the eleventh century - c.1136) and Abraham ibn ‘Ezra (1092 -1167), both Spaniards, were the first to compose treatises in these domains in Hebrew. Although very different in their personal histories, their intellectual activities, and their perceptions of science and religion, their contributions, while important for the advance of medieval science in general, thoroughly transformed

Jewish science in the Middle Ages.[23] While Abraham bar Ḥiyya had little interest in the medical sciences, Abraham ibn ʻEzra employed medical knowledge particularly in his attempts to demonstrate the necessity of studying "foreign sciences" in order to understand the Holy Scripture and God's commandments.[24] However, the only truly medical treatise attributed to Ibn ʻEzra is *Sefer ha-nisyonot* (The Book of [Medical] Experiences), which is, in fact, an enlarged Hebrew version of ʻAbd al-Rahmân ibn al-Haitham's Book of

---

[23] We know almost nothing about the biography of Abraham bar Ḥiyya, but from the few remarks in his scientific works we may learn the he was born in Barcelona to an important Jewish family (as attested by his title: *ha-Nassi*, the Prince). He had intellectual exchanges with scholars, Jewish and non-Jewish alike in Spain and southern France concerning scientific and religious matters. (For more details see M. Steinschneider, *Abraham Judaeus, Savasorda und Ibn Esra zur Geschichte der mathematischen Wissenschaften im 12. Jahrhundert* , in: *Gesammelte Schriften*, I, Berlin,1925, pp. 327-387). Most of his work was dedicated to mathematics, geometry, astronomy and cosmography. He probably wrote a book on astrology, which has been lost, and dedicated a long chapter to this art in his *Meguillat ha-Megalleh* (The Revelator Scroll), in which he attempted to foresee the Day of Redemption of the people of Israel. In addition, he wrote a long apologetic epistle, vindicating the study and the use of astrology, addressed to Rabbi Yehudah Barzilai of Barcelona. On his works and their impact on Jewish and Christian scholars, see J. Ma. Millás Vallicrosa, "La obra enciclopédica de R. Abraham bar Ḥiyya", in his *Estudios sobre historia de la ciencia española*, Barcelona, 1949, vol. I, pp. 219-262 (a new facsimile edition, Madrid, 1987); Abraham bar Ḥiia, *Llibre Revelador, Meguillat Hamegallé*, Segons l'edició del text revisat i prologat per J. Guttmann, versió de l'hebreu per J. Millás Vallicrosa, Barcelona, 1925, pp. I-LVII.

Abraham ibn ʻEzra was undoubtedly one of the most original medieval thinkers and had a wide range of intellectual interests. He wrote poetry - religious as well as profane, treatises on astronomy, astrology and the astrolabe on the one hand, and religious matters on the other. This combination is revealed especially in his commentary to the Bible, in which he used different domains of science, and in his *Sefer yesod mora* (Book on the Foundation of the [Lord] Fear), aimed to demonstrate that it is impossible to have a real understanding of God's commandments without the study of science. Unlike bar Ḥiyya, Abraham ibn ʻEzra never tried to apologise for his scientific activities (concerning astrology, see R. Barkaï: "Astrologie juive au moyen âge: aspects théoriques et pratiques", *Le moyen âge*, 93 (1987), pp. 323-348). It is impossible to reproduce here the essential bibliography on Ibn ʻEzra, but the last published collective work may give the reader an impression, although a partial one, on his literary activity: F. Díaz Esteban (ed.), *Abraham ibn Ezra and his Age*, Proceedings of the International Symposium, Madrid, Tudela, Toledo, February 1-8, 1989, Madrid, 1990.

[24] See for example *Sefer yesod mora*, Jerusalem, 1970, p. 11 (Hebrew); Ibn ʻEzra Commentary to Exodus, 23:25. (Hebrew)

[Medical] Virtues.[25] In any case, the only evidence that Ibn ‘Ezra practiced medicine dates from 1588, and his authorship of *Sefer ha-nisyonot* seems to me very doubtful.[26]

C. The Early Scientific Hebrew Translations

From the end of the eleventh to the beginning of the sixteenth century, about two hundred Jewish scholars completed approximately one thousand (!) translations of Arabic scientific texts into Hebrew. We have no estimate of the number of Hebrew translations from Latin and other European languages, but we can safely assume that the total number may be more than double.[27] Moreover, almost all the original works written by Jews at this time, in all the sciences, were composed directly in Hebrew. This phenomenon is even more astounding if we bear in mind that in the twelfth century, the Hebrew language almost totally lacked a scientific terminology.

It appears that the translators were well aware of the inferiority of the Holy Language as a vehicle for expressing scientific ideas, especially when compared to Arabic. As stated by Yehudah ibn Tibbon, the most illustrious translator of the twelfth century: "[Arabic] is in fact an extensive language, full of resources concerning every subject. It satisfies the necessities of all those who speak or write this

---

[25] The original Arabic treatise has been lost and only its Hebrew translation exists. For a critical edition of both texts, see *Sefer Hanisyonot, The Book of Experiences Attributed to Abraham ibn Ezra*, Edited, translated and commented by J. O. Leibowitz and S. Marcus, Jerusalem, 1984. It is of interest to note that some of the gynaecological treatments mentioned in these texts reappear in later gynaecological treatises. See R. Barkai, "A Medieval Hebrew Treatise on Obstetrics", *Medical History*, 33 (1988), pp. 111-112.

[26] The literary style of *Sefer ha-nisyonot* is completely different of the other writings, and surely written by Ibn ‘Ezra. Although the editors of the text are uncertain, they do not remove the possibility that Ibn ‘Ezra was indeed its author: "During the Middle Ages, Jewish sources did not mention Abraham ibn Ezra as a physician, extolling him rather as a commentator, poet, and astronomer. Nevertheless, we may report one item [reference], without lending it too much weight, in support of his having been a physician, a fact which would lend some credence to the hypothesis of his authorship of our treatise", *Sefer Hanisyonot, The Book of Experiences Attributed to Abraham ibn Ezra*, p. 31.

[27] On these assessments, see A. S. Halkin, "Translations and Translators", *Encyclopaedia Judaica*, vol. 15, 1971, cols. 1318-1329; but the essential work is still that of Steinschneider, *Die hebraeischen Übersetzungen*, see especially pp. XV-XXIV.

language. Its expressions are exact and clear, and it reaches at the heart of all questions, much more than is possible in Hebrew. For what has remained of the Hebrew language is not more than the Biblical Books, and these are not sufficient to our needs...".[28]

The inevitable question is, then, why did the Jews of the Latin West prefer to use Hebrew for their scientific works, given that this language lacked the comprehensiveness of Arabic, Latin or even the Romance vernaculars during the Middle Ages? It seems that various factors contributed to the reemergence of Hebrew as a dominant element in medieval Jewish culture. In the first place, most of the Jews did not have linguistic access to the Latin scientific literature which had begun to circulate in Western Europe at the end of the eleventh century. This was especially true of the Jews who had immigrated from Muslim Spain, despite their being the intellectually most active community among medieval Jewry. Indeed, as stated above, the first scientific works written in Hebrew were composed in Christian Spain, and the first Hebrew translations made in Southern France and Northern Italy were accomplished by translators of Spanish origin. Moreover, this Jewish intellectual élite in Christian lands (Spain, France and Italy) continued to write poetry in Hebrew, a fact attesting to their fluency as well as their attachment to the language.[29] Also, we have to recall that a large number of Jews in the Middle Ages had acquired Hebrew in communal schools or within the family. The reason for this phenomenon was purely religious, i.e., the duty of every father to teach his sons Hebrew, so that they would be capable of reading the Bible and reciting the prayers; but this knowledge enabled them, of course, to read profane literature, such as medical texts.

The second explanation for the use of Hebrew in scientific writing stems from the professional life and legal status of the Jews in medieval Europe. In general, Jews were prohibited from studying medicine or any other profession within the framework of the Christian higher education system, i.e., the *studia* and the universities. On

[28] Introduction to his Hebrew translation of Beḥyah ibn Paquda's, *Sefer ḥovot ha-levavot*, Zifroni edition, Jerusalem, 1969, p. 2.

[29] The best examples of these intellectuals are Judah al-Ḥarîzî (thirteenth century), who wrote rhymed prose in the Arabic *maqâma* style, as well as a poem on *regimen sanitatis* (Refu'at ha-gviyah), and Joseph ben Me'ir Zabarah who wrote, in the same century, the maqâma *Sefer ha-sha'shu'im*, in which he included important medical materials particularly concerning gynaecology (Berlin, 1925, pp. 112-113;121).

the other hand, they could gain a *Licentia curandi et practicandi* from the Christian authorities if they passed the formal examinations. Based on medieval documentation, we learn that most Jews who wished to practice medicine studied the theoretical and practical aspects of this art almost exclusively within the private, or "open", system as defined by García Ballester.[30] They thus received their education in a one-to-one relationship, between a physician-tutor and his (or her) student or, even more frequently, in the family circle, where the medical profession was transmitted from father to son.[31]

Furthermore, as may be inferred from the introductions to Hebrew translations and original Hebrew works, the motivation for writing in Hebrew was eminently practical. These introductions, themselves a distinct literary genre frequently appearing in Hebrew scientific writings, teach us that their authors specifically intended to supply Jewish physicians and other practitioners with an accurate classical and current medical literature in order to assist them in improving their professional skills.[32] Due to the legal and social restrictions

---

[30] I borrowed this expression from his remarkable work on the moriscos' medicine. For political, social and cultural reasons, that minority, living in sixteenth century Spain, did not have access to the universities and continued to transmit medical knowledge within the family or in private circles organized by well-known physicians. See L. García Ballester, *Los moriscos y la medicina. Un capítulo de la medicina y la ciencia marginadas en la España del siglo XVI*, Barcelona, 1984, esp. pp. 140-143.

[31] J. Shatzmiller, "On Becoming a Jewish Doctor in the High Middle Ages", *Sefarad*, 43 (1983), pp. 239-250. In some exceptional cases, Jews were admitted as students of medicine in the framework of the universities, see *idem*, "Etudiants juifs à la faculté de médecine de Montpellier, dernier quart du XIV siècle", *Jewish History*, 6 (1992), pp. 243-254.

[32] An excellent analysis of the translations' introductions, including those to medical treatises, was made by: J.-P. Rothschild, "Motivations et méthodes des traductions en hébreu du milieu du XIIe à la fin du XVe siècle", *Traduction et traducteurs au Moyen Age*, Actes du colloque international du CNRS, Paris 1986. Textes réunis par G. Contamine, Paris, 1989, pp. 279-302. On the utilitarian aspect, see esp. pp. 291-292. The medical treatise *Guerem ha-ma'alot*, by the abovementioned Spanish Jew Joshua ha-Lorki was written according to the same logic: "To compose a short treatise in order to pave a road and a path for the physician's community; to study the composition of the major medicaments and drugs, and to discover their components, in order to prevent any error". But ha-Lorki preferred to write the treatise "in Arabic, the sweet and the pure language, in which he was fluent. As his words were for some of the readers like a "sealed book", for they were not proficient in that language, adds the translator, the author ordered me to translate it into our holy and sanctified tongue, so that it would be useful for all". Paris, Bibliothèque Nationale, ms. héb. 1143, f. 86r.

imposed on the Jews in the Middle Ages, the learning of professions such as medicine, astrology etc., which they could practice within Christian as well as Jewish society, was indeed their main option for social mobility. This explains the fact that the number of Jewish physicians in Christian and Muslim lands far exceeded their proportion in the society.

Last but not least, many of the translators and authors of Hebrew texts emphasize the cultural and even "nationalistic" aspect of their efforts. The Hebrew language served as a symbol of their cultural identity in the broadest sense of the term. In their confrontation with the extensive Arabic literature and the burgeoning Latin scholarship, the Jewish élite was eager to prove to the gentiles (and to themselves) that their own ancient language was not inferior, and it could be as accomplished and useful as Arabic and Latin.[33]

One of the first to express these sentiments was the Italian Jew, Nathan ha-Méatî. In the introduction to his translation to Ibn Sînâ's treatise *Kitâb al-Qânûn fi al-ṭibb* (completed in 1279), the great translator states that he had learned many languages in his numerous travels, and in particularly he had deepened his knowledge in Hebrew and Arabic. He also related how incensed he was to hear the Christians mocking the Jews because they have no medical literature. Knowing that such a literature from the times of King Solomon had been lost after the exile, he decided to translate into Hebrew every book which seems to him of importance. Hence, utilitarian and apologetic approaches are frequently combined in the expository introductions to his and other's translations. An instructive example may be found in the introduction to the Hebrew translation of John of Burgundy's treatise on the plague (1349): "And I, little in quality and merits, Benjamin son of Rabbi Isaac Qarqasani [of Carcassonne], the translator, I have seen this treatise closed and sealed in the treasuries [of the Christians], and it has been examined and verified by noteworthy physicians. So, I have made all efforts to gain access to it and to translate it from their language into the Holy Tongue, so that it will be of help and benefit to us and to our successors as well...".[34]

Even more explicit is the statement made by Solomon ha-Rofé (the Physician) ben Moses Shalom the Spaniard (14th century), in the introduction to his Hebrew translation of Antonius Guainerius'

---

[33] Rothschild, "Motivations et méthodes des traductions", pp. 289-290.

[34] Paris, Bibliothèque Nationale, ms. héb. 1191, f. 142r.

De febribus. The interesting point here is the translator's justification for using non-Hebraic terms, which, of course, was a common phenomenon in medieval Hebrew medical works. In the beginning, the translator states that he had read the treatise several times and had been impressed by its quality. Although this might well serve as a sufficient cause for the translation, he adds: "I have heard many Christian sages boasting and bragging of this treatise, while maligning us by saying that we can never reach perfection in curing fevers, as did Ibn Sînâ, Galen, Hippocrates and other ancient sages... Therefore, seized with internal torment and great envy, I undertook the mission to translate it to the best of my ability into our Holy Tongue..".[35]

As to the linguistic aspect, the translator apologizes for the use of foreign terms, giving two reasons for their necessity. The first is the lack of appropriate terms "...in our Holy Tongue. In fact," explains the Jewish physician, "all these terms once existed in Hebrew, but were lost during the many generations in which the language remained in disuse". Moreover, even if such terms were available in Hebrew, they would be "utterly strange" for a contemporary reader, since their origin lies in the Rabbinical Hebrew of the Talmudic period. For that reason, concludes the translator, the use of these Hebrew terms is unjustified, even for a Jewish physician familiar with Biblical and post-Biblical Hebrew, and certainly for a physician ignorant of the ancient language, "of which there are a countless many". Attempting to use the work, he would never understand it; rather, he would be like one conversing with a Greek or with a German without knowing their languages.[36]

D. The First Translations of Latin Medical Texts

The oldest testimony available of a well-designed and comprehensive project for the translation of medical works from Latin into Hebrew dates from the end of the twelfth century, the author of which remains anonymous to this day. The sole known manuscript of this document is found in a codex conserved in the Bibliothèque Nationale in Paris, and is followed by two medical treatises translated from

[35] Parma, ms. 1365/7, f. 23r.
[36] *Ibid.*

Latin into Hebrew: the *Isagoge Iohanitii*,[37] and Philaretus' work on pulses.[38] From the remaining two folios of the text it is quite clear that the document is an introduction to the medical books which the anonymous author has translated from Latin into Hebrew, and in which he explained the motives for such a huge project and the reasons for his selection of the texts. As to the first issue, he states: "I have seen groups of the Holy [the Jews] hasten to the gentiles' doors, seeking [remedies] for their illnesses and for the sicknesses of their sons and daughters. They receive from the [gentiles'] hands every remedy, although they do not differentiate between the pure and the impure; into their compound medicines they mix libation wine [forbidden to Jews] with pure wine, unclean meat and milk and blood. None escapes the prohibited nor the abhorrent. For this reason I decided to translate all the erudites' books on theoretical and practical medicine into the Holy Tongue".[39]

In the last part of the document, the author specifically refers to the formation of the profession of medicine within the Jewish society, citing the words of the old Sages of Israel: "A man should teach his son the Torah, [but also] he should teach him a craft".[40] The study of medicine, according to our author, is especially recommended "since in the entire world there is no other art so pure".[41] This statement hints at the polemic then conducted within the Jewish communities concerning the study of non-religious subjects, a stronger echo of which can be found in his defence of the study of "foreign sciences". Replying to the traditional argument that a Jew "should study the Bible day and night" (Ps. 1:2) and do other things when there is neither day nor night, the author says: "They did not mean the whole day or the whole night, since when would he [the

[37] Paris, Bibliothèque Nationale, ms. héb. 1190, f. 46v-110v; incipit: "Introductory book on the art of medicine, written by Ḥanan ben Yiṣḥaq [*sic*], in the form of question and answer... Ḥanan said: into how many parts medicine is divided? Into two [parts]. What are they? The theoretical and the practical"; explicit: "Ended and completed, glory to the God of the world".

[38] *Ibid*, ff. 111r-118r; incipit: "The book on pulse written by the sage Philaret [*sic*]. We decided to explain in this treatise, in a brief way the theory of pulse..."; explicit: "And the learneds will shine as the sky's splendour... completed the book which gives beautiful saying". Note that the first part of the concluding formula is taken from Daniel, 12:3, and appears also at the end of *Sefer ha-toledet*, see *Les infortunes de Dinah*, p. 223.

[39] Paris, Bibliothèque Nationale, ms. héb. 1190, f. 44r.

[40] *Babylonian Talmud*, Kidushin, 32b.

[41] Bibliothèque Nationale, Paris, ms. héb. 1190, f. 45v.

father] have the time to teach him [his son] a craft... The study of the Bible is the essence of life but the [study of] other sciences is a way of making a living".[42] He thereby precisely reinforces his stated purpose, i. e., to supply Jews interested in studying medicine with the best, most up-to-date theoretical and practical texts to be found in the Christian environment.

A careful study of the books listed by the translator leads to the conclusion that the rich library on medical matters he had at his disposal was essentially that of the medicine School of Salerno. Several of the medical books he enumerates seem to be taken from the *Articella* or *Ars medicinae*, - a collection of medical treatises that served as a basic curriculum, most of which are Latin translations of Arabic medical works made by Constantine the African and others.[43] By the second half of the twelfth century, this corpus of medical writings was in circulation in Provence, where the Hebrew translations were made. Due to the exceptional importance of the document, it seems appropriate to reproduce the entire list of the translated texts and the author's evaluation of these writings:

> These are the titles of the books I have completed translating in the seventeenth, eighteenth and nineteenth years of the two hundred sixty-first cycle [of the moon = 1197-1199]. The first theoretical book I translated is *Sefer Ḥaguan*, which is an introductory book to the honourable book written by Galen called *Tegniugs*. It is indeed an introduction to the theoretical books and called *Guanis* by the erudites of the nations.[44] After-

[42] *Ibid*, f. 46r.

[43] P. O. Kristeller, "The School of Salerno: Its Development and Its Contribution to the History of Learning", in his *Studies in Renaissance Thought and Letters*, 2nd ed., Rome, 1969, pp. 495-551; *idem, Studi sulla scuola medica salernitana*, Naples, 1986; D. Jacquart et F. Micheau, *La médecine arabe et l'occident médiéval*, Paris, 1990, pp. 118-129; H. Schipperges, *Arabische Medizin im Lateinischen Mittlalter*, Heidelberg, 1976. I have used the Spanish translation (*La medicina árabe en el Medioevo Latino*, Toledo, 1989), pp. 106-109.

[44] The author is referring to the Latin translation of *Kitâb al-mudkhal fi al-ṭibb,* written by Ḥunain ibn 'Isḥâq (died in 873 or 877), based essentially on Galen's works. The Latin translation was made by Constantine the African at the end of the eleventh century, and was known under various titles: *Isagoge Iohannitii, Isagoge Iohanicii ad Tegni Galieni, Liber Introductorius in medicinam*. There is another Hebrew translation of this treatise, also from the Latin version, called *Sefer iohanitio*. See Paris, Bibliothèque Nationale, ms. héb. 1116, ff. 1r-12r. Cf. Steinschneider, *Die hebraeischen Übersetzungen*, p. 712. On the treatise itself and its Latin transla-

wards I translated the book called *Tegni,* which I entitled *Sefer ha-me'asef le-kol ha-maḥanot* (The Collected Book of All the Fields), wherein lies its significance.[45] Then [I translated] *Sefer Agor*, which was written by the wise and pious Hippocrates. This book contains much material, in abridged form, and is called in their language *Anforismis.* This book is really a delight, and I have put its contents into alphabetical order so it will be easier for the learned to conserve and remember it.[46] Afterwards, I translated *Sefer ha-ḥidot ve-ha-hashgaḥot* (The Book of Enigmas and Observations), which is called *Pronosticas* in their language. The book was written by the learned Hippocrates and is like a splendid crown on the heads of those who read it.[47] Then [I translated] the Book on Urine, whose author is Taufoli the Philosopher, which illu-

---

tion, see Sezgin, *Geschichte des arabischen Schrifttums*, Band III, pp. 247-251; Jacquart et Micheau, *La médecine arabe et l'occident médiéval*, pp. 96-107.

45 The *Tegni*, also known under other various titles (*Ars medica, Ars parva, Microtechne*), is the Latin version of Galen's brief treatise. See P. G. Ottosson, *Scholastic Medicine and Philosophy, A Study of Commentaries on Galen's "Tegni" (ca. 1300-1450)*, Naples, 1984. The same titles, as they appear in this manuscript, are found at the end of the Hebrew translation of the above-mentioned work: "Finished the first book on medical science, written by the erudite, the well-versed in both foreign languages: Greek and Arabic, called *ḥagukhan* [*sic*], and it was written as an introduction to Galen's treatise called *Tit* [*sic*], which means *me'asef le-kol ha-maḥanot* [The Collected Book of All the Fields]", Paris, Bibliothèque Nationale, ms. héb. 1116, f. 12r. This note leads us to the conclusion that it is indeed a copy of the translation made by our author. Cf. Steinschneider, *Die hebraeischen Übersetzungen*, p. 651.

46 Sezgin, *Geschichte des arabischen Schrifttums*, Band III, pp. 28-32. Both this treatise and Galen's *Tegni* were translated into Latin from Greek and transmitted to the West via Byzantium. See Jacquart et Micheau, *La médecine arabe et l'occident médiéval*, pp. 171-172. The explanation of the Hebrew title given by the translator is to be found in one of the manuscripts of this translation: "[*Sefer agor*] means a short treatise which contains much", Paris, Bibliothéque Nationale, ms. héb. 1116, f. 12v. We find the same translation bearing the same title in another Hebrew codex, but according to the scribe, that translation was made from the Arabic (Paris, Bibliothèque Nationale, ms. héb. 1191, ff. 103r-124r). Cf. Steinschneider, *Die hebraeischen Übersetzungen*, p. 651.

47 The translator refers to Hippocratic treatise *Prognostikon*, translated into Arabic under the title: *Taqdimat al-ma'rifa.* See Sezgin, *Geschichte des arabischen Schrifttums*, Band III, p. 32; B. Alexanderson, "Die hippokratische Schrift Prognostikon", *Studia Graeca et Latina Gothoburgensia*, 17 (1963), pp. 156-170. A copy of a Hebrew translation, bearing the same title, exists in Paris, Bibliothèque Nationale, ms. héb. 1191, ff.124r-134r. This book was also translated by Nathan ha-Méatî, but was made from the Arabic version and it is entitled *Sefer haqdamat ha-yedi'ah* [Book on Introductory Knowledge]. See Paris, Bibliothèque Nationale, ms. héb. 1106, ff. 141r-202r. Cf. Steinschneider, *Die hebraeischen Übersetzungen*, pp. 662-663, 665-666.

minates the physicians' eyes.[48] Later [I translated] the Book on the Pulse, written by Pilart the Learned. It is indeed a very precious and important book.[49] Then [I translated] a book containing the whole [wisdom of medicine], called *Pantegni*, written by the learned Muḥammad al-Râzî.[50] It is a great book due to its immense quantity and its excellent quality. These are the seven books on medical theory used by them [the gentiles], and I have made every effort and employed all my intelligence to translate them. Praised be the God of my life.

The following are practical books I have translated: The first is *Sefer ha-kibusim ve-ha-taharot ha-gufaniyot* (Book on Purgations and Purifications of the Body), a sublime and wonderful [work].[51] Then, *Sefer ha-sheten* [Book on Urine], written by the learned physician Yiṣḥaq ha-Yisraeli.[52] Then, *Sefer ha-seter* (Book on Hidden [Place]), referring to

---

[48] The deformed name in the Hebrew manuscript refers to Theophilus, a Byzantine author, who wrote a treatise on urine, which was translated into Latin at the end of the eleventh century. See Jacquart et Micheau, *La médecine arabe et l'occident médiéval*, p. 101. A copy of this Hebrew translation is found in Paris, Bibliothèque Nationale, ms. héb. 1165, ff. 103r-108r. Cf. Steinschneider, *Die hebraeischen Übersetzungen*, p. 833.

[49] Philaretus, another Byzantine author whose book on pulses was translated into Latin at the same time as Theophilus' treatise on urine, see Jacquart et Micheau, *La médecine arabe et l'occident médiéval*, p. 101. For the Hebrew translation see Paris, Bibliothèque Nationale, ms. héb. 1190, f.111r.

[50] The *Liber Pantegni* is in fact the Latin translation made by Constantine the African of the great encyclopaedic Arabic work *Kâmil al-ṣinâ'a al- al-ṭibbîa*, written by 'Alî ibn al-'Abbâs al-Majûsî in the tenth century. The book became one of the most popular medical treatises in the Latin West during the Middle Ages. As far as we know there is a Hebrew translation only of the anatomical chapter of the book, which was made from the original Arabic and not from the Latin translation. It is possible, of course, that the translation mentioned here was lost. See R. Barkai, "The Hebrew and Judeo-Arabic Versions of al-Majûsî", in C. Burnett and D. Jacquart (eds.), *Constantine the African and 'Alî ibn al-'Abbâs al-Majûsî*, Brill, Leiden, New York and Köln, 1994, pp. 57-70. Cf. Steinschneider, *Die hebraeischen Übersetzungen*, p. 723. On the treatise and its translation into Latin, see Jacquart et Micheau, *La médecine arabe et l'occident médiéval*, pp. 101-107; Sezgin, *Geschichte des arabischen Schrifttums*, Band III, pp. 320-322.

[51] There are two Hebrew translations bearing the same title: the first is attributed to Hippocrates and Galen (Paris, Bibliothèque Nationale, ms. héb. 1120, f.1r-24v), and the second one to Gerard de Dontis (Paris, Bibliothèque Nationale, ms. héb. 1128, ff. 128r-165v). Both translations were made from the Latin, but the translator probably refers to the first one. Cf. Steinschneider, *Die hebraeischen Übersetzungen*, p. 792.

[52] See notes 5-6. On this specific treatise see E. Fontana, "Il capitolo sulle urine del 'Fasciculo de medicina'", *Pagine di storia della medicina*, 13 (1969), pp. 37-42; J. Peine, *Die Harnschrift des Isaac Judaeus*, Berlin, 1919. The treatise was indeed

women's hidden parts and cosmetics.[53] Afterwards, *Sefer ha-mis'adim* (Book on Foods), also written by Yiṣḥaq ha-Yisraeli, which explains the virtue of every category of food we eat and beverage we drink. It is called in their language *Diatespratikol.*[54] And *Sefer ha-tòledet* (Book on Generation), on conception, the womb, and pregnancy. They call it *Gynesias.*[55] And *Sefer ha-ém 'al Galynus* (Galen's Book on the Womb), which is very good.[56] And *Sefer le-ḥazeq et bedeq ha-bayit* (Book on [How] to Improve the Maintenance of the House). This book describes the various parts of the human body, the illnesses which could afflict these parts, and the appropriate treatment for each sickness.[57] Each book of this category is called *Practica.* Every one of them was written by a learned physician. As I have chosen to translate the most distinguished of these works, I continued and translated the *Sefer ya'ir nativ* (The Shining Road Book), called *Viatiq*, written by the learned Yiṣḥaq ha-Yisraeli. It is the most precious [f. 45v] since it concerns the strengthening of the body.[58] And *Sefer ha-madvim* (Book on Illnesses), written by Galen and

---

translated from Latin into Hebrew; one copy from the fourteenth century is conserved in Paris, Bibliothèque Nationale, ms. héb. 1125.

[53] The translator refers to one of the three texts which form the treatise traditionally attributed to Trotula. John Benton, adopting the incipit, entitled this text *Cum auctor*; Monica Green, however, identified its own title when it was circulating independently: *Liber de sinthomatibus mulierum* (LSM). We know only of a fragmentary Hebrew translation of this text which, based on my English translation, Monica Green identified as the version 3 of the treatise. See below, p. 30.

[54] On this treatise see Sezgin, *Geschichte des arabischen Schrifttums*, Band III, p. 296; concerning the Hebrew translation from the Latin version, see Steinschneider, *Die hebraeischen Übersetzungen*, pp. 755-756. The Hebrew title of the book is a deformation of the Latin one: *Liber diaetarum universalium et particularium.* The same treatise was also translated from the original Arabic into Hebrew. See Paris, Bibliothèque Nationale, ms. héb. 1128, ff.1r-33r.

[55] This is the first evidence of the translation of the Latin version of Soranus' *Gynaecia* into Hebrew. For a further discussion, see below, pp.30-31.

[56] The work was mistakenly attributed to Galen. In fact, it was identified by Monica Green as a translation of the *De passionibus mulierum* (Version B), a minor treatise on gynaecology derived in part from Muscio's Latin version of Soranus' treatise on gynaecology. See Hanson and Green, "Soranus of Ephesus: *Methodicorum princeps*", pp. 1054-1055. Cf. below p. 46.

[57] For the origin of the Hebrew title, see 2 Kings, 22:5. According to the description of the content given by the translator, it might be Constantine's *Practica.* Steinschneider identified it with a work written by Platearius, see *Die hebraeischen Übersetzungen*, p. 821.

[58] For the origin of the Hebrew title, see Job, 41:24. The author refers to the treatise *Zâd al-musâfir wa-qût al-ḥâdir*, written in the tenth century by Ibn al-Jazzâr, who was a disciple of Yiṣḥaq ha-Ysraeli, and not by ha-Ysraeli himself, as the translator claims. The work was translated into Latin by Constantine the African under the title *Viaticum peregrinantis*, mentioned in our text. There are in fact two

called *Pasionsi*, which is of great importance.[59] And *Sefer ha-qadaḥat* (Book on Fever), also written by Yiṣḥaq ha-Yisraeli, which is a precise and wonderfully profound book.[60] And *Sefer shnei ha-shemot* (Book on the Double Names), called *Synonimos.* [61] And *Sefer ha-ma'alot* (Book on Qualities), which explains the qualities of herbs and seeds their qualities of heat and cold, humidity and dryness, a very important book.[62] And *Sefer hashlamat ha-teva' ve-ha-mezeg* (Book on the Perfection of Nature and Temperament), which is good and useful.[63] And *Sefer ha-riquaḥ ha-qatan* (An Abridged Book on Pharmacology), called *Antidotary.*[64] And

---

other translations into Hebrew: the first one was made from the Latin version in the twelfth century, and the second, in 1259, from the original Arabic by the famous Moses ibn Tibbon under the title *Zeidat ha-derakhim* (Provision for the Ways). See Sezgin, *Geschichte des arabischen Schrifttums*, Band III, p. 305; Steinschneider, *Die hebraeischen Übersetzungen*, p. 761.

[59] The deformed Latin term mentioned by the translator probably refers to the treatise *Passionarius*, written in the middle of the eleventh century by Gariopuntus, and often attributed to Galen. See Jacquart et Micheau, *La médecine arabe et l'occident médiéval*, p. 120; Steinschneider, *Die hebraeischen Übersetzungen*, p. 791.

[60] It is *Kitâb al-ḥummayât*, translated into Latin by Constantine the African *(De febribus)*. On its translations into Latin and Hebrew, see M. Steinschneider and H. Friedenwald, "Manuscript Copies of the Medical Works of Isaac Israeli", in *The Jews and Medicine*, Essays I, Baltimore, 1944, p. 187. Cf. P. J. Llamas, *Ishaq Israeli: Tratado de las fiebras*, edición de la versión castellana y estudio, Madrid, 1945; D. J. Latham, "Isaac Israeli's Kitâb al-ḥummayât and the Latin and Castilian Texts", *Journal of Semitic Studies*, 14 (1969), pp. 80-95; Jacquart et Micheau, *La médecine arabe et l'occident médiéval*, p. 113-114. Another Hebrew translation of this treatise was made from the original Arabic, see Paris, Bibliothèque Nationale, ms. héb. 1126. Cf. Steinschneider, *Die hebraeischen Übersetzungen*, p. 761.

[61] I could not identify the treatise. For various Hebrew translations of this genre, see Steinschneider, *Die hebraeischenÜbersetzungen*, pp. 839-840.

[62] The translator refers to Ibn al-Jazzâr's work *Kitâb 'i'timâd al-adwiya al-mufarada*, translated into Latin by Constantine the African under the title *Liber de gradibus.* See Sezgin, *Geschichte des arabischen Schrifttums*, Band III, pp. 304-305; cf. M. Wack, "'Alî ibn al-'Abbâs al-Magûsî and Constantine on Love, and the Evolution of the *Practica Pantegni*", in Burnett and Jacquart (eds.), *Constantine the African and 'Alî ibn al-'Abbâs al-Majûsî*, pp. 178-184. Cf. Steinschneider, *Die hebraeischen Übersetzungen*, pp. 703-704.

[63] Actually, there is a treatise bearing the same title. See Paris, Bibliothèque Nationale, ms. héb. 1171, ff. 5r-29r. Steinschneider identified it with Galen's *De virtutibus simplicium medicinarum*, see: *Die hebraeischen Übersetzungen*, p. 790.

[64] Since the translator follows the work of Constantine in most cases, it would reasonable to suppose that he refers to the *Pantegni* antidotary, which appears in the tenth book of the *Practica.* On this text and its sources, see Wack, "'Alî ibn al-'Abbâs al-Magûsî an Constantine on Love, and the Evolution of the *Practica Pantegni*", pp. 184-194. However, we cannot exclude other possibilities, such as the second part of the second book by John of Damascus, translated into Latin and then

Sefer ha-'asavim (Herbal Book), which describes the herbs' forms, qualities, and habitats; it is a precious and graceful book.[65] Another herbal book, called *Maser*, after the name of its author, refers to herbs neglected by other authors.[66] And *Sefer ha-'ofot ha-tofsim aḥerim* (Book on Birds of Prey), such as the *Avotor,* the *Falcon* and others. This book refers to the sicknesses which might afflict these birds. I liked it very much.[67] The total number of practical books which I have translated is seventeen, with seven more on medical theory...[68]

The authenticity of the information given in this personal testimony has been verified by a large number of known translations which bear the same titles as those listed by the author. It is true that the Hebrew author cites some of the author's names erroneously, but this kind of error was quite common in the Middle Ages, given the long period during which translations were made from Greek into Arabic, from Arabic into Latin, and from Arabic and Latin into He-

---

into Hebrew (see: Paris, Bibliothèque Nationale, ms. héb. 1128, ff. 60r-94v); or the *Antidotarius magnus*, complied around 1100, or the *Antidotarium Nicolai.* On these two treatises, see A. Lutz, "Der verschollene frühsalernitanische Antidotarius magnus in einer Basler Handschrift aus dem 12. Jahrhundert und das Antidotarium Nicolai", *Die Vorträge der Hauptversammlung der Internationalen Gesellschaft für Geschichte der Pharmazie*, XVI, Stuttgart, 1960. Steinschneider, however, identified this translation with the *Antidotarium Nicolai* (*Die hebraeischen Übersetzungen*, p. 812). The Hebrew introduction to this translation, made by Jacob ha-Qatan, was published by S. Muntner in his "Ya'qob ha-Qatan, the Anonymous Translator of the 13th Century", *Tarbitz*, 18 (1947), pp. 192-193. (Hebrew)

[65] According to the description given in the manuscript, it has to be an illuminated herbal book, but we do not have any clue which can help in its identification. Perhaps he refers to Dioscorides' *Materia medica*, which was available from the end of the eleventh century in an enlarged and alphabetized Latin version. See J. M. Riddle, "Dioscorides", in *Catalogus translationum et commentariorum: Medieval and Renaissance Translations and Commentaries*, edited by P. O. Kristeller et al., Washington, D. C., IV (1980), pp. 6-8.

[66] The author refers to one of the most popular medieval herbal called *Macer Floridus*, written in the eleventh century and attributed to Odo Magdunensis. See B. Flood, "The Medieval Herbal Tradition of Macer Floridus", *Pharmacy in History*, 18 (1976), pp. 62-66. Cf. Steinschneider, *Die hebraeischen Übersetzungen*, pp. 808-809.

[67] Medieval Jews did not take part in bird, or other animal hunting for two main reasons: most of the hunted animals were forbidden according to Jewish dietary laws; furthermore, their social and environmental situation did not allow them to participate in such leisure activities. So, except for pure curiosity, I do not see any reason to translate a treatise on falconry into Hebrew. Cf.: Steinschneider, *Die hebraeischen Übersetzungen*, p. 969.

[68] Bibliothèque Nationale, Paris, ms. héb. 1190, ff. 44r-46r.

brew, which resulted in authors' names being omitted, added or deformed. Moreover, in some cases he simply repeated the errors made in the Latin texts he translated. Therefore, this document stands as authentic evidence to the powerful impulse to translate into Hebrew major medical treatises which existed amongst the Jewish communities at that time. It is undoubtedly a direct source of information on what had come to be considered an indispensable corpus of medical literature. No less instructive is the fact that three gynaecological works were included in the list, as we shall see.

The Hebrew translator faithfully follows the new conceptions of medical science finding a foothold in the West under the influence of Latin translations of Arabic medical works. "Arabic Galenism" clearly distinguished between the *Theory* and the *Practice* of medicine. This division gave rise to encyclopaedic works, composed according to the two distinct themes, and, to a certain extent, to specialised practical treatises. This explains the Hebrew translator's insistence on the separation of the two domains - he was following the Arabic tradition in its Latin version. This perspective may explain why the first work he translated was the *Isagoge Iohanitii*, a fragmentary Latin translation of Ḥunain ibn Isḥâq's *Masâ'il fi al-ṭibb* which is a general introduction to the art of medicine, in form of questions and answers, and is based on the division between theory and practice.[69] We should note that the title of the treatise given in the Hebrew text, *Guanis*, is, of course, a deformation of the Latin *Iohannitius*, itself a deformation of the Arabic name Ḥunain in its Latin transliteration.[70] The Latin translation of the *Isagoge*, probably made by Constantine the African, is somewhat inaccurate, although it remains a systematic treatise, with comprehensive sections on anatomy, physiology, pathology, and therapeutics. Many Latin medieval manuscripts describe this work as an introduction to Galen's important medical treatise, *Tegni*, and it had a permanent place at the head of the *Articella*.[71] The Hebrew translator concurs with this as-

---

[69] Jacquart et Micheau, *La médecine arabe et l'occident médiéval*, pp. 46-54.

[70] A modern edition of the *Isagoge* was published by Gregor Maurach in his article "Johannicius: Isagoge ad Techne Galieni", *Sudhoffs Archiv*, 67 (1978), pp. 148-174. Cf. F. Newton, "Constantine the African and Monte Cassino: New Elements and the Text of the *Isagoge*", in Burnett and Jacquart (eds.), *Constantine the African and 'Alî ibn al-'Abbâs al-Majûsî*, pp. 16-42.

[71] On the development of the *Articella* see P. O. Kristeller, "Bartholomaeus, Musandinus and Maurus of Salerno and other Early Commentators of the *Articella*

sessment, describing the *Isagoge* as an introduction to other theoretical texts, which was indeed its role within the *Articella*.

Constantine the African is the author of other major translations from Arabic into Latin which are included in the Hebrew list. Two of them, Galen's *Tegni* and the *Prognostics*, attributed to Hippocrates, can be readily identified. On the other hand, the Hebrew author claims to have translated Hippocrates' *Aphorisms*, traditionally called *Sefer Agor* in Hebrew medieval literature, whereas as far as we know, Constantine translated the *Expositio Aforismi*, Galen's commentary to the Hippocratic work.[72]

The second discrepancy concerns one of the most important Latin translations of an Arabic medical work, the *Pantegni*, translated by Constantine the African from 'Alî ibn al-'Abbâs al-Majûsî's book *Kâmil al-sinâ'a al-ṭibbiya.* Divided into two parts, *Theorica* and *Practica*, this treatise was the natural complement to the *Isagoge.*[73] The Hebrew translator mistakenly attributed the treatise to another major Muslim physician, Muḥammad al-Râzî. This error demonstrates how faithfully the Hebrew translator followed the Latin tradition, which sometimes attributed the work to "Rasis".[74]

As stated, seventeen books appear in the section on the "practice" of medicine. Three were written in Arabic by the Jewish physician and philosopher Isaac ha-Yisraeli, and translated into Latin by Constantine: *De urinis*, *De dietis* and *De febribus*. Ha-Yisraeli is the only author whose name Constantine cited in his Latin translations. Some historians are inclined to believe that Constantine retained ha-Yisraeli's name due to his religious affiliation: "Il ne peut en effet s'agir d'une simple coïncidence si le seul auteur cité en clair a, inscrite dans son nom, son appartenance à la religion juive".[75] In any case, there can be no doubt concerning the enthusiasm of the Hebrew translator toward his co-religionist: witness the explicit references in

---

with a Tentative List of texts and Manuscripts", *Italia medioevale et umanistica*, 19 (1976), pp. 57-87.

[72] Another Hebrew translation of Galen's commentary was made in the thirteenth century by Nathan ha-Méatî. See Sezgin, *Geschichte des arabischen Schrifttums*, Band III, pp. 29-30.

[73] On the various historical, philological and medical problems regarding this translation, see *Constantine the African and 'Alî ibn al-'Abbâs al-Majûsî.*

[74] On the Latin manuscripts which attribute the treatise to al-Râzî, see M. Jordan, "The Fortune of Constantine's *Pantegni*", in *Constantine the African and 'Alî ibn al-'Abbâs al-Majûsî*, pp. 293-294.

[75] Jacquart et Micheau, *La médecine arabe et l'occident médiéval*, p. 114.

the introduction, the inclusion of three authentic works by ha-Yisraeli, and the attribution of the *Viaticum* to him. This treatise was actually written by ha-Yisraeli's Muslim disciple, Ibn al-Jazzâr (d. 1009), and was among the Arabic medical works translated by Constantine. It is worth noting that copies of our anonymous translator's Hebrew version were immensely popular in the Middle Ages.[76]

Regarding the history of medieval Hebrew gynaecological texts, this introduction is of great importance for two major reasons: Clear testimony is presented of the availability of at least three gynaecological texts in the Hebrew medical corpus namely, *Sefer ha-toledet, Sefer ha-ém 'al Galynus* and *Sefer ha-seter*, as early as the end of the twelfth century; second, we can determine with certainty the origin of these texts, as well as the time and circumstances of their translation from the Latin.

Of the two first texts *(Sefer ha-toledet, Sefer ha-ém 'al Galynus)*, several manuscripts exist which bear the same titles indicated in the document;[77] however, none have been discovered with the heading *Sefer ha-seter*. The translator is probably referring to the Latin gynaecological text entitled *Liber de sinthomatibus mulierum* (*Lsm 3*) or, according to its incipit, *Cum auctor*, which was one of the three components of the treatise attributed to Trotula.[78] The fact that the Hebrew translator mentioned cosmetics as an item in the treatise may be a further indication that he was indeed referring to this text.[79] A fragment of a manuscript of the Hebrew *Lsm 3* exists in the same codex in which the two other treatises are preserved.[80] An examination of the manuscript has revealed that five to nine leaves are missing between fols. 59 and 60,[81] that is to say, the end of the previous text (*Sefer ha-ém 'al Galynus*) and the beginning of *Sefer ha-seter* have been lost.[82]

As noted above, *Sefer ha-toledet* is the Hebrew adaptation of Muscio's Latin version of the *Gynaecia* written by Soranus of

---

[76] Steinschneider, *Die hebraeischen Übersetzungen*, pp. 703-705.

[77] See Table I.

[78] On the treatise, its components and authorship, see Monica H. Green, "The Development of the *Trotula*", *Revue d'Histoire des Textes*, 26 (1996), pp. 119-203.

[79] The tract on cosmetics, beauty aids, etc. in the compilation is entitled *De ornatu mulierum*, see *ibid.*, pp. 139-143.

[80] London, Jews' College, Montefiore Ms. 440.

[81] See: M. Steinschneider, "Medicinische Handschriften im Besitz des Herrn Halberstam", *Magazin für die Wissenschaft des Judenthums*, 1883, p.108.

[82] See also below, pp. 62-63.

Ephesus.[83] In the critical edition of this text, appearing in the second part of *Les infortunes de Dinah, ou la gynécologie juive au moyen âge*, the hypothesis was raised that the Hebrew version was written in the first half of the thirteenth century, probably by Solomon ibn Ayyub, a Jewish physician who had immigrated from Granada to Béziers.[84] However, a close comparison of this treatise with *Sefer ha-ém 'al Galynus* (the Hebrew translation of the minor Latin gynaecological treatise *De passionibus mulierum*, Version B, derived in part from Muscio's *Gynaecia*) demonstrates that the assumptions underlying this hypothesis were wrong. Both translations were undoubtedly made by the same author, who committed the same errors in comprehension of the Latin texts and employed exactly the same terms while rendering the Latin into Hebrew.[85] Perhaps the most striking example is the employment in both texts of the Occitan term *breç*, for "rocking bed".[86]

Nevertheless, there is one important difference between these three Hebrew texts: While the translation of the two minor works - *Sefer ha-ém 'al Galynus* and *Sefer ha-seter* - parallel the original Latin almost word by word, the translator "dressed" Muscio's *Gynaecia* with Jewish garments. This transformation was accomplished by adding the translator's own introduction to the treatise, by inserting Biblical and Talmudic quotations and expressions, and by revising the whole work as a dialogue between two Biblical personalities, namely, the patriarch Jacob and his daughter Dinah.[87]

Why did the translator take such pains to "Judaize" only Muscio's *Gynaecia* ? Since the author himself says nothing on the matter in any of the documents, including the *Gynaecia*, we may offer two possible explanations: the first is that the "Jewish" introduction and happy ending, together with the Biblical and Talmudic references, were added later by another author; the second is that the translator himself Judaized the treatise in order to facilitate its circulation among the Jewish communities. The latter seems the more likely answer for the following reasons: formally, the entire treatise is written in the same medieval Hebrew style; more significantly, the

[83] Steinschneider, "Medicinische Handschriften im Besitz des Herrn Halberstam", pp. 157-158; cf. *Les infortunes de Dinah*, pp. 117-128.
[84] *Les infortunes de Dinah*, pp. 127-128.
[85] See below p. 56.
[86] See: *Les infortunes de Dinah*, pp. 285.
[87] See: *Les infortunes de Dinah*, pp. 129-132.

translator probably realised that this text, in addition to its size and comprehensiveness, was also a normative pillar of the Latin medical corpus of his time, one he intended to render available to the Hebrew reader.[88]

The intriguing question is, of course, who was this translator and where did he conduct this enormous project? Moritz Steinschneider, the first to understand the critical importance of this document for the history of medieval Hebrew translations and Jewish medicine, has identified most of the translated treatises.[89] In his attempt to locate the site where the translations were undertaken, he identified the translator with the author of "The Treatise on Procreation Called the Secret of Conception" (see below, pp. 76-79, 212-222), who lived in Orange in southern France. As already demonstrated by Neubauer in his catalogue of Hebrew manuscripts kept in the Bodleian Library, this identification is incorrect inasmuch as the last treatise mentions the names of Arnold of Villanova and Robert King of Naples, indicating that the treatise was written in the fourteenth century and not in the twelfth, the period in which the other translations mentioned in the document were written.

Suessman Muntner has suggested that our laborious translator was Rabbi Jacob ha-Qatan (c. 1230-1290), who translated Averroes' medical treatise *Kitâb al-kullîyyât fi al-ṭibb* from Arabic into Hebrew.[90] His argument is based on a medical text called *Sefer ha-yosher*, written by Jacob's brother.[91] The author of this treatise, whose name is unknown, mentions some translations made by his brother Jacob ha-Qatan, which Muntner tried to identify with the list supplied by the anonymous translator. The accuracy of Muntner's identification seems doubtful due to the striking fact that the translator does not include Averroes' treatise in his list. If Jacob was indeed the translator, why did he omit this title? Moreover, *Sefer ha-yosher* mentions a gynaecological text called *Sitrei nashim*, which Muntner refers to as if it was identical to the *Sefer ha-seter* which appears in

---

[88] On the dominance of Muscio's *Gynaecia* and its derivative texts up through the twelfth century, see Hanson and Green, "Soranus of Ephesus: *Methodicorum princeps*", pp. 1055-1057. I am indebted to Monica H. Green for many of these conclusions.

[89] Steinschneider, *Die hebraeischen Übersetzungen*, pp. 712-714.

[90] A critical edition of the treatise was published by J. M. Fórneas Besteiro and C. Alvarez de Morales, Madrid, 1987 (2 vols.).

[91] S. Muntner, "R. Ya'qob ha-Qatan the Anonymous Translator of the 13th Century", pp. 195-199.

the list of translations. The fact that words based on the Hebrew root "s-ṭ-r" appear in both titles does not prove that the works are identical. In other cases, the author of *Sefer ha-yosher* mentions titles of translations in fact listed by the anonymous translator; however, he does not state that these texts were translated by his brother. Muntner's last argument deals with the date of the translations: Contrary to Muntner's assumptions, Steinschneider's reading of the date appearing in the document (1197-1199) is correct. It seems, then, that the issue of the identity of the translator has yet to be resolved.

The anonymous translator represents, in fact, an excellent example of the role of personalities in history: Unquestionably he was an intellectual product of his time, a Jew who was fluent in Hebrew as well as in Latin, anchored in Jewish culture but deeply interested in the Latin one. And yet he, as an individual made the specific choices of what to translate into Hebrew; by doing so, he marked the course of Jewish medicine in general and of gynaecology in particular. The consequences of his decisions may be illustrated by the fact that his Hebrew translation of Muscio's *Gynaecia* rendered it the most popular gynaecological work among Jewish physicians during the Middle Ages.

Another interesting question is to what extent the Hebrew translator fulfilled his intention, made in the introduction, to avoid the cure of Jews by gentile physicians because their therapies included methods and ingredients which contradict Jewish Law? The use of impure medicaments was not censored at all in the three translated gynaecological texts; thus, medical treatments involving the use of materials such as pork fat frequently appear within them.[92] On the other hand, he omitted some important paragraphs and significantly changed others in *Sefer ha-toledet*, the translation of Muscio's text. While Muscio, following Soranus, affirmed that perpetual virginity was salubrious, the Hebrew author only recommended the prolongation of virginity; again, guided by the same religious precepts, he eliminated the paragraph claiming that pregnancy is noxious to a woman's health.[93]

[92] The use of "impure" materials and prohibited practices was common phenomenon in Jewish medical and magical writings during the Middle Ages, see Barkaï, *Les infortunes de Dinah*, pp. 99-104.

[93] For a comparison of the Hebrew text with the original Latin, see *ibid.*, pp. 137-138.

The difference between the two cases is evident: Medieval Jewish medical treatises rarely censored the use of impure curative materials. The Biblical and Talmudic commandment to heal the sick was considered a cardinal religious duty, and medieval Jewish physicians followed this commandment even if it involved a transgression of the Purity Laws. On the other hand, Soranus' medical conceptions of virginity, sexual relations and pregnancy diametrically contradict Jewish Law concerning the creation of new lives ("Be fruitful and multiply...", Genesis I: 28), and the translator was thereby obliged to amend Soranus' text.

To summarize, our anonymous translator certainly played a decisive role in the development of medieval Hebrew medicine, a role comparable to that of Constantine the African in Latin medicine at the end of the eleventh century. During a turning point in medieval Jewish culture, when the use of the "Holy Tongue" in writing philosophical and scientific works, expressing ideas and thoughts taken from foreign cultures (considered hostile to Judaism), and creating a comprehensive scientific corpus became permissible, he undertook the challenge to make the most important Latin medical literature of the twelfth century available to the Jewish intellectuals and practitioners. It was indeed an enormous task, not only because of religious-cultural barriers, but also due to the sheer quantity of material. His achievement is especially monumental when we consider the fact that the Hebrew language of the period lacked the necessary medical lexicon.

E. The Formation of the Hebrew Medical Corpus

The translation project accomplished by the anonymous author at the end of the twelfth century was a pioneering work, which was followed by other translators and writers until a corpus of Hebrew medical texts was created, equal in quantity and quality to the Arabic and the Latin. By the thirteenth century, a large number of medical works had already been translated into Hebrew directly from the original Arabic by a number of translators residing in southern France, Christian Spain and Italy.

The first major translations from the Arabic were made by Moses ibn Tibbon, who well illustrates the extraordinary medieval phenomenon of families of physicians and scientific translators. His grandfather, Judah ben Sha'ul ibn Tibbon, was born in Granada and emigrated (c. 1160) to Lunel in southern France, were he practised medicine and translated some minor medical texts from Arabic into Hebrew. Judah transmitted his medical knowledge and the Arabic language to his son Samuel, who, in turn, became a famous physician and translator. This lineage attained its height with the son of Samuel ibn Tibbon, Moses, the "Prince of Translators", who also practised medicine in Montpellier, were he completed his most important translations from Arabic into Hebrew.[94]

Due to his great prestige as a physician and commentator on Jewish Law, it is not surprising that almost the entire medical corpus written in Arabic by Maimonides, was translated into Hebrew by the end of this century, some treatises were even translated twice, and by different authors. As early as 1244, Moses ibn Tibbon translated Maimonides' *Regimen sanitatis*[95] into Hebrew; shortly afterwards, he successively translated the *Aphorisms* of Hippocrates, based on the Arabic version by Ḥunain ibn Isḥâq, and Maimonides' Commentary to this work.[96] Moses ibn Tibbon also translated Maimonides' treatise on Poisons and their Antidotes, also entitled "The Treatise to the Honoured One"[97] (a second Hebrew translation was made by Zeraḥiah ben Shaltiél), and the treatise "On Hemorrhoids".[98] In addition to the Maimonidian medical corpus, Moses ibn Tibbon dedicated his energies to translating a number of major medical treatises such as Ḥunain ibn Isḥâq's *Masâ'il fî al-ṭibb* or *al-Mudkhal ilâ al-*

---

[94] D. Bercovy, "Un nome illustre parmi les médecins juifs de Provence: Ibn Tibbon", *Revue d'histoire de la médecine hébraïque*, 20 (1967), pp. 169-176.

[95] Steinschneider, *Die hebraeischen Übersetzungen*, p. 769. Cf. *Maimonides Medical Works, Vol. I: Regimen sanitatis*, ed. S. Muntner, Jerusalem, 1957, pp. 20-21 (Hebrew).

[96] We may learn of the importance of this genre of medical writing in Hebrew medicine from the fact that apart from Ibn Tibbon's translation, Hipppocrates' Aphorisms with Galen's Commentary were translated twice from the Arabic (by Nathan ha-Méatî and Zeraḥiah ben Shaltiél Gracian) and once from the Latin by the same above mentioned anonymous author. There are more than 40 Hebrew manuscripts of Hippocrates' Aphorisms, most of them also include the Commentaries of Galen and Maimonides. See *Maimonides' Medical Works, Vol. III: Commentary on the Aphorisms of Hippocrates*, ed. S. Muntner, Jerusalem, 1961, pp. XXVI-XXIX. (Hebrew).

[97] See S. Muntner edition, Jerusalem, 1942.

[98] The Hebrew translation of Maimonides' work *On Hemorrhoids* was attributed to Nathan ha-Méatî as well, but since this translator worked in Rome and the translation was made in Provence, it is more likely that Ibn Tibbon wrote it. See *Maimonides' Medical Works,* Vol. IV, Jerusalem, 1972, p. 10 (Hebrew).

ṭibb[99]; *Kitâb taqsîm al-'ilal* and *Kitâb al-aqrâbâdîn* written by al-Râzî[100]; and finally, Ibn al-Jazzâr's treatise *Zâd al-musâfir wa-qût al-ḥâdir*, completed in 1259.[101]

Moses ibn Tibbon was followed by another great translator, Nathan ha-Méatî, also called *Nagid ha-metarguemim* (The Prince of Translators) or "the Italian Tibbon". A native of the Italian city Cento, the source of his surname ha-Méatî (Cento = hundred, in Hebrew Méah), he worked as a translator in Rome between 1273-1283. In his introduction to the translation of Ibn Sînâ's *Qânûn*, Nathan ha-Méatî considered himself the follower of the Tibbons, who had "redeemed" this literature from the Arabs. Of Maimonides' medical works, he translated the "(Medical) Aphorisms of Moses" in 1283 (six years after Zeraḥiah ben Shaltiél Gracian accomplished his translation of the same work, also in Rome).[102] This work attracted great interest during the Middle Ages and in modern times. Not only did Maimonides expound on his medical views and conceptions in this piece, he also stated his critical position regarding Galen - the "Sacred War Against Galen".[103] In addition he translated various treatises of the Hippocratic corpus from the Arabic: The Aphorisms, including the commentary of Galen *(al-fusûl)*;[104] the Prognostic *(Taqdimat al-ma'rifa)*;[105] On Acute Diseases *(al-Amrâd al-ḥâdda)*;[106] and Book on the Airs, the Times, the Waters and the Countries *(Kitâb al-ahwiya wa-l-azmina wa-l-miyâh wa-l-buldûn)*, to which his son Solomon ha-Méatî added a Hebrew translation of Galen's commentary.[107] Furthermore, he translated a number of original treatises written in Arabic by Muslim physicians: 'Ammâr al-Mausilî's book on the eye, its diseases and their remedies *(Kitâb al-muntakhab fî 'ilm al-'ain wa-'ilalihâ wa-mudâwâtihâ bi-l-adwiya wa-l-ḥadîd)*,[108] the surgical treatise of al-Zahrâwî (Abulcasis): *Kitâb al-tasrîf li-man 'ajiza 'an al-tasnîf)*, (which was also translated by

---

[99] Steinschneider, *Die hebraeischen Übersetzungen*, pp. 709-711.

[100] *Ibid.*, pp. 729-730.

[101] *Ibid.*, p. 703

[102] *Maimonides' Medical Works, Vol. II: (Medical) Aphorisms of Moses in Twenty Five Treatises*, ed. S. Muntner, Jerusalem, 1972, pp. XXII-XXIII (Hebrew).

[103] *Ibid.*, 323-398.

[104] Steinschneider, *Die hebraeischen Übersetzungen*, p. 659.

[105] *Ibid.*, p. 663.

[106] *Ibid.*

[107] *Ibid.*

[108] *Ibid.*, p. 670.

Shem-Tov ben Isaac of Tortosa)[109] and finally, Ibn al-Jazzâr's treatise On Oblivion.[110]

We see, then, that in a relatively short space of time after the commencement of the "second Renaissance" of medieval Hebrew, Jewish physicians and scholars, had at their disposal the major works of Arabic Galenism in a Hebrew rendition and, in several cases, even various translations of the same work. These translations, which encompassed all the major trends of Arabic (from Ḥunain to Averroes) and Latin medicine (based on Greek authors ignored by the Arabs or Latin versions of Arabic texts) available at the time. These enabled Jewish physicians to be well versed in the medical science of the era and to practice this art on a high level.[111] Other than the professional-practical impact of these translations, they also prepared the ground for a rich, genuinely Hebrew medical literature, to be written from the end of the twelfth to the fifteenth centuries, since they provided the medical lexicon previously absent in the Hebrew language. The huge quantity of Hebrew medical manuscripts - whether translated from Latin and Arabic or in the original Hebrew - which cover all aspects of medieval medicine, presents undeniable evidence that the "Holy Tongue" had become a written scientific language in Latin Europe.

Furthermore, these translations provide clear indications that medieval Jewish culture developed in close interaction with other cultures. In order to understand the role of this interaction in the formation of the Hebrew gynaecological literature as well as the differences between this corpus and the Arabic and the Latin, I present to the reader a general overview of the Arabic and Latin gynaecological texts in the next chapter.

---

[109] Paris, Bibliothèque Nationale, ms. héb. 1163. Cf. *ibid.*, pp. 740-741.

[110] Steinschneider, *Die hebrischen Übersetzungen*, p. 752. S. Muntner published this Hebrew version in: *Ha-rofé ha-'ivri*, New York, 1953.

[111] Unfortunately, there is not any comprehensive study of medieval Hebrew medicine based on a detailed examination of the available translated and genuine manuscripts. Such a study might enable us to understand the choices made by the translators and the scientific trends that prevailed in the Jewish communities. Thus the great significance of the finding that Ibn Sînâ's Qanûn was not only translated twice from Arabic into Hebrew, but also circulated in Jewish European communities in one hundred and eleven partial or complete manuscripts. See B. Richler, "Manuscripts of Avicenna's Kanon in Hebrew Translation: A Revised and Up-to-date List", *Koroth*, 8 (1982), pp. 145-168 (Hebrew).

CHAPTER TWO

THE SPECIALIZED ARABIC AND EARLY MEDIEVAL LATIN GYNAECOLOGICAL TREATISES

A. The Greek Heritage

The sources of medieval medicine, whether Arabic, Latin or Hebrew, are to be found in ancient cultures, and particularly in Greek science. Some Greek medical texts were translated into Latin and circulated in the West as early as the sixth century, but only with the rise of the Muslim Caliphate was a systematic and comprehensive translation of Greek sciences accomplished.

In the first two centuries of the existence of the Caliphate, the early Muslim regime was highly open to "foreign" influences, especially of those cultures with which it had come in contact as a result of the creation of the Muslim Empire, from China in the East to Spain in the West. The rich literatures of the various nations subjected to Muslim power were soon translated into Arabic and widely disseminated. In the domain of medicine, between the eighth and the ninth centuries, Greek authors especially were translated into Arabic. The medical ideas and conceptions of Galen and Hippocrates soon came to dominate Arabic medicine.[1]

However, Greek medicine was by no means monolithic; it needs to be understood in its larger context, namely, as part of the various contemporary philosophical schools which interpreted medical conceptions of illness and therapy as elements in a global vision. Generally speaking, we may distinguish three main schools of thought: the Dogmatic, the Empiricist, and the Methodist. The Dogmatic approach, represented notably by Hippocrates and Galen, assumed that anatomy, experience and observation could supply a solid basis for

---

[1] M. Ullmann, *Islamic Medicine*, Edinburgh, 1978, pp. 7-40; F. Sezgin, *Geschichte des Arabischen Schrifttums*, Band III, 1970, pp. 20-171.

the development of a general medical theory (such as the theory of humours). Thus, the learned physician, by rationally evaluating the causes of an ailment, can treat it efficiently.[2]

As opposed to this rationalistic and optimistic view, there was the sceptical attitude, which gave rise to the Empiricist or experimental school of medicine. This school doubted the capacity of human reason to understand nature's secrets, such as the functioning of the human body, by means of observation and rational analysis. Thus, the physicians who belonged to this school concluded that the only valid medical methodology was personal experience of the physician, and the practical knowledge accumulated by physicians and other medical practitioners over the generations. Experience, and not a general theory, was thus deemed the sole source of information on ailments, only by accumulating experience could the physician respond correctly.[3]

The third group - the Methodist identified primarily with Soranus, - totally rejected the conceptions of the preceding two schools. The Methodists claimed that appropriate medical treatment had nothing to do with anatomical knowledge nor with a general theory of the body's nature. In addition, they claimed that experience could not serve as the only, or even the principal basis of medical treatment. According to this "most radical of sects", the physician should know the three general conditions of the human body, namely, the "lax" *(solutio, fluens)*, the "constricted" *(strictura, adstrictum)*, and the "mixture" *(complexio)* of the two.[4] To this general consideration of

---

[2] Two medical authorities represent the rationalistic, "Dogmatic" attitude in medicine: Hippocrates (c. 460 - c. 370 B. C.) and Galen (c. 130-c. 200). We usually refer to the *Hippocratic medical corpus* as a whole since research has not been able to identify which of these texts were written by Hippocrates himself and which by his disciples. See G. E. R. Lloyd, "The Hippocratic Question", *Classical Quarterly*, 25 (1975), pp. 175-192. On Hippocratic medicine, women's ailments and their cure, see *idem*, *Science, Folklore and Ideology*, pp. 58-86. Cf. W. D. Smith, *The Hippocratic Tradition*, Ithaca and London, 1979. On Galen and his medical conceptions, see O. Temkin, *Galenism: The Rise and Decline of a Medical Philosophy*, Ithaca and London, 1973; L. García Ballester, *Galeno, en la sociedad y en la ciencia de su tiempo*, Madrid, 1972.

[3] Lloyd, *Science, Folklore and Ideology*, pp. 182-188.

[4] *Soranos d'Éphèse, maladies des femmes*, p. XIII. The authors note that: "Les expressions de *status strictus, status laxus* et *status mixtus*, choisies par l'érudition moderne, ne figure ni dans Celse ni dans Caelius Aurelianus", *ibid.* Cf. O. Temkin, "Celsus' 'On Medicine' and the Ancient Medical Sects", *Bulletin of the Institute of the History of Medicine*, 3 (1935), pp. 249-264.

the states of the body, they distinguished between two different situations of the ailment itself, *chronic* and *acute*, upon which the physician should base adequate treatment. An additional, third principle characterized Soranus' medical attitude to gynaecological therapy: He insisted on external treatment rather than internal interventions, which might be brutal and harmful.[5]

Undoubtedly, Soranus was one of the most distinguished representatives of the Methodist trend and his gynaecological works exercised a profound influence on both Latin and Jewish women's medicine. From the little information on the life of this important physician, we know that he was born in the middle of the first century A. D. in Ephesus, in Asia Minor, and studied medicine in Alexandria. He practised his profession in Rome, from the end of the first to the beginning of the second century.[6] From Soranus' *Gynaikeia* we can learn that he possessed more precise knowledge on female anatomy than that which had been available to the Hippocratic school. This was due primarily to the anatomical studies, which were based on the dissection of human corpses, carried out by Herophilus at the Alexandrian School in the third century B. C.[7]

Some scholars have remarked upon the inconsistency in Soranus' theoretical system, which on the one hand rejected any general theory of medicine yet, on the other, relied on some theory when dwelling on aetiology and therapy. It is especially instructive to follow G. E. R. Lloyd's conclusions, based on a detailed analysis of Soranus' gynaecology: "When tensions between Methodist or sceptical principals and actual medical practice arise, they are resolved by Soranus, in several of the cases we have considered, in favour of practice, in the sense that the purity of some of the principles is sacrificed, or the principles more or less drastically modified, in the course of his discussion of what were, after all, often obscure and

---

[5] Lloyd, *Science, Folklore and Ideology*, pp. 182-200; M. H. Green, *The Transmission of Ancient Theories of Female Physiology and Disease Through the Early Middle Ages*, Ph. D. dissertation, Princeton University, 1985, pp. 24-36.

[6] Hanson and Green, "Soranus of Ephesus", pp. 969-1005.

[7] It should be noted that even in the Alexandrian School, human dissections were rare, and the description of female's genital members was based essentially on the study of animals. See P. Porter, "Herophilus of Chalcedon; An Assessment of his Place in the History of Anatomy", *Bulletin of the History of Medicine*, 50 (1976), pp. 45-60; H. von Staden, *Herophilus. The Art of Medicine in Early Alexandria*, Cambridge, 1989. Cf. Hanson and Green, "Soranus of Ephesus", p. 982.

complex issues. This makes Soranus a better gynecologist, but a less interesting exponent of a particular philosophy of science".[8]

Learned medicine in the Middle Ages, Arabic, Latin as well as Hebrew generally followed the rationalistic school of Hippocrates and Galen. Nevertheless, the Empiricist trend retained certain influence in medieval medicine, as may be attested from both "practical" texts and the criticism against this school made by rationalistic authors. On the other hand, the impact of Methodism was limited to Latin and Hebrew Gynaecology.

B. Arabic Gynaecology and Obstetrics

The Greek medical texts were introduced to the Arabic speaking élite of the Caliphate *via* two main paths: Syriac translations and essentially original Greek texts found in the Byzantine Empire. The latter path provided the Muslim world not only with the content of Greek medicine, but also with its manner of presentation: Generally speaking, Arab authors of medical works had a preference for the encyclopaedic format, which encompassed medical knowledge, theoretical as well as practical, in its entirety, in one comprehensive text. This genre, corresponded perfectly to the social and intellectual needs of Muslim society. The comprehensive medical manual, organized in a rigid rational pattern, could serve equally well physicians who wished to have, in one portable book, the whole of medical knowledge; students of medical sciences who could learn the various aspects of this art with the aid of one consistent approach; and last but not least, educated laymen, for whom medicine and biology formed an integral part of general education. This trend was well described by D. Jacquart and F. Micheau: "On rédige quantité d'ouvrages à caractère encyclopedique; qui pretendent tout embrasser et ne rien négliger des connaissances tenues pour indispensables à l'honnête homme d'alors. En un même volume et sous une form maniable, ils réunissent les informations les plus diverses, jusque-lâ dispersées. Par leur contenu étendu et par leur forme soignée, ils témoignent des curiosités et des goûts de toute une société".[9]

---

[8] Lloyd, *Science, Folklore and Ideology*, p. 200.
[9] Jacquart et Micheau, *La médecine arabe et l'occident médiéval*, p. 56.

However, a survey of Arabic medical literature shows that Muslim physicians also wrote specialized practical treatises on almost every branch of the medical arts. And yet, within the expanse of their specialized medical texts, very little was written by them on gynaecology and obstetrics. This characteristic was already discernible during the "age of translations" from Greek and Syriac. Thus, out of the rich ancient literature on these specializations, only a few minor treatises were translated into Arabic. For example, of the entire Hippocratic corpus on gynaecology, only two lesser texts were translated: *Perì epikyêsios* (On Superfoetation),[10] and *Perì partheniôn* (On Diseases of Virgins).[11]

Furthermore, the texts by Soranus of Ephesus, whose Methodist gynaecology played an important role in Latin and Jewish medicine, were almost entirely neglected by Arab translators and medical writers. In fact, medical historians are still debating whether one of his minor gynaecological texts, *Gynaikeia kat' eperôtêsin* (Gynaecology, According to Questioning), was ever translated into Arabic.[12]

The evidence thus leads to the impression that Muslim medicine was preoccupied, at least from the perspective of practicality, in caring for pregnant women, newborn babies and young children, and

[10] The Arabic title is *Kitâb Buqrât fî ḥabl 'alâ ḥabl*; for an edition of the Arabic text see *Hippocrates: On Superfoetation*, edited and translated with introduction, notes and glossary by J. N. Mattock, Cambridge, 1968. Cf. M. Ullmann, *Islamic Medicine*, p. 11; Sezgin, *Geschichte des arabischen Schrifttums*, Band III, p. 42. The Hippocratic work deals with cases in which the woman bears more than one foetus in her womb.

[11] Ullmann, *Islamic Medicine*, p. 11; M. H. Green, *The Transmission of Ancient Theories*, pp. 75-76.

[12] "Perhaps more remarkable than the lack of any Hippocratic gynecological texts is the absence of any definitive proof of a translation of Soranus' *Gynecology* into Arabic. According to Ullmann's research, the Arabs had only a slight knowledge of this Methodist physician... Diepgen's assertations that al-Majûsî used such a translation of Soranus in his *Kâmil aṣ-ṣina'a*, and likewise Ibn Sînâ in his *Qânûn*, are apparently unfounded. There is some possibility that Soranus' smaller gynecological work, the *Gynaikeia kat' eperôtêsin*, was transmitted to the Islamic world... Ullmann has suggested that this catechism is represented in Arabic by the *Kitâb al-qawâbil* ("Book of Midwives"), attributed to an otherwise unknown Mîsûsun. Yet even Ullmann is not at all secure in this identification... Sezgin, on the other hand, attributed this text to yet another ancient physician: the Methodist Mnaseas, who lived in the first century B. C.", Green, *The Transmission of Ancient Theories*, pp. 75-76; cf. P. Diepgen, *Frau und Frauenheilkunde in der Kultur des Mittelalters*, Stuttgart, 1966, pp. 33-34; M. Ullmann, *Die Medizin im Islam*, pp. 77-78; Sezgin, *Geschichte des arabischen Schrifttums*, Band III, p. 56.

not with gynaecological problems *per se*. Witness that only two important Arabic works were written on this subject in the early Middle Ages. Although these cannot be considered gynaecological treatises in the classical sense of the term, they do contain some references to the subject. The first, *Kitâb ḥalq al-janîn wa-tadbîr al-ḥabâlâ wa-l-mawlûdîn*, (Book on the Creation of the Foetus and the Treatment of Pregnant Women and the Newborns), was written in the mid tenth century by the Al-Andalusian polygraph 'Arib ibn Sa'îd.[13] Ibn Sa'îd used quite disparate sources, such as Hippocrates, Galen, Arabic traditional medicine, as well as Egyptian and Indian female informants, to compile his treatise, which he wrote in a logical format.[14] Considering that only one manuscript of the work and its *resumé*, have been preserved,[15] as well as the absence of citations and references in later Arabic medical texts, we may conclude that the treatise was not very popular in Muslim Lands. On the other hand, the text attracted the attention of Jewish physicians for it was translated twice into Hebrew.

The other treatise, *Kitâb tadbîr al-ḥabâlâ wa-l-atfâl* (Book on the Treatment of Pregnant Women and Young Children), was written in the Orient by Abû al-'Abbâs Aḥmad b. Muḥammad b. Yaḥyâ al-Baladî, at the end of the tenth Century. It seems that this text was by far more popular than the first, for at least five manuscripts are available.[16]

In fact, most ancient conceptions of female anatomy, physiology and pathology were integrated within the Arabic medical encyclopaedias. But, as stated by Monica Green: "...there was a significant change in genre from the way the ancient world (with the notable

---

[13] On the author and his rich literary activity, see A. C. López, "Vida y obra del famoso polígrafo cordobés del s. X 'Arîb ibn Sa'îd", in *Ciencias de la naturaleza en Al-Andalus, textos y estudios*, ed. E. García Sánchez, Granada, 1990, pp. 317-347. The article was reprinted in French translation in *Chrétiens, musulmans et juifs dans l'Espagne médiévale*, R. Barkaï (ed), pp. 77-101. For the treatise itself, see *Le livre de la génération du fœtus et le traitement des femmes enceintes et des nouveau-nés*, publié, traduit et annoté par H. Jahier et A. Noureddine, Algier, 1956. The treatise was also translated into Spanish, see A. Arjona Castro, *El libro de la generación del feto, el tratamiento de las mujeres embarazadas y de los recién nacidos de 'Arib Ibn Sa'id* (Tratado de obstetricia y pediatría hispano árabe del siglo X), Córdoba, 1983.

[14] For a detailed list of Ibn Sa'îd's sources, see López, "Vida y obra del famoso polígrafo cordobés del s. X 'Arîb ibn Sa'îd", pp. 335-337. On the logical structure of the work, see Ullmann, *Die Medizin im Islam*, pp. 139-140.

[15] F. Sezgin, *Geschichte des Arabischen Schrifttums*, p. 385.

[16] Sezgin, *Geschichte des Arabischen Schrifttums*, Band III, p. 318.

exception of Galen) had customarily addressed the diseases of women. Whereas ancient authors, in writing specialised treatises, had relegated gynaecology to a separate existence as a medical sub-speciality, the Byzantine and Arabic encyclopaedists included discussions of gynaecological and obstetrical matters within a rigid organizational pattern as a necessary complement to the treatment of afflictions of the male sexual organs - necessary, that is, for reasons of completeness which was, of course, the encyclopaedists' main goal".[17]

C. Latin Gynaecology

In contrast to Arabic and Byzantine medical traditions, the medical corpus which circulated in the Latin West during the early Middle Ages was extremely rich in specialized gynaecological treatises. The basic components of the disparity between the two medical traditions can be summarized as follow: (a) Since late Antiquity and the beginning of the Middle Ages, the medical tradition prevailing in the Latin West was dominated by the writings and medical conceptions of Soranus "because [the Latins] considered them more practical and accessible than the prolix, theory-laden works of Galen".[18] At the same time the Latin West was also familiar with parts of the Hippocratic corpus, due to the translations of some important works from Greek to Latin between the fifth and the seventh centuries.[19] (b) Latin medicine preferred the genre and format of specialized texts to encyclopaedic ones, which dominated Arabic medical writings. (c) Until the end of eleventh century, Latin medicine was essentially concerned with practical aspects of this art, while Arabic medicine, from its inception, also highly estimated its theoretical dimensions.

The translations of Greek medical texts into Latin were undertaken during the early Middle ages in two main centres, namely North Africa and the northern Italian city of Ravenna. Together, they

---

[17] Green, *The Transmission of Ancient Theories* , p. 83.

[18] *Ibid.*, p. 131. The *résumé* given here is based mainly on chapter three: "The Transmission of Ancient Gynecology Through the Early Medieval Latin West", in Green, *The Transmission of Ancient Theories.*

[19] *Ibid.*, pp. 141-149. Cf. P. Kibre, "Hippocrates Latinus: Repertorium of Hippocratic Writings in the Latin Middle Ages", *Traditio*, 31 (1975), pp. 99-126; 32 (1976), pp. 257-292; 33 (1977), pp. 253-295; 34 (1978); pp. 193-226; 36 (1980), pp. 347-372.

supplied the Latin West with numerous gynaecological works. A major focus of this effort, at least until the twelfth century, was the translation of the works of Soranus and the drafting of their Latin derivatives. Soranus' *Gynaikeia*, his most important text on the subject, was in fact rendered into Latin by three translators-adaptors: Theodorus Priscianus, Caelius Aurelianus and Muscio, each one of whom followed the original to different degrees of fidelity.[20] We are especially interested in Muscio's version because "... the influence of his 'Genecia' was profound. Thirteen complete or near-complete copies of Muscio's 'Genecia' are still extant.... The 'Genecia' was exploited, moreover, by later compilers for its gynaecological and especially obstetrical material which had no equal in other texts available in the West before the translation of major Arabic texts like those of al-Majûsî (Haly Abbas), az-Zahrâwî (Abulcasis), or Ibn Sînâ (Avicenna) in the eleventh and twelfth centuries".[21] Consequently, due to the close relations between the Hebrew medicine and the Latin, its influence on Jewish gynaecology was considerable.

When comparing Muscio's version to Soranus' *Gynaikeia*, Monica Green concluded that although the Latin translator omitted considerable doxographic material from the original Greek, he "nevertheless maintained the theoretical integrity of Soranus' work in most of its essential points. Muscio's Methodism is particularly apparent in 'Genecia' II, on pathological conditions".[22] Thus, he kept the distinction between lax and constricted conditions, and the cure of chronic illnesses by metasyncretic and cyclic remedies. Even more important from the standpoint of its influence on Jewish gynaecology, is his fidelity to Soranus' ideas that for certain categories of women, amenorrhea is salubrious and that virginity is healthful while coitus and pregnancy are harmful.[23] However a critical deviation from Soranian physio-pathological conceptions regarding uterine suffocation appears in Muscio's version: While Soranus completely rejected the idea of the wandering womb, Muscio held this notion as the cause of the disease. In this respect he followed

[20] On these translations-adaptations and their different attitudes toward the original text, see Green, *The Transmission of Ancient Theories* , pp. 135-139; Hanson and Green, "Soranus of Ephesus", pp. 1045-1054.

[21] Hanson and Green, "Soranus of Ephesus", p. 1054.

[22] *Ibid.*, pp. 1050-1051.

[23] On the challenge that these Soranic medical conceptions presented to Jewish Law and ethics, see Barkaï, *Les infortunes de Dinah*, pp. 122-123.

Hipppocrates[24], whose ideas were popular in the Middle Ages. Strangely enough, as regards the cure of the disease, he did not accept the Hippocratic therapy, namely, the use of foul and sweet odorous which repel and attract the uterus, but echoes Soranus' rejection of such a remedy.

We know of at least three medieval Latin adaptations whose main source is the 'Genecia'. The first, *De passionibus mulierum*, Version B (hereafter Dpm B), was probably written in southern Italy in the eleventh century. Of the twenty-six chapters of this treatise, which deals exclusively with gynaecology, seventeen were drawn, though in a summary manner, from Muscio's Latin version.[25] The second work, entitled according to its incipit *Non omnes quidem*, is based almost entirely on Muscio's gynaecology. In contrast to the Dpm B, it includes gynaecological, obstetrical and post-partum materials. In summarizing the attributes of these treatises, Monica Green says: "Obviously some of the deletions from the 'Dpm B' and 'Non omnes quidem' can be explained by factors that characterized most early medieval medicine: an emphasis on symptoms and therapy, with little interest in more subtle details of etymology and the niceties of diagnosis. Some of them, too, are due to a simple desire to abbreviate. The absence (or misunderstanding) of the basic Methodist principles of lax/constricted and acute/chronic may have been due to the physically disintegrated state in which Muscio's text probably reached both compilers... But there is no question, especially in the case of the 'Non omnes quidem' that the compiler deliberately excised material that he could not understand... Whatever the reasons for the compiler's lack of comprehension, both the 'Dpm B' and the 'Non omnes quidem', therefore, can be called 'Soranian' only in the most limited sense: Both texts preserve the original categorization and many of the essentials of the therapy, but the reader of either texts would be hard-pressed to discern that there lay behind these brief works anything like a 'Method' of medicine".[26] The third adaptation, *De naturis mulierum* (On the Nature of Women), was proba-

[24] On the Hippocratic conception and other Greek texts, see Lloyd, *Science, Folklore and Ideology*, pp. 83-84; on the ambiguous conceptions of Galen, see Green, *The Transmission of Ancient Theories*, pp. 151-152. For Soranus and Methodist rejection of this notion, see Lloyd, *op. cit.*, pp. 171-172.

[25] Hanson and Green, "Soranus of Ephesus", p. 1054. This text was translated into Hebrew. For more details on its characteristics, see below, p. 62.

[26] *Ibid.*, pp. 1055-1056.

bly composed in the later thirteenth century, when the 'Genecia' had become somewhat "old-fashioned" in the Latin West. It reveals also that the main interest in this text was due to the obstetrical materials it contained.[27]

Consistent with this line of interest in specialized texts on women's medicine, a major portion of the Hippocratic corpus was translated into Latin in the early Middle Ages, including the two important gynaecological works, *Diseases of Women I* and *Diseases of Women II*. The first treatise was probably translated in Ravenna in the sixth century; its fullest rendition is found in an early medieval compilation, the *Liber ad Mecenatem*.[28] The compiler included a large part of the first chapter, in which the essential Hippocratic notions on women's physiology are disclosed, omitted the following six chapters, which were dedicated to menstruation, and concentrated on selections dealing mainly with conception, pregnancy and their respective problems.[29] In spite of the omissions and the changes made by the translator/compiler, "...we can conclude that the *De conceptu* represents a relatively faithful transference of the Hippocratic tradition (as expressed in *Diseases of Women I)* to the Latin world".[30] Sections of the second major Hippocratic gynaecological text, *Diseases of Women II*, are dispersed among four different treatises. The largest of these, *De diversis causis mulierum*, "seems to have the most direct correspondence with the original [Greek] text...".[31] With these two texts and other Latin translations such as the Aphorisms, transmission of the fundamental theories and prac-

---

[27] For a description of the text, see *ibid.*, pp. 1056-1057.

[28] On the Hippocratic gynaecological texts, see H. Grensemann, *Hippokratische Gynäkologie: Die gynäkologischen Texte des Autors C nach den pseudohippokratischen Schriften De mulieribus I, II und De sterilibus*, Weisbaden, 1982. Cf. A. E. Hanson, "Hippocrates: "Diseases of Women I", *Signs*, I (1975), pp. 567-584; Green, *The Transmission of Ancient Theories* , pp. 13-22.

[29] For the Latin text and its comparison to the original Greek, see I. Mazzini and G. Flamini, *De Conceptu: Estratti di un'antica traduzione latina del Peri Gynaikeion pseudoippocratico libro I*, Introduzone di I. Mazzini, testo critico di G. Flammini, revisto da I. Mazzini, Bologna, 1983.

[30] Green, *The Transmission of Ancient Theories* , p. 146.

[31] *Ibid.* The title was given by Walter Brütsch according to the incipit, of which the opening words are missing (*De diversis causis mulierum...*, Freiburg, 1922). The correct reading, based on another manuscript, is given by Augusto Beccaria: "Potio utilis valde ad universas causas mulierum" *(I codici di medicina del periodo presalernitano (secoli IX, X e XI)*, Rome, 1956, p. 258).

tices of the Hippocratic gynaecology to the West was accomplished.[32]

In addition to the gynaecological treatises composed by the masters of Greek medicine, a number of other gynaecological texts, either translated into or composed in Latin, circulated in the Latin West during the early Middle Ages.[33] One of the most original and popular works was *Gynaecia Cleopatrae*, a book on women's diseases, conception, birth, contraception and voluntary abortion, attributed either to the Egyptian queen or to Theodote, a female physician in her service.[34] Two other gynaecological texts are affiliated - though to differing degrees - to that work. The first, *De pesis cleopatrae*, is in fact a collection of pessaries designed to cure various women's diseases; the second, *Liber geneciae ad Soteris obsetrix*, is apparently more directly related to Cleopatra's *Gynaecia* since it reproduces its preface and includes a pessary to promote conception attributed to the Egyptian queen. Another important characteristic of this text is its clear relation to Soranus' gynaecological works: the first book of the treatise is composed in the form of a dialogue between Soteris the midwife and Soranus himself. Comparing this text to the other Latin versions of Soranus' gynaecology, Monica Green concludes that this text "may even represent a *third* tradition of Soranus' catechism into Latin".[35]

Also of great interest is the eleventh-century Vendôme 175 codex, including five different gynaecological texts which have not been thoroughly examined to date.[36] Of these texts, most noteworthy is the one entitled by Wickersheimer as *De matrice et de menstruis.* As noted by Monica Green, *De matrice* is "quite novel and seems to have no strong ties to any of the other early medieval gynaecological treatises".[37] The text methodically deals with the anatomy of the

---

[32] Green, *The Transmission of Ancient Theories* , pp. 147-149. On Hippocratic gynaecology, see Lloyd, *Science, Folklore and Ideology,* pp. 62-94.

[33] For a general survey of these gynaecological texts, see Green, *The Transmission of Ancient Theories* , pp. 155-170.

[34] For a description and preliminary analysis of the treatise, see *ibid.*, pp. 156-160.

[35] *Ibid.*, p. 161.

[36] See H. Sigerist, "Early Medieval Medical Texts in Manuscripts of Vendôme", *Bulletin of the History of Medicine*, 14 (1943), pp. 68-113; Green, *The Transmission of Ancient Theories* , pp.162-164.

[37] Green, *The Transmission of Ancient Theories* , pp.162.

womb, the reproductive life of women, and the various afflictions which may befall them.

Due to this richness, it is no wonder that Jewish gynaecological literature flourished in the bosom of Latin medicine. The circulation of these Latin gynaecological texts continued during the High and Late Middle Ages and became the essential resource nourishing and shaping the Hebrew literature on this subject. Out of fifteen known Hebrew treatises, eleven flowed directly from Latin sources and fourteen were written in Christian lands. And similar to the vein of the Latin texts, most of the Hebrew gynaecological writings are practical in nature and show limited interest in the theoretical aspects of this art. These elements, however, were discussed at length in Hebrew medical encyclopaedias, which were profoundly influenced by the Arabic medical literature translated into Hebrew or Latin.

CHAPTER THREE

HEBREW TRANSLATIONS OF LATIN AND ARABIC GYNAECOLOGICAL TREATISES

As we have seen above, the translations from Latin and Arabic into Hebrew were the first steps in the creation of a specifically Jewish medical corpus. I have already stressed elsewhere, that we can not speak of medieval "Jewish science" (and certainly not of a "modern Jewish science") since, basically, the Jews shared the same scientific body of knowledge as did the Christians and the Muslims of their time.[1] However, these translations furnished Jewish physicians and scholars a scientific language of their own. Thus, this process responded to both necessities: indispensable scientific knowledge (both theoretical and practical), on the one hand, and cultural self-assertion, on the other. Moreover, it seems to me that the cultural transmission of medieval gynaecology was indeed a more delicate matter than in other areas of medical science because occasionally challenged Jewish Law and tradition. Therefore, in conjunction with the historical examination of the translated texts, we should pay special attention to the manner in which these translations rendered into Hebrew the ideas and conceptions taken from a foreign culture.

Of the rich gynaecological literature which circulated in European Jewish communities, fourteen texts were written in Hebrew and one in Judeo-Arabic (Arabic written in Hebrew letters). The latter is included in a Judeo-Arabic codex of medical texts, probably compiled in the thirteenth century.[2] Although it contains three pages written in Judeo-Arabic, the text's heading and colophon are written in Hebrew. The Hebrew title reads *Sefer Dinah le-khol 'inyan ha-reḥem ve-ḥolayehah* [*sic*] (Dinah's Book on All that Concerns the Womb and its Sicknesses). The first striking element is, of course, the name of Dinah, which appears in the title. Dinah, the daughter of Jacob

[1] R. Barkaï, *Les infortunes de Dinah*, p. 7

[2] London, British Museum, or. 10539/4.

and Leah, is the unfortunate heroine of the Biblical story about a young Jewish woman who fell in love with the Gentile Shekhem ben Ḥamor, who later raped her. At the moment of reconciliation between the two families, the Gentile and his tribe are massacred by Dinah's brothers (Genesis, 34).

Both the Biblical myth itself and the post-Biblical exegesis are written from the male viewpoint and completely ignore the sentiments and thoughts of the female protagonist. Symbolically, some *Midrashim* (homiletic interpretations of the Bible) even tell that finally she was married to the most unfortunate of Biblical personae: Job.[3] Surprisingly, Dinah evolved into the principal spokeswoman of her sex in medieval Jewish gynaecological literature. Thus, the book entitled *Trotula* was also attributed to Dinah by a Hebrew commentator. In another Hebrew gynaecological treatise *Sefer ha-toledet*, Dinah represents all women who wished to acquaint themselves with their anatomy, conception and childbirth, along with the range of women's disorders and their treatment.[4] It would have been reasonable to expect from Jewish compilers/authors to give this role to one of the "Nation's mothers" mentioned in the Bible, or even more - due to the nature of these texts - to Shifrah and Pu'ah. These two women, who took part in the Moses' delivery and took care of him after his birth, were considered in Jewish tradition as the prototypes of midwives. But Dinah was chosen, probably because she, more than other distinguished women, represented the fate and the suffering of her own sex in the eyes of these (male) authors.

The colophon of this Judeo-Arabic text, which is supposed to give the reader some information both about the author and the treatise itself, relates the following: *"Tam ve-nishlam shevaḥ le-boré 'olam, sefer msvh ve-'imo gam liqutim aḥerim"* (Finished and Completed, Praise be to God the Creator of the World, Msvh's Book and other Extracts). Since the author's name is not vocalized (the vowels usually being dropped in Hebrew script, nevertheless, some medieval authors kept them when employing non-Hebrew names or terms), it is impossible to establish its correct pronunciation. We might expect that the name of Dinah, which appears in the heading, would help us identify the origin of this text. This identification is

---

[3] See for example *Genesis Rabba*, 57, 4. For a more detailed analysis of this myth, see R. Graves and R. Patai, *Les mythes hébreux*, Paris, 1987, pp. 234-239.Cf. R. Barkaï, *Les infortunes de Dinah*, p. 127.

[4] Barkaï, *Les infortunes de Dinah*, pp. 129-284.

possible primarily by relating *Sefer Dinah* to the above-mentioned *Sefer ha-toledet*, which is composed in a form of a dialogue between Dinah and her father. As we have seen, *Sefer ha-toledet* is, in fact, a Hebrew version of Muscio's *Gynaecia*, there even being a similarity between the two names, *Msvh* (the author of *Sefer Dinah*) and *Muscio*, for in the Hebrew form, only the letter *yod* was omitted. Indeed, an examination of the content of *Sefer Dinah* demonstrates that it is composed of thirty-three *pessaria*, of which twenty-six were taken from the *Pessaria Muscionis*, appended to the last part of his Latin text. As may be gleaned from a review of the critical edition of *Sefer Dinah*, the *pessaria* in the Judeo-Arabic version appear in an order different from the Latin original; furthermore, of the sixty original prescriptions, only twenty-six are integrated into the Judeo-Arabic text. However, it is impossible to determine whether these significant changes, together with some modifications in the content of the prescriptions, are the result of the translator's selection and rearrangement or whether the text known to us is the original translation or a later version.

Nor does the manuscript of *Sefer Dinah* provide any clues about the identity of the translator, or the time and the place of its accomplishment. Nevertheless, some terms appearing in the *materia medica* demonstrate that the text was written in a Spanish milieu: all the non-Arabic terms are Romance. Thus, for example, the author mentions the Arabic name of the plant *mulukhiya*, saying: "this is *malbabis*", which is the Castilian synonym for *malva visco*.[5] The name of a solid resin, colophony, frequently appears in its Romance form: *qalafonia* (from the Latin Colophonia).[6] The same may be observed concerning the name of the plant known in Arabic as *khirwa'*, which appears in the manuscript under its Romance name -

---

[5] This is the exact transliteration of the term used in medieval Castilian medical texts. See, for example, "Para estos conuiene los vañosen esta guisa, con agua tiuia en que aya cozido maluauisco e violetas...", *Menor daño de la medicina de Alonso de Chirino*, edición crítica y glosario, por M. Teresa Herrera, Salamanca, 1973, p. 162. Cf. p. 287.

[6] The Spanish medical texts give both forms: calafonía and colofonía, *ibid.*, p. 259.

risin (ricino).[7] Finally, the term for pine resin is transcribed exactly in its Romance form - *trebentina.*[8]

With regard to the author's identity, in the critical edition of *Sefer ha-toledet*, the question was raised whether the Hebrew adaptation of Muscio's *Gynaecia* was made directly or through an intermediary, Judeo-Arabic version known to us only by way of the pessaries comprising the *Sefer Dinah.* It would appear that at this stage of the research, we can argue with certainty that the Hebrew adaptation of Muscio's *Gynaecia* was anonymously translated directly from the Latin between 1197-1199, and not from a Judeo-Arabic version. However, the question remains: Since both use the name of Dinah, which of the two versions is older?

We have noted above the significant role the Hippocratic gynaecological texts fulfilled within the Latin corpus and the insignificant impact they had on Arabic medicine. Jewish gynaecology, however, although it owed its beginnings and development to Latin medicine, followed the Arabic tradition in this respect and showed little interest in these gynaecological writings. The fact that most of the Hebrew gynaecological works were composed in the Latin West from the end of the twelfth century, and that by this time the early medieval Hippocratic texts on gynaecology were out of circulation, may explain why none of these texts were incorporated in the Hebrew medical corpus. The distinctive Hebrew translation of Hippocrates' Book on Pregnancy, *Sefer le-Abûqrât be-herayon*, was translated from the Arabic version, and we know of only one manuscript of the work, in Hebrew-Spanish handwriting, made in the fourteenth century by Pinkas ben Solomon of Lundel, in Provence.[9] The colophon, written in rhymed prose, reads as follows: "Thus ends the Book on Pregnancy and the Book on the Womb, [written by] Abuqrat. At the end of his work, the author glorifies Him, Who created everything by His wisdom. He is our God and there is no other, blessed be Him and blessed be His gift, which He gave to His people and His community, on the Mount of Sinai, in His honourable and glorious

[7] Maimonides already identified this form as Spanish: "Khirwa' , it is *târtqah*, also called kiki and in the Spanish language *rijinah*", in Meyerhof, *L'explication des noms de drogues*, p. 41.

[8] In the Spanish medieval texts we find two forms: *trebentina* and *trementina*, see *Menor daño de la medicina de Alonso de Chirino*, p. 305.

[9] Parma, ms. 3040 (Rossi, 150/4), ff. 26r-30v.

[presence]. He will send redemption to the exiled of Israel and the Redeemer will come to Zion".[10]

It is impossible to conclude either from the introduction or from the colophon whether Pinkas ben Solomon translated the work or if he simply copied it. However, there is no doubt that the Hebrew translation was based on the Arabic version of the Hippocratic work On Superfeotation, mentioned above (see p. 42). Other than external indications, such as the appearance of the name of Hippocrates in its Arabic form, numerous additional signs lend weight to this conclusion: The prevalence of Arabic terms transliterated into Hebrew letters; the use of the Hebrew word *reḥem*, which is very similar to the Arabic *raḥim*, to designate the womb, (in most translations from Latin the preferred term is é*m* [= mother], a literal translation of *matrix*, a term employed in medieval Latin texts to designate the womb or the vagina, whose linguistic root is the Latin: *mater* [=mother]).[11]

Furthermore, comparison of the two texts demonstrates that the Hebrew faithfully follows, almost word-by-word, the Arabic. Thus for example, the Hebrew text begins with the phrase : "אמר בקראט כשתהר האשה על הריון העובר הראשון אם יהיה באמצע הרחם יצא העובר השני חוצה כי הראשון ידחנו". (Hippocrates said: When a woman becomes pregnant over [a previous] pregnancy, if the first foetus is in the middle of the womb, the second foetus will be ejected out because the first will push it). This translation is not only verbatim, but even the Arabic syntax has been "imposed" on the Hebrew phrase: "قال ابقراط اذا حبلت امراة حبلا علي حبل فان كان الجنين الاول في وسط الرحم خرج الجنين الثاني الي خارج لان الولد يدفعه".[12] Even more significant is the fact that the two Semitic translations provide the same contradictory meaning to paragraph 13 of the original Greek: "If a pregnant woman has sexual relations, it eases her childbirth". The Hebrew translator, following the Arabic one, states that "If a woman has sexual relations with her husband during her pregnancy, it eases her childbearing".[13] Finally, the same phrases and paragraphs are missing in both the Arabic and the Hebrew texts. All

---

10 *Ibid*., f. 30v.

11 On the confusion resulting from the use of these terms in gynaecological texts see D. Jacquart and C. Thomasset, *Sexualité et savoir médical au moyen âge*, pp. 32-36; R. Barkai, "A Medieval Hebrew Treatise on Obstetrics", *Medical History*, 33 (1988), pp. 107-108.

12 Parma, ms. 3040 (Rossi, 150/4), f. 26r; Mattock, *Hippocrates: On Superfoetation*, p. 1

13 Parma, ms. 3040, f. 26v; Mattock, *Hippocrates: On Superfoetation*, p. 7.

these elements leave no doubt regarding the origin of the Hebrew translation of the Hippocratic treatise.

Nonetheless, this unique translation appears to have played only a minor role in the complex of Jewish gynaecological literature parallel to its status within Arabic medical literature. Evidence for its marginality rests on the fact that only one sole manuscript survives, and that the treatise is hardly mentioned in the medieval Hebrew medical corpus. Other indications of its peripheral status include its abridged form, which leads us to conclude its purpose was strictly practical. However, there are no indications that it was addressed to midwives: witness the masculine form of its instructions; and the occasional appearance of the term *rofé* (physician) as the authority in charge of the medical operation.

A. Soranus in Hebrew

The most significant characteristic of Jewish gynaecological literature in the Middle Ages is undoubtedly the dominant role exercised by Soranus' gynaecology through its Latin versions.[14] While Muslim medicine almost entirely ignored these works, and although their influence declined considerably in Latin medicine from the thirteenth century on,[15] their influence flourished in Hebrew medicine from the twelfth to the fifteenth centuries.

---

[14] For an up-to-date bibliography on Soranus and his medical works, see Hanson and Green, "Soranus of Ephesus", pp. 1061-1071.

[15] After a careful examination of all available manuscripts of Soranus' works transmitted to the Middle Ages, Monica Green arrived at the following conclusion: "The chronological distribution of Muscio's 'Genecia', the 'Dpm B', the 'Non omnes quidem', and Theodorus Priscianus' 'Genecia' shows a peak in copying in the twelfth and thirteenth centuries, a period which saw a profusion of copying classical texts in general. Even in the thirteenth century, which produced six new copies of Muscio's 'Genecia', there was already something old-fashioned about the texts: only one of the six copies of the 'Genecia' (the New York ms.) appears with recently composed or recently translated treatises..." Green goes on stating that : "It fell completely from favor in the fourteenth century when it was not copied, apparently, even once." The reason for this phenomenon, given by Green, is that: "By the late twelfth century, the various Latinizations of Soranus' 'Gynaikeia' had come into competition with an ensemble of gynecological and obstetrical material, composed in the twelfth century at the southern Italian medical centre of Salerno. Two treatises, often called the 'Trotula major' and the 'Trotula minor', began to circulate outside of Italy in the late

As we have already seen, Soranus' principal work, the *Gynaecia*, in Muscio's Latin version, was translated into Hebrew and "dressed with Jewish clothes" at the end of the twelfth century. As noted above, the Hebrew adaptation, entitled *Sefer ha-toledet* (Book on Generation), was written as a dialogue between Jacob and his daughter Dinah. In order to stress the Jewish character of the treatise, the author not only ignored the names of its foreign authors, but also added a beautiful introduction, written in Biblical Hebrew, and embroidered the text as a whole with Biblical and Talmudic citations. The Hebrew version, originally written in Southern France, attested to by the frequent use of Occitan terms,[16] circulated among the European Jewish communities. In fact, three known Hebrew manuscripts were written in Provençal, Spanish, and Italian script[17]. These remaining manuscripts date from the fourteenth and the fifteenth centuries, the earlier manuscripts apparently having been lost. The number of the manuscripts and their geographical dispersion demonstrate well the great popularity the work acquired in the Jewish medical milieu.

The second Hebrew translation affiliated to a Soranian work bears the title *Sefer ha-ém el Gâlinus hû ha-niqra Genicias* (Galen's Book on the Womb, Which is Called Genicias). While attributing the text to Galen, the Hebrew translator faithfully followed the heading appearing in the Latin manuscript he was using.[18] Two Hebrew manuscripts have been preserved: one in Spanish script, the other written in an Ashkenasi hand,[19] both composed at the end of the fourteenth or the beginning of the fifteenth century. There are some slight differences between the two versions in the main body of the work, which is based on Muscio's text, probably the result of copyist errors during the more than two centuries of its transmission. Thus, for example, the term *Genicias* is replaced by *Oficias* in the Parma

twelfth century, and by the middle of the thirteenth century they could be found all over Western Europe", *ibid.*, pp. 1056-1057.

[16] At least 88 terms are Occitan transliteration in Hebrew letters, see Barkaï, *Les infortunes de Dinah*, pp. 285-286.

[17] Vatican, heb. 360; London, Jews College, Montefiore, 440, ff. 25v-53r; Vatican, 366, 4.

[18] This text is attributed to Galen in the following thirteenth-century Latin manuscripts: Madrid, Biblioteca Nacional, Ms. 4234, ff. 12v-16v; Oxford, Ms. Rawlinson C. 671, ff. 19v-23v. I owe this information to Monica Green.

[19] Respectively: London, Jews' College, Montefiore, 440, ff. 53v-59v; Parma, 1316/7, ff. 47r-51r.

manuscript. Unfortunately, several folios of both manuscripts are partially damaged: the Montefiore manuscript, which is the more reliable of the two, breaks off at the bottom of folio 59v (the following ten leaves being lost); the Parma manuscript is damaged at the upper binding in all the folios.

As noted above (see p. 31), a gynaecological treatise bearing the title *Sefer ha-ém el Gâlinus* was translated into Hebrew between the years 1197-1199.[20] We may thus conclude with certainty that the history of this particular translation begins at that point, and that the anonymous translator was indeed referring to this text. The question then is what Latin treatise served the translator ? Moritz Steinschneider, in his preliminary study of this Hebrew translation, argued that it is identical to "Pseudo-Galen's *De Gynacaeis sive de passionibus mulierum* or to the *De mulierum morbis sive de matricis*, written by Constantine the African".[21] The considerable advances made in the study of Latin medieval gynaecology during the last decade, thanks largely to the comprehensive and rigorous work of Monica Green, enables us to identify the source of this Hebrew translation with greater precision. In fact, the Hebrew text *Sefer ha-ém el Gâlinus* is the translation of the previously mentioned Latin treatise, *De passionibus mulierum*, Version B (Dpm B). This eleventh-century Latin text composed in southern Italy, "is a strictly gynecological text in twenty-six chapters, four of which are drawn from a full version of the 'De passionibus mulierum'..., five from some version of the 'Genecia Cleopatrae', and the rest from Muscio's Genecia'".[22]

However, we should note some important variations between the two Hebrew manuscripts of this translation: The Parma manuscript alone incorporates three prescriptions for the facilitation of conception between chapters 25 (De nimio feruore) and 26 (De uulneribus in matrice) of the Dpm B, and adds a chapter on inflammation of the womb, two prescriptions to provoke menses, one to "enlarge" the

---

[20] Note that the translator's title says: *'al Galinus*, while in both manuscripts appears: *el Galinus*.

[21] M. Steinschneider, "Medicinische Handschriften im Besitz des Herrn Halberstam", *Magazin für die Wissenschaft des Judenthums*, 1883, pp. 108-112; cf. *ibid.*, *Die hebräischen Übersetzungen des Mittelaters*, p. 415. On the gynaecological text printed among Constantine's Opera omnia in the sixteenth century, see M.H. Green, "The De Genecia attributed to Constantine the African", *Speculum*, 62 (1987), pp. 299-323.

[22] Hanson and Green, "Soranus of Ephesus", p. 1054.

womb, another to eliminate uterine pains and illnesses, and still another to stop bleeding to the original Latin text.

This Hebrew translation, in both manuscripts, faithfully follows the twenty-six chapters of the Dpm B with only insignificant omissions. Some of the Latin terms for pharmaceutical ingredients, pathologies and anatomy were transliterated into Hebrew letters and correctly vocalized in the Montefiore manuscript; in the Parma manuscript, on the other hand, no vocalization signs whatsoever are indicted. One remark in the Parma manuscript leads us to conclude that it is a later version of this translation: Referring to a "cradle", the anonymous translator employed the Occitan term *Breç* (he used the same word in his *Sefer ha-toledet*, the Hebrew adaptation of Muscio's *Gynaecia*), to which the author of Parma manuscript adds his own explanation: "and it is called in the Calabrian language *nakn*".[23] Based on this remark, we can deduce not only that the Parma version was composed subsequent to the Montefiore, but also that it was written in the Calabria region, of southern Italy.

Traces of Muscio's gynaecology may also be discerned in a medieval Hebrew treatise on obstetrics, *Miqoshi ha-ledah* (On the Difficulties of Birth), published in 1988.[24] Two manuscripts of this text have been preserved: one in the British Library, the other in the Bibliothèque Nationale in Paris.[25] Some important disparities differentiate between the two manuscripts: from a review of the content of the British Library manuscript (which dates from the fourteenth century), it is clear that the scope of its subject matter was not limited to women's medicine although it was obviously one of its main topics. Aside from the chapter on the difficulties of parturition, it contains a chapter on the extraction of the placenta after birth and a chapter devoted to uterine diseases. The Paris manuscript, on the other hand, is written in the form of an independent specialized treatise, conserved in a codex including other fourteenth and fifteenth century medical works. Irrespective of its textual discrepancies, the Paris manuscript is of considerable importance to the history of Hebrew obstetrics as it is accompanied by sixteen drawings describing pathological presentations of the foetus within the womb. Similar drawings may be found in the Latin gynaecological literature, beginning with Muscio's *Gynaecia*. It may be assumed that such

---

23 Parma, 1316/7, f. 47r.

24 R. Barkai, "A Medieval Hebrew Treatise on Obstetrics", pp. 96-119.

25 Respectively: Ms. or. 10766, ff. 9r-9v; Ms. héb. 1122, ff. 66r-67r.

drawings also accompanied Soranus' work, but it is not clear whether they were originally included in his *Gynaikeia* or in his shorter gynaecological text, the *Cateperotiana*.[26]

This incorporation of these illustrations, a phenomenon common in Latin Europe had no parallel in Muslim medical literature, and the illustrations appended to the Paris manuscript are the only ones known in Hebrew medical works. The sixteen drawings represent the pathologies in a manner similar to those found in several Latin treatises of this kind. However, their artistic style, the structure of the womb, and the detailed drawing of the foetus, especially its hair, are startlingly similar to those of a thirteenth-century Latin manuscript. In the latter treatise, which begins "*Incipit genecea cleopatre ad deodatam*... ",[27] i. e., the gynaecological text attributed to Cleopatra (see above, p. 48), the illustrations were added to the bottom of the text by a later hand. Finally, it should be noted that in this particular Latin as well as in the Hebrew manuscripts, there is no direct connection between the text and the drawings.

Besides the drawings, the text itself expresses some important Soranian medical ideas. Thus, for example, the Hebrew text differentiates between three types of birth: *natural birth*, or normal labour; *unnatural birth*, where delivery involves pathological presentations; and *difficult birth*, where delivery causes suffering to the mother or the foetus. The sources of this differentiation may be found in ancient and early medieval medical treatises. However, these three types of births are described in the very same terms by Muscio's Latin version of Soranus work: *adversa et contra naturam; secundum naturam; cum difficultate*, respectively.[28] In fact, these ideas were transmitted to the author indirectly, since most of this specific text probably originated from Bernard of Gordon's medical treatise *Lilium medicine*.[29]

---

[26] Hanson and Green, "Soranus of Ephesus", p. 1024. The total number of medieval manuscripts that include these diagrams is 22; for a list of these manuscripts see *ibid.*, p. 1073.

[27] Paris, Bibliothèque Nationale, Ms. lat. 7056, ff. 87r-89r.

[28] Barkai, "A Medieval Hebrew Treatise on Obstetrics", p. 115; Rose, *Sorani Gynaeciorum*, p. 79.

[29] *Lilium medicine*, Venice, 1521, Book 7, ch. 16. Cf. L. Demaitre, *Doctor Bernard of Gordon: Professor and Practitioner*, Toronto, 1980. I am grateful to Dr. Aoibheann Nic Dhonnchadha, School of Celtic Studies, Dublin for offering me this information.

However, the Hebrew author integrated medical ideas and treatments completely alien to the Methodist master into the Hebrew treatise. The most salient of these are the theory of astrological influences on the development of the foetus during pregnancy and the employment of magical devices in order to facilitate parturition.[30]

The presence of Soranus' medicine or its echoes in Jewish gynaecological literature may be traced, as we have seen, to a large variety of treatises. For a start, there is the *Sefer ha-toledet*, the Hebrew adaptation of Soranus' major gynaecological work, which was incorporated *via* its Latin version. There were also minor treatises, such as *De passionibus mulierum* (version B) bearing the Hebrew heading *Sefer ha-ém el Galinus*; finally, we have the shorter Jewish texts, such as *Sefer Dinah* (Muscio's *Pessaria*) and *Miqoshi ha-ledah* (On the Difficulties of Birth).

Based on this information, we may conclude that Latin adaptations of Soranian medicine, on theoretical as well as practical issues, comprised the mainstream of Jewish specialized treatises on gynaecology. But this conclusion is to be taken with some reservation: As attested to by the Hebrew texts themselves, their translators and the physicians who used them misunderstood some of the fundamental ideas of Soranus' and Muscio's Methodism. A prime example is the translator's misunderstanding of the concept of *metasyncrisis*, which he mistook for a name of medicament rather than of a general therapeutic program. Not less significant are the many omissions of such Methodist concepts as the "differentiation between lax and constricted conditions" and "the distinction between 'crisis' *(accessio)* and resolution *(dialimma)*".[31] Monica Green has accurately formulated the problematics involved with the transmission of the Soranian work to Jewish gynaecology: "Even though on the whole he [the translator] retains most of the basic Methodist therapies (controlled diet, massage, passive exercises. etc.), he clearly had no idea that he was adhering to the Method... Despite its notable deletions, therefore, the Hebrew tradition was distinctive in preserving as much of Muscio, and through him of Soranus, as it did".[32] Taking this reservation into account, we may insist that Jewish midwives and physicians, who were engaged in curing women, had at their disposal an important corpus of gynaecological texts profoundly

[30] Barkai,"A Medieval Hebrew Treatise on Obstetrics", pp. 101-104, 111-113.

[31] Hanson and Green, "Soranus of Ephesus", pp. 1059-1060.

[32] *Ibid.*, p. 1060.

influenced by the Soranian work. Not less significant is the fact that this school of medicine enjoyed great popularity within Jewish gynaecology between the twelfth and the fifteenth century, a lapse of time during which Latin gynaecology was almost entirely dominated by gynaecological texts attributed to Trota.

B. The "Trotula" Texts in Hebrew

In the early decades of the twelfth century, a new group of gynaecological Latin texts, probably originating in the medical centre of Salerno, began to circulate in Italy. Towards the end of the century, they crossed the Alps, and by the middle of the thirteenth century they were already widespread in Western Europe. Compiled in the form of paired treatises, namely, *Trotula major* and *Trotula minor*, they became the most popular writings on gynaecology, obstetrics and women's cosmetics in the late medieval and early-Renaissance Europe. The issues concerning the origins of these texts and their authorship, which were until recently the subject of vivid polemics among scholars, began to be clarified about ten years ago, with the publication of the late John Benton's study on the subject.[33] Benton demonstrated that what was traditionally attributed to Trota, the female physician from Salerno, actually consisted of three different works, none of them written by her. He identified these tracts according to their incipits as the following: *Cum auctor, Ut de curis* and *De ornatu.*[34] At the same time, Benton concluded that a woman doctor named Trota had indeed written a gynaecological treatise, whose incipit is *Practica secundum Trotam.* This work apparently did not achieve the great popularity enjoyed by the treatises wrongly attributed to her, since we know of only one sole manuscript of the text.[35] Monica Green, continuing the initial ground-breaking work of John Benton is able now to offer a comprehensive work to the reader interested in the history of women's medieval medicine as well as gender history.[36] Based on her extensive study of a large number of

[33] J. Benton, "Trotula, Woman's Problems, and the Professionalization of Medicine in the Middle Ages", *Bulletin of the History of Medicine*, 59 (1985), pp. 30-53.

[34] *Ibid.*, pp. 32-35.

[35] *Ibid.*, pp. 41-45.

[36] The work includes four distinct studies: "The Development of the Trotula", *Revue d'histoire des textes*, 26 (1996), pp. 119-203 (a survey of the complicated development of the three independent Trotula texts and the conjoined ensemble,

known manuscripts, she reveals that each of the three texts constituting the "Trotula" treatise has its own history and, when circulated independently, its own title. Therefore, the correct title of the text identified by Benton as the *Cum auctor* is actually *Liber sinthomatibus mulierum.* Moreover, she demonstrates that this text existed in three distinct versions, which she has numbered 1, 2 and 3.

As we have seen above, the anonymous Jewish author mentioned three gynaecological texts he had translated, *inter alia,* from the Latin by at the end of the twelfth century. We have already identified *Sefer ha-toledet* (Muscio's *Gynaecia*) and *Sefer ha-ém el Galinus* (*De passionibus mulierum* version B). The work of Monica Green enables us to identify the third, namely *Sefer ha-seter* (Book on Hidden [Places]). As already mentioned, some leaves of the Montefiore codex, between folios 59v and 60r, are missing, that means the last leaves of *Sefer ha-ém el Galinus.* The remaining fragment begins with a history relating Galen's treatment of a woman suffering from uterine suffocation: "Galen told of a woman [who suffered from this disease][37] in her blood; she had no pulse and nor any exterior signs of life. But nature left some [small amount of heat near] her heart. Most physicians consigned her to the dead. Galen himself came, took a piece of soft, pure wool, and placed it near her mouth. Thanks to its movement he recognized that she was alive".[38] On the basis of my English translation of the Hebrew text, Monica Green positively identified this fragmentary translation with the *Liber sinthomatibus*

---

with an exhaustive list of manuscripts); *The Diseases of Women According to Trotula*: Edition and Translation, (forthcoming), (an edition of the mid-thirteenth-century "standardized" Trotula ensemble, i. e., the text that was most commonly known to medieval readers); *Women and Literate Medicine in Medieval Europe*, Cambridge University Press (forthcoming), (a social-historical study of the larger significance of Trota and the Trotula; including an edition of Trota's Practical Medicine); *Salernitan Medicine for Women*: Critical Editions of the 'Liber de sinthomatibus mulierum', De curis mulierum' and 'De ornatu mulierum' (tentative title), (critical editions and extensive historical commentary on the original forms of the three Trotula texts). I am very grateful to Monica Green for permitting me to read and use her pre-published work.

[37] [...] signifies lacunae in the manuscript.

[38] Compare to the Latin text: "Galyenus refert de quadam muliere que ita patiebatur et amiserat pulsum et vocem et erat quasi defuncta, quia exterius nullum signum uite apparebat, sed tamen circa cor natura adhoc parum caloris retinuerat. Vnde quidam iudicabant eam mortuam. Galyenus uero lanam bene carpinatam naribus et ori eius apposuit, cuius motu eam uiuam cognouit".

mulierum 3.[39] And indeed, this piece ends at the same place where the *Liber simpthomatibus mulierum* 3 terminates. The Hebrew compiler added at this point: "Ended and completed. Thanks be to God of the Universe".[40]

The corpus of medieval Hebrew medical treatises also includes the mention of another gynaecological text, called *Sitrei nashim*, which we may translate as "The Hidden [Places] of Women" or "Secrets of Women". It is possible that the Jewish authors were referring to yet another translation of the *Trotula* texts. Monica Green found that the *Trotula* texts themselves, the Latin as well as the vernacular versions, occasionally circulated under the title 'Secrets of Women'. This hypothesis should be considered with an important reservation: We do not, in fact, have any Hebrew text, or even fragments, which bear this title. It is possible, of course, that such a text existed and was lost, but only the discovery of a manuscript with the same title and the examination of its content would permit us to assess such a possibility.

The name "Trota" is explicitly mentioned in only one Hebrew medical text: a Provençal compilation from the fourteenth century. The manuscript has been erroneously identified as a translation of Arnald of Villanova's work. It is, in fact, a comprehensive treatise, dealing with theoretical and practical aspects of medicine, and based on ancient and medieval authorities whose names are frequently mentioned.[41] Trota's name is cited once, in the chapter on the differences between the pathological phenomenon called *mola*, and pregnancy. The passage begins: *ve-katav Dinah be-sefer ha-niqra Trotilla* ("and Dinah wrote in a book called Trotilla").[42] Strangely, the Jewish compiler, who undoubtedly was familiar with the Biblical name of Jacob's daughter, refers to her in the masculine form. On the other hand, he precisely cites the initial title of the *Trotula* ensemble: "The Book Called Trotula", which demonstrates that he was familiar with the treatise; nonetheless, it is impossible to say whether he knew the original Latin or whether he used a Hebrew translation. Moreover, the passage cited is in fact taken from Muscio, not from the "Trotula". Based on the extant data, we may conclude that at least a portion of the "Trotula" texts was known to Jewish physicians

---

39 Personal correspondence, February 13, 1995.

40 See below, pp. 191.

41 Oxford, Bodleian Library, ms. or. 2133, ff. 157r-197v.

42 *Ibid.*, f. 184r.

but that their circulation within the Jewish medical milieu and their impact on Jewish gynaecology were limited. Undoubtedly, this is a surprising finding when taking into consideration the immense popularity of these texts in the Latin West,[43] especially the fact that medieval Hebrew gynaecological literature was born and developed in the bosom of the Latin tradition.

C. Arabic texts translated into Hebrew

Medieval Arabic gynaecology also left its traces on the Hebrew specialised treatises dedicated to women's health. In fact, we know of only two Arabic texts translated into Hebrew in the High Middle Ages: the work of ʻArib ibn Saʻîd on obstetrics (see p 43), and selected paragraphs on gynaecology culled from Maimonides' Aphorisms. Of the first, only two fragments are known to date, both conserved in Munich.[44] One of these fragments includes some recipes, relayed by "ʻArib the Physician" but attributed to King Solomon; the other is in fact the translation of the twelfth chapter of ʻArib ibn Saʻîd's work on the treatment of young children.[45] The most interesting question is, of course, whether the whole Arabic treatise was translated, or only a few fragments. I am inclined to believe that there originally existed a complete Hebrew translation (or even two different translations), probably composed in Christian Spain or in Southern France, but I must admit that the known manuscripts do not supply any evidence to support such an hypothesis.

D. Maimonides on Gynaecology and Obstetrics

That Maimonides enjoyed great prestige as a physician in Jewish medieval society is evidenced by the degree his medical works circulated in the Orient as well as in the Latin West, and by the fact that Jewish authors of medical texts frequently referred to him as a great authority on medicine. Further proof of his stature lies in the translation into Hebrew, from Judeo-Arabic, of almost all his medical cor-

---

43 Green, "The Development of the Trotula", pp. 119-123.

44 Munich, Ms. 295, ff. 30v-32v; Ms. 220, ff. 64v-65r.

45 On these two fragments, see Steinschneider, *Die hebräischen Übersetzungen des Mittelalters*, p. 671.

pus quite early in the first half of the thirteenth century.[46] Maimonides himself did not write any specialized treatise on gynaecology or obstetrics, but material on these subjects was dispersed among his various works, especially in the sixteenth chapter of his *Aphorisims.* The treatise was originally written in Arabic (1187-1190) under the title *Fusûl mûsî* (Moses' Chapters), then translated into Hebrew by Nathan ha-Méatî in the thirteenth century. The material on gynaecology and obstetrics was accumulated by an anonymous compiler under the heading: *Liqutei Rabbenu Moshéh be-'inyanei vesset veherayon* (Our Rabbi Moses' Compilations on Menses and Pregnancy). It is difficult to say whether the compiler used the Nathan ha-Méatî translation or whether he composed his own translation of this chapter, for some paragraphs are omitted and substantial changes have been introduced in the language he employed. It is even more difficult to date the compilation as we know of only two versions of the text among medical codices from the fourteenth and the fifteenth centuries, one conserved in Parma, the other in the Bodleian Library, Oxford. Neither version provides any hint regarding the compiler himself, the place where he worked, nor the date of the text's completion.[47]

As has already been demonstrated, Maimonides was not only perfectly acquainted with Galen's theoretical and practical medicine, he also heavily relied on Galen's medical views when propounding his own. The fact that this great Jewish physician was critical of Galen's medicine as well as his "philosophy" does not contradict the profound "Galenization" of Maimonides' medicine.[48] This characteristic is especially evident in Maimonides' *Aphorisms*, in which "the Rambam [Maimonides] quotes his sources... particularly passages scattered here and there in the books of Galenus, so that his book

[46] On Maimonides medical works, their translations and circulation, see: above, pp. 35-36.

[47] Parma, Ms. 1339/2 {3169}, ff. 185r-186v.

[48] J. Schacht and M. Meyerhof, "Maimonides Against Galen on Philosophy and Cosmogony", *Bulletin of the Faculty of Arts*, Cairo, vol. V (1937), pp. 53-88. Cf. R. Walzer, *Galen on Jews and Christians*, Oxford, 1949. Maimonides was not, of course, the only medieval physician to criticize Galen nor was he the first to do so. See S. Pines, "Razi, critique de Galien", in *International Kongress der Geschichte der Naturwissenschaften*, 7 (1953), pp. 480-487; J. Chr. Brügel, *Averroes, contra Galenum*, Göttingen, 1967. But, it seems, Maimonides' critique was the most severe; see S. Muntner's introduction to the *Aphorisms of Moses*, Jerusalem, 1992, pp. XV-XX. [Hebrew].

[*Aphorisms*] served from the thirteenth century to the fifteenth century as the most widely known and wanted repertorium of Galenus. Iohannes de Tornamira (1329-1396), a famous physician at Montpellier, recommends this book for study, calling it 'Flores Galieni'".[49]

Maimonides' Galenism is clearly revealed in his two salient works: the "Summary of Galen's Books" *(Mukhtasar)*[50] and the "Commentary on Hippocrates' Aphorisms". When dealing with important issues such as the definition of the male as "active" and the female as "passive", the theory of their respective contributions to the creation of the foetus and the double seed theory, Maimonides faithfully followed Aristotle's ideas.[51] On the other hand, in the sixteenth chapter of his *Aphorisms*, dedicated to women's anatomy, physiology, menstruation, pregnancy, illnesses and disorders, his conceptions were taken exclusively from Hippocrates and Galen.[52] Suessmann Muntner, in his critical edition of the Hebrew translation of Maimonides' *Aphorisms*, examined the sources used in every passage. From his examination we learn that most of the references are to Galen's original works or to his commentary to the Hippocratic treatises in their Arabic translation. Thus, for example, his description of female genitalia as anatomically parallel to those of the male but located inside her body is based on Galen's "Book on Sperm", translated into Arabic by Ḥunain ibn Isḥâq.[53] The aetiology, symptoms, and cure of uterine suffocation are taken, respectively, from Galen's commentary to the Hippocratic treatise on "Diseases of Women" and Galen's *"De locis affectis"*.[54]

This compilation, then, is the only one among the specialized Hebrew gynaecological treatises from the Middle Ages that represents,

---

[49] S. Muntner's English introduction to the *Aphorisms of Moses*, p. XIII. Cf. idem, "Galen's Books Listed by Maimonides in His Aphorisms", in *Homenaje a Millàs-Vallicrosa*, Jerusalem, 1956, vol. II, pp. 119-130. [Hebrew].

[50] See Sezgin, *Geschichte des arabischen Schrifttums*, Band III, p. 120.

[51] Barkaï, *Les infortunes de Dinah*, pp. 29-30,61,74-76.

[52] See W. Steinberg and S. Muntner, "Maimonides' Views on Gynecology and Obstetrics - English Translation of Chapter Sixteen of his Treatise 'Pirke Moshe' (Medical Aphorisms), *American Journal of Obstetrics and Gynecology*, 91 (1965), pp. 443-448. Cf. D. Bercovy, "Quelques reflexions sur la gynécologie et l'obstétrique dans l'Aphorismes de Maïmonide'", *Revue d'histore de la médecine hébraïque*, 19 (1966), pp. 123-129.

[53] *Aphorisms of Moses*, pp. 207-208; Sezgin, *Geschichte des arabischen Schrifttums*, Band III, p. 113.

[54] *Aphorisms of Moses*, pp. 208-209; Sezgin, *Geschichte des arabischen Schrifttums*, Band III, p. 90-91.

completely and comprehensively, the school of Hippocrates and Galen or, even more precisely, "Arabic Galenism" on women's medicine. While others, as we shall see below, were influenced by this conceptual framework, none provides such a faithful and coordinated reflection of this school as does the text taken from Maimonides' *Aphorisms*.

The translations of gynaecological texts from Latin and Arabic as early as the end of the twelfth and the beginnings of the thirteenth century provided Hebrew medicine, from the first formative phases, with both a specialized medical corpus and a scientific lexicon. It is true that throughout the Middle Ages, the "Holy Language" as it was used in medical writings did not achieve the degree of perfection attained by Arabic and Latin. The frequent employment of foreign terms, in Arabic, Latin and the vernacular, attested to by the texts found in the second part of this book, is one of the salient characteristics of medieval Hebrew medicine (in medicine more than in other branches of medieval science). Nevertheless, from the thirteenth century on Jewish authors wrote some important original Hebrew gynaecological treatises (to be examined in the following two chapters). However, it should be noted that out of nine known genuine Hebrew texts, only three are dedicated to gynaecology *per se*, while the others concentrate on fertility and giving birth. Therefore it seems that translated treatises, notably *Sefer ha-toledet* and *Sefer ha-ém el Galinus* (both originating from the Soranian oeuvre), continued to serve as standard texts in Hebrew gynaecology up to the end of the Middle Ages.

CHAPTER FOUR

GENUINE HEBREW TREATISES ON FEMININE AND MASCULINE GENITAL DISEASES

The treatment of male and female genital diseases in one specialized treatise is a rare phenomenon in medieval medicine. Usually, these problems were attended to within the general and comprehensive medical texts which represented the encyclopaedic conception of this genre, meant to supply information on every known medical issue. Therefore, special interest lies in the Hebrew manuscript called *Zikhron ha-ḥolayim ha-hovim bi-khlei ha-herayon* (Record of the Diseases Occurring in the Genital Members),[1] which appears as an independent and specialized treatise containing two parts: The first deals with male genital diseases, and the second with female problems and sicknesses.[2] The manuscript is included in the codex that contains three other gynaecological works, mentioned previously: the "Book on Generation", "Galen's Book on the Womb", and the "Book on Hidden [Places]". The *Zikhron ha-ḥolayim ha-hovim bi-khlei ha-herayon* was written in fifteenth-century Hebrew Spanish script by the same scribe who copied the whole codex. But, in contrast to the three other gynaecological texts, which were directly translated from the Latin, this treatise originated in an environment where the Arabic language prevailed. The manuscript itself does not furnish any indications concerning the identity of its author, or the place and time of its writing, but a close examination of its language and glossary of medical terms may yield important information on these issues.[3]

The treatise was probably written in Christian Spain in the second half of the twelfth century or at the beginning of the thirteenth cen-

---

[1] London, Jews College, Montefiore, 440, ff. 15v-25r.

[2] *Ibid.*, respectively: ff. 15v-19v; 19v-25r.

[3] On the basis of the Arabic terms employed, M. Steinschneider raised the possibility that it is a translation from Arabic. See "Medizinische Handschriften", *Magazin für die Wissenschaft des Judentums*, 10, 1883, p. 103.

tury, by a Jew who had either immigrated from Al-Andalus to Castile, or who was a descendant of immigrants, judging from his Hebrew, which is profoundly influenced by Arabic terminology, syntax and style. Moreover, he intermittently uses Hebrew, Arabic, Castilian and Latin terms, although quantitatively Arabic terms dominate. It is evident that the author of the Hebrew text did not depend upon the Hebrew lexicon available to him: He frequently added Arabic synonyms, or even used exclusively Arabic terms in Hebrew transliteration. Thus, for example, among the chapter headings we may find such phrases as: "Abundance of menses, which it is the disease called *nazf*";[4] "suffocation of the womb, which is a disease similar to *ṣar'* , which is epilepsy";[5] "*al-raḥa*, which is a disease causing the woman to seem pregnant or swollen from bad water".[6] Even if the chapter headings are the work of a later scribe, they faithfully reflect the dominant presence of Arabisms in the text.

In order to relay the flavour of the text, a number of examples may be cited. For instance, parallel to the current medieval Hebrew term *leḥah*, indicating the "humours", the author employs, from time to time the Arabic word *khalt*, the source of the Arabic derivations designating the four cardinal humours: *khalt dammî* (sanguine bile); *khalt aṣwadî* (*sic*! the correct Arabic term is *sauda'* or *suwaida'* , black bile); *khalt ṣafrawî* (yellow bile); *khalt balghamî* (phlegm).[7] Similarly, most types of medicaments appear under their Arabic names: *ma'jun* (electuary); *duhn* (oil); *marhani* (*sic*! for *marham* , pomade). However, in this particular sphere of medical terminology, the influence of the Romance vernacular is also attested: The author regularly employs the Romance form *asharab*, derived from the Arabic *sharab* (beverage).[8] Another Romance term, this time an original one, *pilulas* (for *pildolas, pildoras*, pills), may be found throughout the treatise.[9] On the other hand, Hebrew medical terms originating in the thirteenth and the fourteenth centuries do not appear in the manuscript. Thus, when referring to arteries, the author

---

[4] Montefiore, 440, f. 22v.

[5] *Ibid.*, f. 21v.

[6] *Ibid.*, f. 20r.

[7] See for example *ibid.*, f. 17r.

[8] *Ibid.*, f. 17r. Cf. C. Vázquez de Benito and Ma. T. Herrera, *Los arabismos de los textos médicos latinos y castellanos de la edad media y de la modernidad*, Madrid, 1989, p. 194.

[9] See for example Montefiore, 440, f. 19v. On the Romance forms, see *Menor daño de la medicina de Alonso de Chirino*, p. 294.

uses the ambiguous Talmudic term *guid*, which also means sinew, vein, tendon, and penis;[10] while under the Arabic influence, felt from the thirteenth century on, the accepted Hebrew terms became *'oreq dofeq* ("beating artery") and *'oreq bilti dofeq* ("unbeating artery" = vein).

We may conclude, therefore, that the three languages - Hebrew, Arabic and Castilian - are considered as legitimate means of expression by the author. Not only are terms taken from the three languages employed when prescribing certain compound medicines but, most interestingly, the author at one point refers to Romance as a foreign language (*la'az*): "*'ushnân* [the Arabic term for salsola kali] which is called in the foreign language *erba deshawaq [herba de shawaq]*"[11] and, at another, Arabic is considered a foreign language: "*sabinah* [savin], which is called in the foreign language *al-abhal"*,[12] (*abhal* is indeed the Arabic term for savin). In this regard, historians of Jewish medicine and the Hebrew language can use this text as a valuable reference for the further study of developments in both areas.

It appears that the few examples mentioned strongly support the two important points noted in the opening of the discussion, i.e., the treatise was written in a Christian-Castilian environment that sanctioned the use of the Arabic language, and it is one of the first medical works originally written in medieval Hebrew.

If these contentions are correct, the *Zikhron ha-ḥolayim ha-hovim bi-khlei ha-herayon* treatise may have played an important role in the history of gynaecology in the Iberian peninsula, whether directly or indirectly, as the source of the chapters on male and female genital diseases contained in two other major medical works, written in Arabic and medieval Castilian. Concepción Váquez de Benito and María Teresa Herrera, in a study published in 1981,[13] compared chapters on genital diseases from these two treatises: the*'Amal man ṭabba lî-man ḥabba*, written by Muḥammad ben 'Abd Allâh b. al-Khatîb of Granada (1313-1373)[14] and an anonymous fifteenth-

[10] See for example, Montefiore, 440, f. 17v.

[11] *Ibid.*, f. 24v.

[12] *Ibid.*, f. 20v.

[13] C. Vázquez de Benito and Ma. T. Herrera, "Dos capítulos ginecológicos: árabe y castellano", *Asclepio: Archivo iberoamericano de historia de la medicina y antropología médica*, 33 (1981), pp. 183-241.

[14] *El libro del 'Amal man ṭabba li-man ḥabba de Muhammad b. 'Abdalllah b. al-Jatîb*, ed. C. Vázquez de Benito, Salamanca, 1972.

century Castilian medical text, the *Tratado de patología general.*[15] From this comparison they concluded, convincingly enough, that: "...if [the Arabic] was not the only source [of the Castilian], it could well be one of the most important axes of the work, to which the Castilian author, perhaps in order to make it more clear and complete, added the medical knowledge prevailing at that time".[16]

Nonetheless, there is an important categorical difference between the Hebrew text and those studied by Vázquez de Benito and Herrera: The Hebrew is written as an autonomous specialized treatise, while the others are chapters integrated into comprehensive volumes on general medicine. In Ibn al-Khatib's work, Chapter seventeen is dedicated to male genital diseases and Chapter eighteen to female pathologies. Yet, there is a clear similarity in the internal form and content of the texts. Thus, all three begin with a definition of the malady, followed by its causes and symptoms, and concluding with its treatment, which is also organized in a well-defined format: popular compound medicaments; more sophisticated compound medicaments; sympathetic remedies; nutrition; prevention.[17]

The first part of the Hebrew treatise, on diseases afflicting male genital members, is of some importance to our subject since various diseases described therein also afflict female genitalia. A number of these sicknesses are mentioned as well by Ibn al-Khatib and the anonymous Castilian. The Hebrew text opens with an enumeration of the causes of male sterility, evidence, among many other indications that contrary to the opinion of some historians, medieval physicians did not believe that women alone were responsible for failure in conception.[18] The author points out two major causes of male sterility: "scantity of sperm and deficiency of [sexual] desire";[19] in other words, the quality and quantity of male sperm and the lack of sexual potency.[20]

---

[15] Madrid, Biblioteca Nacional, Ms. 10.051.

[16] Vázquez de Benito and Herrera, "Dos capítulos ginecológicos: árabe y castellano", p. 184.

[17] *Ibid.*, pp. 185-186.

[18] See for example V. L. Bullough, "Medieval Medical and Scientific Views of Women", in *Sex, Society and History*, New York, 1979, p. 55. For an excellent discussion of the issue, see J. Cadden, *Meanings of Sex Differences in the Middle Ages. Medicine, Science*, 1993, chapter 5.

[19] Montefiore, 440, f. 15v.

[20] Compare this to the opinion expressed in the *Trotula* ensemble: "Conceptio impeditur tam uicio uiri quam mulieris", followed by a description of the causes of

The second and the third chapters of the first part of the Hebrew text are dedicated to male sexual pathologies other than sterility. The prior one is devoted to "excessive [sexual] desire",[21] a flaw generally attributed to women in medieval Latin moral and medical literature,[22] and only attributed to men in the present Hebrew treatise. The later deals with an equally unpleasant pathology: "permanent erection of the penis without [sexual] desire".[23] Diseases afflicting both men and women are described in the remainder of the first part of the treatise. These are essentially various types of inflammations, such as "hot inflammation", "cold inflammation", and "watery inflammation", as well as skin diseases, which have the same generic name in Hebrew and in Arabic: *garab.*

In the second part of the Hebrew text, dedicated to female problems and diseases, the main topics are parallel to most of those appearing in the Arabic and Castilian texts: sterility and impediments to pregnancy (Arabic: nonexistent; Castilian: Ch. 21); *Al-raḥa,* a disease in which the woman's condition resembles pregnancy or dropsy (Arabic: Ch. 2; Castilian, Ch. 19); difficulties of parturition and removal of the dead foetus (Arabic: Chs. 6-7; Castilian: Chs. 27-29, 40); suffocation of uterus (Arabic: Ch. 1; Castilian: Ch. 30); excessive menses (Arabic: Ch. 3; Castilian: Chs. 35, 16, 13); on retention of menstruation and scantity of menstrual blood (Arabic: Ch. 5; Castilian: Ch. 33). Other pathologies discussed in both the Arabic and Castilian texts in the chapters dedicated to female medicine are mentioned in the first part of the Hebrew treatise as referring to men's diseases although the author indicates that they may also afflict women.

Beyond these similarities, the Hebrew text is distinguished by two main characteristics. First, its descriptions of pathological phenomena are more detailed; and second, the text is more vivid, since the author incorporates information gained from his own medical experience. Furthermore, some textual differences appear between the

---

male's sterility: " Si uicio uiri impediatur conceptio, aut fit ex defectu spiritus sperma impellentis, aut ex defectu spermatice humiditatis aut ex defectu caloris. Si ex defectu caloris, non appetit coitum", Green (forthcoming).

[21] Montefiore, 440, f. 16r.

[22] The question regarding this issue, as formulated in the treatise *On Human Generation*, is very insructive: "Since woman is naturally cold and moist, how is it that she is more heated in libido than man?", Cadden, *Meanings of Sex Differences in the Middle Ages*, p. 97; cf. pp. 38, 98.

[23] Montefiore, 440, ff. 16v-17r.

Hebrew treatise and its Arabic and Castilian parallels.[24] For example, in the chapter dedicated to the sickness called *mola*, the Hebrew is closer to the Arabic not only because both employ its Arabic term *raḥa* but also because they alone mention, as one of the symptoms, that the sick woman resembles one who is pregnant.[25] The Hebrew text only adds that she may be seem "dropsical". Similarly, only the Hebrew text indicates that the sickness may linger for six or even more years, and that during this period, the woman may suffer from "symptoms similar to giving birth", such as hydrorrhea and labour pains. But unlike a "normal birth", the woman will produce "thick and strong winds" or she will give birth to a formless piece of flesh.[26]

Even more important, the Hebrew text refers to classical theories on conception in order to provide rational explanations to such phenomena: The author incorporates Galen's theory on excessive heat in the womb at the moment of ejaculation and a pseudo-Aristotelian explanation on disturbances which prevent the joining of the female with the male sperm. As a result, the material - the female contribution to conception - lacks the shaping force - the male sperm; hence, the woman produces a formless creature.[27] In addition, this treatise also relates the *mola* phenomenon to the human birth of monsters and animal-like creatures. No less interesting is the very fact of the author's inclusion of this information, based on what he had been

---

[24] On the differences between the Arabic and the Castilian texts, see Vázquez de Benito and Herrera, "Dos capítulos ginecológicos: árabe y castellano".

[25] Montefiore, 440, ff.20r-20v; Vázquez de Benito and Herrera, *ibid.*, pp. 189-190; 214-215.

[26] The Castilian text raises the possibility of giving birth to a piece of flesh or "winds" if the sick woman moves frequently: "E quiçá que se muda de su lugar quando mucho le apretaren e de sy parirá con grandes dolores un pedaço de carne e quiçá no saldrá más que ventosidat", *ibid.*, p. 215. The symptoms described in the Hebrew text are similar to those given in Muscio's Latin adaptation of Soranus: "Valitudo quae appelatur mola duritia matricis est ex praecedente fervore, quae in totum ventrem saepe extensa est, uta ita videatur tamquam praegnans... transactis vero decem mensibus omne corpus earum macie consumitur, venterque et femora in tantum excrescunt ut hydropicam valitudinem mulieri minentur." But such a description of the birth of a formless piece of flesh does not exist in this medical tradition; see R. Radicchi, *La Gynaecia di Muscione*, pp. 128, 130.

[27] On Aristotle's conception, see *De la génération de animaux*, texte établi et traduit par P. Louis, Paris, 1961, pp. 52, 53, 152-155; cf. G. E. R. Lloyd, *Science, Folklore and Ideology*, pp. 53-54.

told by "some just women and midwives".[28] He thus integrated conceptions and ideas originating in popular circles into a learned treatise.

One of the women's diseases frequently described in medieval medical treatises is the suffocation of the womb. In this case, the womb rises up, and presses against the respiratory organs, causing the woman to stop breathing and lose consciousness. Each of the three texts dedicates a chapter to this sickness, and all of them compare this phenomenon to epilepsy, pointing to two possible reasons. In the first case, the menstrual blood is "retained" in the uterus, which corrupts it, causing the physical disturbances; in the second, the suffocation is caused by an accumulation of the woman's own sperm in the womb: The "corruption" of the sperm creates "poisonous vapours", which ascend and afflict her brain.[29] None of the texts explain the reason for the retention of the menstrual blood but they do attribute the second case to a long period of sexual abstinence.[30] Only the Castilian text provides the Hippocratic causal explanation, which was commonly held in the Middle Ages, that claims that the uterus' suffocation is caused by its movement upwards and by the pressure it exerted on the respiratory organs.[31]

The medical treatment for the first cause is actually the same in all three texts: It essentially involves medicaments which stimulate the evacuation of menses and bleeding from the artery called *al-safan* (the Hebrew and Arabic texts employ the same term and the Castilian uses the term derived from Arabic: *la safina)*. Some differences between the texts exist concerning the treatment of the second cause: While they recommend sexual relations as the principal solution, the Hebrew text alone proposes massaging the woman's genitalia by the midwife in cases where sexual relations are impossible. This practice is not even mentioned in the Arabic text, although is recommended by the Castilian treatise in different circumstances.[32]

---

[28] Montefiore, 440, f. 20v.

[29] *Ibid.*, ff. 21v-22r; Vázquez de Benito and Herrera, "Dos capítulos ginecológicos: árabe y castellano", pp.188-189, 228-229.

[30] Lloyd, *Science, Folklore and Ideology,* pp. 83-84; Green, *The Transmission of Ancient Theories*, pp. 19-22, 137. On the history of this disease, called also *hysteria*, see M. S. Micalé, "Hysteria and its Historiography: A Review of Past and Present Writings (1), *History of Science*, 37 (1989), pp. 223-261.

[31] Vázquez de Benito and Herrera, "Dos capítulos ginecológicos: árabe y castellano", p. 228.

[32] *Ibid.*, p. 229.

Only the Hebrew text adds, as an integral part of the treatment, that the woman "should shout with an exceedingly great cry".[33]

Significant differences also exist between the three texts concerning theories about the absence of menstruation. Only the Castilian points out that this absence is natural for pregnant and suckling women. The Hebrew text, on the other hand, indicates that some women either do not have any menses, or do so only in small quantities, as a result of their natural physiology and anatomy, as in the case with women whose bodies resemble those of men. It thus indicates that the phenomenon should not be considered pathological and, therefore, does not require any medical treatment.[34]

This formulation is taken, directly or indirectly, from the medical theories of Soranus of Ephesus.[35] The influence of Soranus may be also found in the chapter On Difficulties in Birth (*"la graveza del parto"*) of the Castilian treatise, which distinguishes between "natural" and "unnatural birth", as well as the ways proposed to handle the various difficulties arising during childbirth.[36] The contents of this chapter are quite different from those appearing in the Hebrew and Arabic texts, but are surprisingly similar to the Hebrew text "On Difficulties of Birth", mentioned above. At this stage, it is difficult to state with certainty whether the Hebrew treatise indeed served as one of Ibn al-Khatib's sources and whether, through him, it also influenced the Castilian text. In any case, it is important to note that similar medical ideas circulated within the three cultures in medieval Spain.

The Hebrew text is also significant concerning the conception of sex differences. In this regard, one peculiar aspect should be emphasized: the author's decision to treat maladies and disorders of both male and female genitalia in the same specialized work. Such a fusion is a rare phenomenon in medieval medicine. It is true that some medieval gynaecological texts also contain a number of references to male disorders, especially to sterility, but they remain, in essence, dedicated to women's medicine. By relating to both sexes in one

---

[33] Montefiore, 440, f. 22v.

[34] Vázquez de Benito and Herrera, "Dos capítulos ginecológicos: árabe y castellano", pp. 230-232; Montefiore, 440, f. 23r-23v.

[35] "Quomodo probamus aliquas secundum naturam non purgari? ex eo quod ad integrum sanae sunt et nullam molestiam corporis sentiunt", Radicchi, *La Gynaecia di Muscione*, p. 46.

[36] Vázquez de Benito and Herrera, "Dos capítulos ginecológicos: árabe y castellano", p. 224-226.

treatise, the Hebrew author minimized the "peculiarity" of women's medicine by his emphasis on the common aspects of the genital diseases suffered by both genders.

As to the audience of the text, it is evident that it was intended to serve as a practical manual for the benefit of male physicians: All the instructions are given in a male form and are explicitly directed to a male physician. Nevertheless, the text clearly bears proof of co-operation between the male physician and the female practitioner, especially in cases requiring direct contact with woman's genitalia. In these cases, the text states: "tell the midwife...". Last but not least, on several occasions the author uses the first-person form, relating his own experiences as a physician, and including the medicaments he had tested in treating sick women and the information he had received from others, especially midwives.[37] All these elements enforce the idea that in the Middle Ages, women's health was, in fact, the business of both female and male practitioners.[38]

Another Hebrew text written by a male physician that addresses issues relevant both to men and women, is *Ha-ma'mar ba-toladah niqra sod ha-'ibbur* (The Treatise on Generation, Called the Secret of Conception).[39] It is actually a short work, containing only three folios, dedicated exclusively to the diagnosis and treatment of male and female sterility. Although we cannot identify the author, the manuscript gives important information regarding the place and the time of its composition. The author explicitly indicates that he wrote the text in his "fatherland", which he refers to as *Abringa*, the common medieval Hebrew appellation for the city of Orange, situated in southern France. However, it is difficult to decide whether he was born in that city or whether he found refuge there at a certain moment of his life. The Hebrew text is unclear on this point: the author states that he was "a wanderer" in his fatherland, which he referred to as *eretz manos*. The Hebrew word *manos* may signify either "a refuge", or the Hebrew name of Manosque, an important centre of

---

[37] See Montefiore, 440, ff. 20r; 20v.

[38] The generally accepted idea held by historians is that in medieval times "women's health was women's business". However, Monica Green successfully challenged this idea and demonstrated that women practitioners were engaged in caring for men's maladies and, male physicians were involved in treating women's illnesses; see M. Green, "Women's Medical Practice and Health Care in the Middle Ages", *Signs*, vol. 12 (1989), pp. 434-473.

[39] Oxford, Bodleian Library, Ms. or. 2142, ff. 248v-250(ii)v.

Jewish life in the Middle Ages, located about one hundred kilometres southeast of Orange.[40]

Steinschneider wrongly identified this text as one of the translations made by the anonymous translator between 1197 and 1199 (see pp. 32-33). The treatise was in fact written in the fourteenth century, evidenced by the author's mention of a medicament prescribed by Arnold of Villanova (c. 1235 - 1313) for Robert the Learned, Duke of Anjou and King of Naples (1309 - 1343). In his catalogue of the Hebrew manuscripts kept in the Bodleian Library, Neubauer argued that this text was originally written in Hebrew, and that it is not a translation of a Latin text. The main focus of the debate is the fact that the author himself used a Hebrew verb, *le- ha'atiq*, which has a double meaning in medieval Hebrew, namely: to copy and to translate. It is true that the literary style is very original: In beautiful and fluent language, the author composed the treatise in the form of a letter addressed to his brother-in-law, analysing the reasons preventing the latter's wife (the author's sister) from becoming pregnant, and describing the medical treatments and the sexual conduct that may facilitate conception. The personal and familiar style of the text could indicate that it is indeed an original Hebrew treatise. But this cannot be considered as ultimate evidence, in as much as the study of Hebrew medical treatises written in the Middle Ages has proven that addressing a friend or a family member in the introduction was a frequent topos.[41] However, there are two factors in the present text which deviate from this topos and which may be considered as proof of its originality: The first element is the specific diagnosis of the nature of both the husband and the wife, made by the author at the beginning of the second part. In his judgement, the lack of harmony between the physiological components of the couple is the main reason for their infertility: the wife's "nature" is cold and wet (which is normal) and her husband's is cold and dry, when it should be hot and dry. In other words, we may have here a concrete case of a medical

[40] On the Jewish communities of this region and their medical occupations during the Middle Ages, see J. Shatzmiller, *Médecine et justice en Provence médiévale: Documents de Manosque, 1216-1348*, Aix-en Provence, 1989; *idem*, "Médecins et expertise médicale dans la ville médiévale: Manosque 1280-1348" in *Vie privée et ordre public à la fin du moyen âge: Etudes sur Manosque, la Provence, et le Piémont (1250-1450)*, ed. M. Hérbert, Aix-en-Provence, 1987, pp. 105-117.

[41] On this topos and the use of the verb - *le-ha'atiq* - in Hebrew medieval medical writings, see R. Barkai, "La obra científica del granadino Selomoh ben Yosef ibn Ayyub", pp. 94-95.

diagnosis, a rare event in medieval documentation of sterility. The second element is a prescription which, according to the author, he had prepared for them in the past, and which he repeats in the present text.[42]

While the opening lines and some passages of the text have a distinctly Jewish character, resulting from its Biblical citations, Talmudic references and special literary style, the text itself is clearly influenced by some of the Latin sources used by the author. A significant number of terms appear in their Latin, Provençal and Spanish forms, transcribed in Hebrew letters; in some cases, even words existing in Biblical and medieval Hebrew, such as "spring" and "autumn", appear in their foreign forms. Hence, we may conclude that even though the Hebrew text was written as a real diagnosis by the anonymous physician, he inserted several additional passages from unidentified texts, some of learned medicine, others magical, but all of Latin origin, reworked in a typical Hebrew style.

Each of the two Hebrew texts presented in this chapter is unique: The first one deals with male and female diseases in two separate parts, and yet in a form of a specialized treatise; the second deals with one of the major enduring problems of family life, the inability to generate offspring. Despite their deviation from the "classical" gynaecological treatises in their form and content, they contain important information on gynaecological treatments during the High Middle Ages, and demonstrate that specialized texts for treating both sexes were available during this period. While the *Zikhron ha-ḥolayim ha-hovim bi-khlei ha-herayon* reveals a "balanced" attitude concerning female and male genital disorders and illnesses, the other one, *Ha-ma'mar ba-toladah niqra sod ha-'ibur*, even reveals a considerably sympathetic attitude toward the woman. The author refers to her using delicate and tender expressions, such as "the honourable woman of valor"; "your temple"; "my sister and mistress"; "your pure mate"; "your honourable rib". Not less important is the tender and thoughtful sexual behaviour he recommends to the husband which, according to the author, is the "medical secret" to ensure conception. Thus, in a quite sophisticated way, he combines two different perspectives: the Jewish tradition, expressed in the Talmud, which aimed to avoid brutal and thoughtless sexual conduct on the part of the man ("It is prohibited to come upon your wife when she is sleeping"), and the biological concept prevailing in the Middle Ages,

[42] Oxford, Bodleian Library, Ms. or. 2142, ff. 250(i)r, 250(ii)r.

which declared that conception is possible only by the union of the male and female sperm, and thus pointing to the necessity of the woman's orgasm.

In the previous chapter we have noticed the great importance of Soranian works in the gynaecological corpus translated into Hebrew. The present two treatises, on the other hand, are based on the medical concepts of Muslim medicine (under which influence the first text was written) and which, from the twelfth century also prevailed in Latin medicine (which profoundly influenced the second text). In consequence, the Hippocratic-Galenic "rational school", especially its theory of humours in conjunction to health and sickness, and the four qualities (dry-wet, cold-hot) in matters of physiology guided both texts in their diagnoses and therapies. The two texts thus offer an alternative conceptual and practical gynaecology to the Soranian. However, judging from the quantity of surviving manuscripts, we cannot have any doubt that the treatises derived from the Soranian tradition were the more popular among Jewish physicians during the Middle Ages.

CHAPTER FIVE

EMPIRICAL AND MAGICAL TREATISES

It has been repeatedly stressed in contemporary historiography of medicine that a clear-cut distinction between "rational and learned" medicine on the one hand, and "magical and popular" medicine on the other, existed neither in Antiquity nor in the Middle Ages. It is true that physicians and naturalists such as the Hippocratic writers, Aristotle and Galen seemingly presented themselves as representatives of a comprehensive scientific system, based on *ratio*, but a thorough investigation of ancient texts reveals a more complex reality. G. E. R. Lloyd commented thus in regard to the ancient sciences: "A very considerable body of evidence can be assembled to show how much of Greek science consists in the rationalisation of popular belief. Time and again Greek scientific writings reflect or are based on traditional ideas, with or without the addition of some kind of explanation or justification. Where this is so we have to ask whether there are any good grounds for speaking of this work as *science* as such at all. It would doubtless be wise to speak of the *literate* representation of Greek folklore: and it was not only in Greece, but also in Egypt and Babylon, that our evidence for folk beliefs generally comes from written sources and often from literary texts".[1]

The situation during the Middle Ages was even more intricate due to the importance of "religious medicine" i.e., the attribution of healing powers to the Holy Scriptures, holy objects and holy men , by a large circle of *literati*, Jews, Muslims and Christians alike, as well as the considerable number of active popular practitioners.

Some medieval physicians tried to refute experimental and magical medicine on scientific as well as religious grounds. Maimonides strongly condemned these types of medicine. In his *Mishneh Torah*, in the chapter on idolatry, Maimonides refers to those who practice religious medicine as impious: "He that mutters incantations over a

---

[1] Lloyd, *Science, Folklore and Ideology*, p. 202.

wound and reads [for that purpose] a verse from the Bible; and he, that reads [a verse] to prevent scaring a baby and puts a Bible or *Tefillin* on a little child, in order to put him to sleep - they are not only sorcerers and magicians, but they also deny the Torah, since they transform the word of the Torah into a physical remedy when it is a remedy for the souls".[2]

In the same decisive manner, Maimonides condemns empirical medicine and medical practices based on inexplicable virtues of materials. He admits that the art of medicine is based on experience *(nisayon)* and rational speculation *(heqesh)*, but according to him, a man should rely only "on those physicians who acquired the theoretical and scientific aspects [of medicine], since these domains are the roots while the practice is the branch [of that art]". Therefore, he despises "the mass of the Occident" who advocate "asking the experienced rather than consulting a physician", an attitude that has led them to trust the "traditions of old women" rather than the wisdom of a well-trained physician. Maimonides concludes that "a sick man who puts himself in the hands of an experienced [practitioner], who does not possess medical theory but does as he has observed, is like a seafarer who may accidentally be saved or drowned".[3]

Notwithstanding his scientific and religious authority, Maimonides' conceptions and attitudes in this matter were rejected by the majority of Jewish leaders. Moreover, at the beginning of the fourteenth century, the religious authorities who had prohibited the study of "rational sciences" by students below the age of twenty-five, explicitly permitted and encouraged the use of experimental and magical medicine.[4] These domains were, in fact, very popular within Jewish medieval communities, as they were in Muslim and Christian societies. They may be found integrated into learned medical trea-

---

[2] *Mishneh Torah hu ha-yad ha-ḥazaqah*, Hilkhot 'avodah zarah, ch. 11, 12. (Hebrew).

[3] Maimonides, *On Asthma*, in *Medical Works*, vol. IV, pp. 112-113. (Hebrew).

[4] The polemic on these subjects, which took place especially in the Jewish communities of Christian Spain and Southern France, is strongly expressed in the *Responsa of Rabbi Shelomoh ben Adret from Barcelona* (Benei-Braq, 1968, No. 413-418). Concerning Christian society, see Tony Hunt's introduction to his *Popular Medicine in Thirteenth-Century England*, Cambridge, 1990; R. Jalby, *Sorcellerie, médecine populaire et pratique médico-magique en Languedoc*, Lyons, 1974. For a detailed analysis of this polemic in both Jewish and Christian societies, see my forthcoming work on the magical uses of Psalms in these communities during the Middle Ages and the Renaissance. Cf. Barkaï, *Les infortunes de Dinah*, pp. 99-104.

tises as well as in the form of independent texts. Some of these texts are exclusively dedicated to gynaecology; but they make no attempt whatsoever to present any diagnoses or theories concerning the female body and its problems, or even to offer any rationalisation for the proposed treatment. Characteristically, these magical and experimental texts content themselves with giving the appropriate receipts or incantations for a given illness or problem, only some of which are attributed to a well-known medical authority in order to reinforce their credibility.

An important collection of these Hebrew magical and experimental gynaecological texts is conserved at the Bodleian Library, Oxford. The codex is entirely dedicated to medical works dated from the thirteenth and fourteenth centuries.[5] The texts are short, and successively copied by the same scribe. The first, "The Treatise on Generation, Called the Secret of Conception", described in the previous chapter, is published in this volume. It is followed by a one-page text entitled: *Merqaḥat mo'il le-qabel ha-herayon be-shem ha-rofé Mae. Vidal Debourian* (A Useful Unguent for Conception, Attributed to the Physician Master Vidal de Bourian).[6]

This Jewish physician, who obtained the honourable title of Maestro, was born in the fourteenth century, probably in the city Arles in southern France, and practised medicine in Bourian, a quarter of Arles (called later Bourg Neuf), during the middle of that century. His son Salves [i. e., son of] Vidal de Bourian, following in his footsteps, practised in the same place until the end of the fourteenth century.[7] This single page is the only known text attributed to Vidal. The *Merqaḥat* contains two receipts of compound medicaments to be placed in the womb in order to facilitate pregnancy; a potion to stimulate sexual desire, to be taken by both partners; and finally, an ointment for the same purpose, to be applied on the penis.

The most important gynaecological treatise in this collection is undoubtedly the one attributed to Sheshet (probably Benveniste), ha-Nasi, the head of the Jewish community of Barcelona, who served as *alfakim* (physician) to the kings of Aragon, Alfonso II (1162-1196) and Pedro II (1196-1213). Apart from medical services, Sheshet also fulfilled important roles in the treasury and diplomatic corps of the

---

[5] Oxford, Bodleian Library, Or. 2142.

[6] *Ibid.*, f. 251r.

[7] On the Vidal family of physicians and the texts attributed to them, see E. Renan, *Ecrivans juifs français du XIVeme siècle*, Paris, 1893, pp. 578, 580, 585.

Aragonese court. The level of his social and political status can be inferred from documents of the royal chancellery, which bear his signature (in Hebrew) together with those of the king and other dignitaries.[8]

The opening line of the text in question, called *Maguen ha-rosh* (The Head's Shield), indicates that it has been copied "two [or] three times" by the famous author of Hebrew literary prose *(maqâmôt)*, Jehudah al-Ḥarîzî (1170-1235)[9]. The title's meaning is clarified at the end of the first recipe, which is intended to stimulate conception. The author then adds that it is also useful for stimulating sexual desire, for all pains afflicting the womb and the stomach, and for headaches, "therefore it is called the head's shield".[10] The treatise as a whole is rationally organized according to the various problems and illnesses afflicting the female body. It is homogenous in its Hebrew style but medical terms, and even entire phrases, in Romance and Latin are frequently employed in their Hebrew transliteration.

Two conspicuous qualities raise doubts regarding the attribution of this gynaecological text to Sheshet Benveniste *ha-Nasi*: The first concerns the frequent presence of Christian medicine while the other points to the frequent employment of experimental (or popular) and magical medicine. Thus, we may find in the treatise formulas "for a woman who can not conceive because of sorcery"; an amulet in the form of a scorpion to prevent miscarriage, etc. In one case, the experimental aspect is of special interest. The author, after offering a formula to prevent miscarriage, proposes an experiment on an animal: "If you wish to test if it really works, tie it on the belly of a hen, which will not give birth as long as it is tied to it".[11] Sheshet was after all known as one of the supporters and admirers of Maimonides. When the polemic over Maimonides' writings erupted at the beginning of the thirteenth century, he vigorously defended Maimonides' rationalistic positions on theological issues and saw in the *Misheh Torah* an important innovation on the matter of Jewish Law *(Halakhah)*. His identification with the Maimonidean attitude does not, of course, suit the employment of experimental and magical

[8] Baer, *A History of the Jews in Christian Spain*, pp.94-95, 100.

[9] Born in al-Andalus, he emigrated to Provence, where he translated Arabic literary prose into Hebrew and later composed Hebrew literary prose according to the Arabic modes. See Schippers, *Arabic Tradition and Hebrew Innovation*, pp. 75-77.

[10] Oxford, Bodleian Library, Or. 2142, f. 251v, lines 17-20.

[11] Oxford, Bodleian Library, Or. 2142, ff. 252r, 254r, 253v.

medicine. The only explanation for this contradiction is the eclectic character of the treatise. The author apparently borrowed receipts on various subjects from a number of sources without any rigorous, critical review. Sheshet may have been an important physician and politician indeed, but he was not a distinguished thinker.

Furthermore, the author incorporated some magical receipts which were circulated in medical works in the early and high Middle Ages. By way of illustration, two related sources can be cited: the tenth-century Muslim-Spanish physician 'Abd al-Raḥmân ibn al-Haitham and a medical treatise attributed to the twelfth-century Jewish-Spanish scientist Abraham ibn 'Ezra. As already noted, the Arabic original of al-Haitham's work has been lost, and it exists presently only in its Hebrew translation under the title *Sefer Segulot* (The Book on Virtues). *Sefer ha-nisyonot* (The Book on [Medical] Experiences), attributed to Abraham ibn 'Ezra, is largely based on al-Haitham's treatise, but the later Hebrew text omits some materials while it adds significant novelties, notably many prescriptions beginning with the phrase "The experimenter said".[12] It is difficult to say which of these works influenced the treatise attributed to Sheshet Benveniste since its description of the magic square used to facilitate delivery more closely resembles the one appearing in The Book on [Medical] Experiences;[13] on the other hand, the prescription describing the use of a stone taken from an eagle's nest, for the same purpose, resembles that which appears in al-Haitham's work.[14]

In any case, it is evident that these prescriptions were taken from a Hebrew work since the author does not use any Latin terms in the respective paragraphs, whereas Latin words are in abundance in other parts of the treatise. Undoubtedly, however, a Latin treatise or even various treatises also served Sheshet as the principal source of his work. It appears that he borrowed not only the usual medical prescriptions, but also typically Christian formulas, even if transliterated in Hebrew letters, which seems quite strange within the context of a Hebrew treatise. The most striking example of this transfer from the Christian medical culture to the Jewish one is a prescription for postpartum treatment: After noting the components of the me-

---

[12] *Sefer Hanisyonot, The Book of Experiences Attributed to Abraham Ibn Ezra*, p. 11.

[13] *Ibid.*, pp. 240-242; Oxford, Bodleian Library, Or. 2142, f. 255v.

[14] Oxford, Bodleian Library, Or. 2142, f. 255r; *Sefer Hanisyonot, The Book of Experiences Attributed to Abraham Ibn Ezra*, p. 316.

dicament, the text states: "fiat electuarium ad modum manum Christum" (make an electuary in the form of Christ's hand).[15] Even if the reference is to a particular type of medicine, the fact that the Hebrew text preserved Christ's name is of significance.

In addition, a number of problematic chapters - from the point of view of Jewish Law - appear in the manuscript. They concern medical procedures which are strictly prohibited by Jewish *halakhah* and severely condemned by Jewish ethics, such as abortion and contraception. These practices, which contradict two major commandments: "Be fruitful, and multiply..." (Gen. 1:28), and "Thou shalt not kill" (Ex. 20:13; Dt. 5:17), are described in several Hebrew medieval medical treatises, generally with an added warning not to use them unless the woman's life is in danger.[16] Such a warning does not appear in the gynaecological text attributed to Sheshet.[17] On the other hand, a unique indication of piety appearing in the text is the reference to the appropriate days for conceiving males or females, to which the author adds: "And God, be He blessed, brings whatever He desires".[18]

Typical of experimental medical texts, the author cites very few medical authorities while insisting on the efficacy of the receipts he presents. Thus, he frequently adds expressions like: "tried and tested"; "tested and I guarantee its efficiency"; "it is tested because I myself tried it", and so on. Of special interest is the receipt for facilitating pregnancy in as much as the formula has been proved in an extremely difficult case. The author remarks here: "Undoubtedly she will conceive, since it has been experimented with many women, including one aged fifty years, who never conceived before and became pregnant thanks to this".[19]

Furthermore, the treatise bears evidence that the Jewish practitioner had professional relationships with non-Jewish healers and patients: In one case, he describes a treatment for difficulties during birth, tested and transmitted orally to him by a Muslim woman.[20] In

---

15 Oxford, Bodleian Library, Or. 2142, f. 253v.

16 See: Barkaï, *Les infortunes de Dinah*, pp. 93-94.

17 Joan Cadden underscores the different attitudes between theology and Canon law and medical literature concerning these "delicate" issues in medieval Christianity (Cadden, *Meanings of Sex Differences in the Middle Ages*, p. 269). Cf. Barkaï, *Les infortunes de Dinah*, pp. 91-94.

18 Oxford, Bodleian Library, Or. 2142, f. 252r.

19 *Ibid.*, ff. 252r-252v.

20 *Ibid*, f.254r.

another, the author testifies to the efficiency of a treatment to promote menstruation, thusly: "It is tested, since it provoked [menstruation] in a Gentile woman".[21]

Of the three medical authorities mentioned in the text, all are Muslims, the names of two of which are deformed. To Ibn Sînâ *(Buzina)*, the author attributes a recipe to straighten the opening of the womb. In the name of al-Zahrâwî *(Zahrabi)*, he provides a formula "to remove inflammation of the breasts". Lastly, he attributes to al-Ṭabarî the above-mentioned use of a stone taken from an eagle's nest to facilitate labour.[22] The absence of both Jewish and Christian medical authorities in the text is, of course, very intriguing, for it was written in a Christian environment and influenced by Latin texts and, undoubtedly, Hebrew medical treatises already in circulation in Christian Spain.

---

21 *Ibid.*, f. 252v.

22 *Ibid.*, respectively ff. 254r; 257r; 255r. The tradition related to al-Ṭabarî appears in both al-Haitham's *Sefer segulot* and *Sefer ha-nisyonot*, attributed to Abraham ibn 'Ezra. See *Sefer Hanisyonot, The Book of Experiences Attributed to Abraham Ibn Ezra*, pp. 316, 240. It should be noted that al-Ṭabarî is often cited in Hebrew medieval medical literature, especially in regard to experimental and magical medicine. And, indeed, in the same codex that includes the gynaecological texts, we find a treatise entitled *Sefer segulot el Ṭâbarî* (Al-Ṭabarî's Book of Virtues) (ff. 28v-43r). The sixth part of the treatise, dedicated to gynaecology (ff. 38r-43r), is divided into twelve chapters as follows: 1. "On uterine pain and suffocation"; 2. "On that which prevents pregnancy"; 3. "On that which retains the foetus"; 4. "On that which causes abortion"; 5. "On that which provokes menses"; 6. "On that which prevents delivery"; 7. "On that which facilitates delivery"; 8. "On that which arouses sexual desire"; 9. "On that which prevents intercourse"; 10. "On that which stimulates love"; 11. "On that which aids pregnancy"; 12. "On inflammation of the pubes and their tumors".

CONCLUSION

The extensive Jewish medieval literature on gynaecology raises three major interrelated questions: First, what motivated those medieval Jewish authors in translating foreign treatises as well as producing original works on women's health? Second, why did they prefer certain medical traditions while others exercised only a limited influence upon them? And third, to whom were these treatises addressed, and for what purpose? Regarding the first question, the translators and the authors clearly expressed their motives; unfortunately, they were not, in most cases, very candid about the other two. Moreover, the considerable variety of the known works makes answering these questions even more complex.

Undoubtedly, the creation of the medieval Jewish corpus of gynaecological texts was part of the revival of the Hebrew culture, a comprehensive phenomenon that transpired within the Jewish communities in Latin Europe from the twelfth to the fifteenth centuries. Two major historical factors, unrelated but coincident, contributed to the unprecedented flourishing of poetic, scientific and religious Hebrew literature: The exile of the Jews from Muslim Spain and their consequent settlement in Christian lands, and the transmission of Arabic sciences and philosophy to the Occident. Exiled Jews not only played a decisive role in rendering the Arabic sciences into Latin and vernacular languages,[1] they also comprised the élite in the sphere of Hebrew literary invention. The motivations of those erudites were simultaneously practical and ideological: To facilitate the access to the contemporary body of knowledge for their fellow Jews, and to do so in their common sacred, historical language.

In trying to answer the second question, we have examined all the available Jewish gynaecological texts, and it was striking to discover that out of the rich Hippocratic corpus on women's medicine, only

[1] J. S. Gil, *La escuela de traductores de Toledo y sus colaboradores judíos*, Toledo, 1985; N. Roth, "Jewish Collaborators in Alfonso's Scientific Work", in R. I. Burns, S. J., *Emperor of Culture. Alfonso X the Learned of Castile and His Thirteenth-Century Renaissance*, Philadelphia, 1990, pp. 59-71.

one text has been translated into Hebrew, i.e., the minor work *On Superfoetation*. The Hebrew translation, derived from the Arabic one, clearly did not play an important role in Jewish medieval medicine, evidenced by its omission from the Hebrew encyclopaedic medical treatises and gynaecological works. Moreover, as only one manuscript of this translation is available, it seems fair to conclude that its circulation was limited. Furthermore, only one Hebrew gynaecological work is attributed to Galen but, as we have seen, Galen was not the true author of this text; rather, it is a medieval compilation based on Soranus' works.

Still, the concepts and ideas of the most important classical writers in medieval medicine - Hippocrates and Galen - may be found in one Hebrew gynaecological treatise: *The Compilations of our Rabbi Moses on Menstruation and Pregnancy*. These compilations, taken essentially from *Maimonides' Aphorisms* and from his commentary on the *Hippocratic Aphorisms*, both translated into Hebrew in the thirteenth century by Mosheh ibn Tibbon, are indeed faithful representations of Hippocratic and Galenic medicine. We should bear in mind, however, that the compilations had an exclusively practical aim, evidenced by the compiler's elimination of almost all the theoretical aspects of Maimonides' text and the retention of only the therapeutic elements.

In contrast to the marginal presence of Hippocratic and Galenic medicine in Jewish gynaecological literature, both, and especially Arabic Galenism, played a decisive role in Jewish encyclopaedic medical treatises. Regarding some theoretical issues, such as the role played by women in the process of conception, a number of distinguished Jewish physicians, notably Maimonides, Gershon ben Solomon and Nathan ben Joel Falaquera, preferred Aristotelian notions;[2] but on the whole, we may define Jewish medieval medicine, as in the case of Arabic medicine, as a Galenized art.

A portion of the Hebrew gynaecological treatises entirely ignored the theoretical aspects of women's medicine. These elements, however, are found in some original Hebrew texts, such as: *A Record of the Diseases Occurring in the Genital Members*, *The Treatise on Procreation Called the Secret of Conception*, *On Birth Difficulties*, and in the *Book on Generation*, the Hebrew adaptation of Muscio's *Gynaecia*. This last case is of special interest for us since it was the most popular of the gynaecological texts but, it should be noted,

---

[2] Barkaï, *Les infortunes de Dinah*, pp. 69-77.

neither the translator nor, most probably, his medieval readers knew that it was a Methodist treatise or for that matter what Methodism was.

The author of the Hebrew version of the *Gynaecia* followed Muscio on most issues, even though some of them presented serious religious and moral problems (such as the affirmation that virginity is healthy and that coitus and pregnancy may be harmful), but he presented them in a rather ambiguous form. The Hebrew text adhered to the Latin in its admission that "the more virginity is prolonged, the healthier it is for the woman", but omitted the Latin text's recommendation of perpetual virginity.[3] Similarly, the Jewish author eliminated most of the paragraph in which Soranus claimed that pregnancy was harmful for women's health. He treated the absence of menses in the same manner, following Soranus' position that menstruation caused women to age earlier, but omitted the paragraph in the Latin text that declared that women may be healthy without menstruation. Moreover, contrary to Soranus' view that menopause is healthy for old women (preserved unaltered by Muscio), the Hebrew version stated: "And old women who emit blood are healthy".[4]

After a careful study of the fate of Soranus' writings in the later Middle Ages, Monica Green notes the evident decline of interest in both Soranus' theory and therapy in late Latin medicine. The "transition" transpired between the late twelfth and the first half of the thirteenth century, when the "Trotula texts" gained popularity and eventually replaced the Latinized *Gynaikeia*.[5] However, the Hebrew gynaecology that developed at that time in the bosom of Latin medical culture continued to keep faith with Soranus. The most intriguing question is, of course, why Jewish gynaecological literature preferred to rely on the Soranian medical writings rather than on other treatises, which were becoming at the time far more popular in the Latin West, especially the gynaecological works attributed to Trotula? One must admit that it seems a strange choice indeed, for two essential reasons: In the first place, the content of the texts attributed to Trotula do not pose serious religious and moral problems for a Jewish physician or midwife, while (as we have seen above) it is difficult to reconcile the basic ideas of Soranus with Judaism; sec-

---

[3] Barkaï, *Les infortunes de Dinah*, p. 230.
[4] *Ibid*. For the French translation see p. 137.
[5] Hanson and Green, "Soranus of Ephesus", pp. 1057-1059.

ond, the balance of Jewish medieval medical literature was basically Galenic, a fact endowing an advantage, *a priori*, to the Trotula.

Was this trend, then, the result of theoretical reflection and conscious decision? The evidence we have does not demonstrate that this was indeed the case. As we have seen above, the introduction of the Latin gynaecological texts into Hebrew medicine was the pioneering enterprise of one person, the anonymous translator, at the end of the twelfth century. Not only did he not know that he was translating a Methodist text, but the translation itself shows that he misunderstood some of the fundamental Soranian medical ideas. Moreover, he himself also translated one of the texts attributed to Trota. It appears, then, that he just translated all the texts available to him. In other words, it was a case of what Monica Green has described as "historical circumstances", explaining that "... the Hebrew translator has simply chosen to take advantage of the only intelligent and therapeutically detailed account of women's medicine he could find".[6] Of all the translations he made, he enhanced only Muscio's *Genecia* with a Jewish countenance, a fact that can explain the popularity of the treatise among the Jewish communities in which it circulated until the end of Middle Ages.

Still, one issue remains enigmatic: From the twelfth to the end of the fifteenth century, Jewish translators rendered a large quantity of medical treatises from Latin into Hebrew preferably those which were very popular in Christian society and which were considered important both for acquiring theoretical knowledge as well as for the actual practice of medicine. Undoubtedly, the Trotula texts, most notably the *Liber de sinthomatibus mulierum* and the *De curis mulierum*, perfectly responded to these two requirements. And yet the Trotula texts exerted only an insignificant impact on Jewish gynaecology: There remains only one solitary manuscript of one of these texts; there is also only one vague reference to the "Book of Trotula", in which the author in fact refers not to "Trotula" but to Muscio's discussion of the difference between pregnancy and the pathology called "mola". Even if we adhere to the explanation that the Soranian texts were influential in Jewish gynaecology due to their "severely practical orientation", an argument which I accept, the Trotula texts undeniably were not less practical. Apparently, at the present stage of the research on medieval Hebrew medicine, we have no clue that may help solve this riddle.

---

[6] *Ibid.*

Finally, for whom were the medieval Hebrew gynaecological treatises written? From the sample of texts presented in the second part of this volume, the reader can discern an important difference between the empirical-magical texts and the treatises which included theoretical, aetiologic and symptomatic materials. The latter, although addressed essentially to a male physician, include, in various cases, instructions to the midwife who assists him. Thus, for example, the author of the treatise *A Record of the Diseases Occurring in the Genital Members*, in the chapter on foetus retention, after describing external treatments to be undertaken by the male physician, adds: "You should order the midwife... to sit on her and to anoint her womb with moistening things...".[7] The same attitude, which ascribes treatments involving direct contact with a woman's genitalia to the midwife, also appears in the text concerning uterine suffocation: The role of the male physician is limited to letting blood and prescribing a diet and other medicaments; the midwife's role, on the other hand, is much more radical, she is veritably instructed to masturbate the suffering woman: "If the cause is the sperm, the proper treatment for her is to have sexual relations. If this is not possible for her she should apply drying things... and the midwife should place it in her womb...". Afterwards, says the author,: "... order the midwife to massage the orifice of her womb with the above mentioned materials...".[8]

Only one text, *Sefer ha-toledet*, seems to be addressed directly to women who wish to study gynaecology and obstetrics, given that its author chose Dinah, a well-known female personality, as the student or the recipient of the medical knowledge. Of course, one may argue that the author employed the dialogue between Dinah and her father for stylistic purposes, which undoubtedly is true, but the fact that a woman and not a male physician was explicitly addressed is meaningful. In this respect, the Hebrew version is even more explicit in regard to its intended audience than are its Greek (Soranus' *Gynaekeia*) and Latin (Muscio's version) sources.[9]

---

[7] See the English translation, p. 136.

[8] *Ibid.*, pp. 139.

[9] According to Ann Hanson, "... the work of rewriting the [Soranus'] 'Gynaikeia' into the simpler, Greek catechism that Muscio eventually encounters and Latinizes for midwives is carried out by someone writing at least a generation or more later than Soranus". See Hanson and Green, "Soranus of Ephesus", pp. 1030-1031, cf. p. 1047. We may infer that Muscio was addressing midwives from his own introduction to the Latin version: "His autem multu simplicius volui loqui et ut verius dicam

The short, experimental and magical texts reflect one exclusive interest: to prescribe the appropriate medical treatment for all female diseases and problems. They contain neither theoretical exposition nor attempt to deal with the causes or the symptoms of the illnesses. In other words, they are meant to serve as a practical manual for the practitioner, whether male or female.[10] They provide no conclusive indications as for whom these texts were explicitly destined since all of them use masculine forms of address, which is the standard form in the Hebrew language when addressing groups of men and women. This raises an intriguing question: To what extent does the gynaecological literature reflect the historical reality concerning the medical attendance on women in the Middle Ages? We have to admit that our knowledge of medieval medical practice in general, and on the treatment of women in particular, is very limited.[11] The documentation that could serve as direct evidence on this matter is very rare, and most of our hypotheses are based on illuminations in medical manuscripts and the medical treatises themselves. Thus, for example, various medieval illuminations present male physicians, attending women accompanied by female practitioners, especially in scenes describing delivery.[12] It is even more difficult to draw solid conclusions about the medical roles of women within medieval Jewish communities since such illustrations do not exist in Hebrew medical

muliebribus verbis usus sum, ut etiam inperitae obstetrices licet ab altera sibi lectam rationem facile intellegere possint", Radicchi, *La Gynaecia di Muscione*, p. 36.

[10] This genre of medical texts, written in both Latin and vernacular languages, was popular in Western Europe and, as noted above, some served as sources for the Jewish compilator. In his study on popular medicine, Tony Hunt mentions two gynaecological texts although he published only a part of the first one, see *Popular Medicine in Thirteenth-Century England*, pp. 142, 143, 199-200, 203. For a more detailed study of vernacular gynaecological texts in medieval England, see M. H. Green, "Obstetrical and Gynecological Texts in Middle English", *Studies in the Age of Chaucer*, 14 (1992), pp. 53-88.

[11] Danielle Jacquart, in her *Le milieu médical en France du XIIe au XVe siècle: En annexe 2e supplément au "Dictionnaire" d' Ernest Wickersheimer*, Geneva, 1981, has listed 127 women practitioners, who represent only 1.5% of all practicing physicians at the time. On gynaecological matters see: Diepgen, *Frau und Frauenheilkunde*. A refreshing methodology was put forward in Monica H.Green, "Women's Medical Practice and Health Care in the Medieval Europe", pp. 434-473 (reprinted in J. Bennett et alia, eds. *Sisters and Workers in the Middle Ages*, Chicago, 1989, pp. 39-78).

[12] See for example S. Laurent, *Naître au Moyen Age, de la conception à la naissance: la grossesse et l'accouchement*, Paris, 1989, Fig. 36, 44, 46, 49.

manuscripts nor, more importantly, have any medieval Jewish archives been preserved in the Latin West. In fact, we have only a few, dispersed mentions, most of which have been culled from Christian archives, of Jewish women who were active in the medical professions.[13]

To sum up, from the comments and therapeutic instructions existing in medieval Hebrew medical treatises, we may learn that midwives indeed played an important role in the medical treatment of women, especially in childbirth, but by no means did they exercise exclusivity in these domains.[14] It appears that in this respect, the situation in Jewish society was similar to that in Christian society, as concluded by Monica Green on the basis of Latin and vernacular medical writings: "Although normal childbirth seems to have been almost completely supervised by women, whether or not they were specialist midwives, complicated childbirth as well as routine gynecological care was more contested terrain. Though we do not yet know much about their actual gynecological practice, male physicians and surgeons were not restricted about making expert pronouncements in their medical writings on every kind of gynecological topic".[15]

---

[13] J. Shatzmiller, *Jews, Medicine, and Medieval Society*, pp. 109-112, 131, 135.

[14] Barkaï, *Les infortunes de Dinah*, pp. 88-89.

[15] Green, "Obstetrical and Gynecological Texts in Middle English", p. 57.

PART TWO

JEWISH GYNAECOLOGICAL TEXTS

INTRODUCTION

As mentioned in the Introduction of Part One, one of the major handicaps in the study of medieval Jewish medicine is the fact that the large majority of medieval Hebrew medical texts are preserved in manuscript and are not available to scholars, particularly those who do not read Hebrew. For this reason, and to provide the reader with a representative sample of Jewish gynaecological texts, I offer critical editions of six of the sixteen texts discussed in the present study, in their original Hebrew as well as English translation, in the Second Part. My choice was made according to two criteria: the value of the text to the history of medieval gynaecology, and the interest historians may find in the text itself. *Sefer Dinah* is a unique Jewish gynaecological text, written in a language other than Hebrew: Judeo-Arabic. Furthermore, it is the only known text of a partial Arabic translation of Muscio's *Gynaecia.* In as much as I have repeatedly insisted on the central place of Soranic medicine within Jewish medieval gynaecology, I consider reasonable to publish another Soranian work which was translated into Hebrew, the *De passionibus mulierum* (Version B). The following text is the *Liber de sinthomatibus mulierum* (3), the only one of the Trotula texts translated into Hebrew. The *Record of the Diseases Occurring in the Genital Members* was not only one of the earliest Hebrew texts on gynaecology, but it probably played an important role in the development of gynaecology in medieval Spain, being a major source of later Arabic and Castilian texts. I have edited both parts of this treatise on men's and women's diseases since they form one integral text: The author, when dealing with women's diseases, also referred to those mentioned in the first part on male ailments. The *Treatise on Generation Called the Secret of Conception* has special literary interest due to its form (a letter written by a physician to his brother-in-law) and its linguistic style. It represents the traditional Galenic approach to the problem of sterility, which is based on a temperamental balance between the man and the woman. Finally, it seems to me that the work attributed to Sheshet Benveniste, *The Head's Shield*, has two essential merits: It is based primarily upon experimental and magical medicine, and its sources are Arabic and Hebrew as well as Latin (transcribed into Hebrew letters). This is an exemplary text, one that demonstrates the high degree of cultural exchange and assimilation which existed in medieval Spain as well as the continuity of popular medical treatments through several centuries.

DINAH'S BOOK ON ALL THAT CONCERNS THE WOMB AND ITS SICKNESSES

British Museum, London, Ms. Or. 10539/4.

ספר דינה לכל ענין הרחם וחלייה לידר אל טמת. יוכד גברית חי וגואשיר וגנדברסת וסדאב מוכי וסמן וטרבנתינא ונטרון אחמר מכוי׳ וקתיין שמע י׳ אוי׳ דמאג איל וקיי׳ דהן קדים אל כפאיי ויעמל פרזגה.[1]

ידר אל טמת יוכד סמן ותרבנתינה [sic] ודהן ורד מכוי׳ גזו יכלט ויעמל פרזגה.[2]

ידר אל טמת יוכד נטרון דקיק וזית מכוי׳ גזו [5] וינעמל פרזגה פאנהא תגרב רטובאת כתירה ותדר אל טמת.[3]

ידר אל טמת יוכד כרבק אסוד ומר מכוי׳ גזו יסחק ויכלט בדהן ויעמל פרזגה כאל זיתון.[4]

ידר אל טמת יוכד גלנאר ושמע מכוי׳ ג׳ אוי׳ שחם אוז וזופא מכוי׳ ח׳ דרי׳ טרבנתינה דרהמין עסל ודהן ורד מכוי׳ דרי׳ אסחק ואכלט בעצארת אל אירסא ויעמל פתילה.[5]

ידר אל טמת יוכד רמון מסחוק ומא אל עסל תשרבא בנביד חאר או יעטיהא בנפסג ופלפל ומר מכוי׳ גזו תסחק ותשרב בנביד חאר.[6]

ידר [10] אלטמת. יוכד מלוכיא והיא מלבאביש ותטבך במא ותגלס פיהא.[7]

פרזגה תסכן כל וגע וכל נפך פי אל רחם. יוכד חלבה ובזר כתאן מכוי׳ וקיי׳ דהן לוז חלו וקייתין תטבך אל בזור מסחוקה פי אל דהן אלי אני יפני אל דהן ותגעל פיה שמע וקיי׳ ותזולה מן עלי אל נאר ותגעל פיה דהן בזר כתאן או שחם אוז או מך דמאג איל וקיי׳ ותסתעמל.[8]

---

[1] *Pessaria Muscionis*, (*P. M.*) 2. The comparision with the Latin text is based on: Radicchi, *La Gynaecia di Muscione*, pp. 222-242.

[2] *P. M.*, 29.

[3] *P. M.*, 30.

[4] *P. M.*, 32.

[5] *P. M.*, 28.

[6] *P. M.*, 37.

[7] This *pessarium* is not mentioned by Muscio.

[8] *P. M.*, 9

פרזגה תסכ[ן] וגע אל רחם ותזיל נפכה. יוכד שמע וסמן מכו׳ י׳ דר׳ זופא ושחם איל מכו׳ ח׳ דרא׳ [15] שחם אוז ד׳ דר׳ דהן ורד נצף ותסתעמל.[9]

פרזגה לכל וגע וכל מרץ פי אל רחם. [יוכד] שחם בקר וקונטריון מ[כו]׳ וקיי׳ שחם אוז דרהמין עצארת רמאן וקיי׳ תסתעמל פרזגה.[10]

פרזגה תסכן נפכת אל רחם. יוכד שחם אוז ושחם דגאג ושחם חזיר אלדי עלי אל כלי ודמאג איל ושמע ודהן קנה ודהן לדאן ודהן סרו ודהן נארדין ועצארת זופא מכו׳ ג׳ או׳ טרבנתינה וקיי׳.[11]

פרזגה תסכן נפכת אל רחם. יוכד זעפראן ודהן ורד וזופא מכו׳ דרהמין דמאג איל ג׳ דר׳ טרבנתינה [20] דרהמין שמע ח׳ דר׳ זופא רטב וסמן ז׳ דר׳ זעפראן ודהן ורד מכו׳ ג׳ דר׳ דהן נארדין ושחם כנזיר ואכליל אל מלך וחלבה מכו׳ דר׳ קסט דרהמין מצטכי ודמאג איל ושחם אוז מכו׳ ח׳ דר׳.[12]

פרזגה תסכן נפכת אל רחם. יוכד שחם פאזאן וסמן מכו׳ דרהמין דמאג איל וטרבנתינה מכו׳ ג׳ או׳ שמע וקיי׳ שחם אוז וקיי׳.[13]

פרזגה תרטב גסאות אל רחם ואנגלאקה. יוכד שחם בקר ודמאג איל ושמע מכו׳ ג׳ דר׳ דהן נארדין ד׳ דר׳ עצארת זופא ג׳ דר׳ ונצף ותסתעמל.[14]

[25] **פרזגה** תרטב גסאות אל רחם ואסתרכאה יוכד שמע וקיי׳ דמאג איל וסמן ועצארת חלבה ועסל ודהן סוסאן מכו׳ וקיי׳ דהן נארדין ד׳ או׳.[15]

פרזגה תרטב אל רחם מן גסאותה. יוכד דמאג איל ושחם אוז ודהן נארדין ושמע ושחם דגאג ודהן סרו.[16]

פרזגה תברד אל רחם מן אל חרארה ולוגעתהא. יוכד מלוכיה תטבך ושחם עגל ושחם אוז וטרבנתינה קליל.[17]

פרזגה תברד אל רחם מן אל חרארה. יוכד שמע וסמן מכו׳ י׳ דר׳ זופא ושחם איל מכו׳ ח׳ דר׳ שחם [30] אוז ד׳ דר׳ דהן ורד אל כפאי׳ ותסתעמל.[18]

פרזגה תברד אל רחם מן אל חרארה. יוכד סנבל הנדי י׳ דר׳ שב דרהמין עוד בלסאן ד׳ דר׳ קצב דרירה ו׳ דר׳ זעפראן רב׳ קסט וקנה מכו׳ ג׳ דר׳ יעגן בעסל אל כפאי׳.[19]

---

9 *P. M.*, 23.
10 *P. M.*, 24.
11 *P. M.*, 52.
12 *P. M.*, 27.
13 *P. M.*, 14.
14 *P. M.*, 17.
15 *P. M.*, 47.
16 *P. M.*, 53.
17 This *pessarium* is not mentioned by Muscio.
18 The second part of *P. M.*, 23.
19 *P. M.*,18.

פרזגה תברד אל רחם מן אלתהאב פיה יוכד זעפראן וקיי׳ שמע וקיי׳ שחם אוז וזופא ודמאג איל מכו׳ וקיי׳ עסל דר׳ ביאץ ביץ דר׳ דהן ורד כפאיי.[20]

פרזגה למראה אלדי לם תטהר כמא יגב מן טמתהא בל בצעובה. יוכד גואשיר וסדאב רטב ומר מכו׳ וק׳ [35] תסחק כל שי נחא תם תכלט מעה דהן זיתון כפאיי ותסתעמל.[21]

פרזגה למראה אלדי לם תטהר [f. 1v] מן טמתהא בכפה. יוכד שחם אוז ודהן קדים ושמע ודהן נארדין וטרמנתינה ודמאג איל ועצארת זופא וסמן ולובן מכו׳ וקיי.[22]

פרזגה תבאעד וקת אל טמת יוכד פלפל אביץ וחלבה מכו׳ גזו תסחק ותכלט בעסל ויעטי להא פי מא בין אל חמאם תדכל פיה מרתין פי יום ואחד.[23]

לתסקט אל גנין יוכד דר׳ גואשיר אוקיי׳ תסקט מסרע. או יטעמהא נענע טרי ז׳ איאם עלי אל [5] ריק לם תחמל אבדא.[24]

פרזגה לי גפף רטובת אל רחם. יוכד דר׳ חגר טליאקניש דרהמין לובן דכר ג׳ דר׳ תכלט בעצארת לסאן אל חמל וביאץ ביץ.[25]

פרזגה ליעין עלי חבל. יוכד מיעה קלאמיטה אעני סאילה מסטכי ולדאן ואנזרוט וכיאר שנבר וסנבל וזעפראן אנפחת אל ארנב ותמר ושחם בקר מכו׳ ד׳ דר׳ יסתעמל פרזגה.[26]

פרזגה ליעין עלי אל חבל. יוכד שמע ותריאק וטרבנתינה ושחם אוז וסמן מכו׳ וקיי׳ עסל ודמאג איל ודהן נארדין וזופא [10] רטב ושחם בקר מכו׳ ד׳ או׳ ופי אל ח׳ איאם מן אל שהר תדכל חמאם ג׳ אמראר ותחתמל הדי אל פרזגה ופי אל ט׳ תדכל מע זוגהא ודאלך חקיק.[27]

פרזגה תעין עלי אל חבל. יוכד שחם אוז ד׳ או׳ זעפראן ומר ושחם דגאג ומסטכי ודהן סרו ושמע ודמאג איל ועצארת זופא וטרבנתיי׳ ושחם דב ושחם לבוא מכו׳ וקתיין ותסתעמל פרזגה.[28]

פרזגה תעין עלי אל חבל פי מזאג בארד. יוכד סנבל וקסט וסראג ומר מכו׳ דרהמין מומיי׳ ד׳ דר׳ דמאג איל ושחם אוז [15] מכו׳ ח׳ דר׳ שמע ג׳ דר׳ דהן נארדין וקיי׳ דהן ורד ד׳ דר׳ תסתעמל פרזגה.[29]

---

[20] *P. M.*,13.
[21] *P. M.*, 2, with slight variants.
[22] *P. M.*, 22.
[23] *P. M.*, 39.
[24] This *pessarium* is not mentioned by Muscio.
[25] *P. M.*, 19.
[26] *P. M.*, 57.
[27] This *pessarium* is not mentioned by Muscio.
[28] *P. M.*, 44.
[29] *P. M.*, 21.

פרזגה תעין עלי אל חבל. [יוכד] אפיון פיסידיכו וזרונד מכו׳ דר׳ ודמאג איל ומצטכי ושחם אוז מכו׳ ג׳ דר׳ גואשיר ודהן ורד מכו׳ דר׳ תסתעמל פרזגה ותצב פי אלרחם ול[לי]ל תרקד מע זוגהא.[30]

מיגא אעני פרזגה תיפש אורם אל רחם אל ברדה ותידו אל טמת. יוכד בזר דקו וכרפס ונכאווה ומסתיק אל באן ובורק ארמני ומחלב וסנבילה מכו׳ אגזא מתסוויא תמר מקדר אל כאפיי בדוק מנוסה.[31]

פרזגה אעני פתילה נאפיעה לאסהל אל צפראי ואל בלגמי ואל זיחיר יוכד מר צאפי ובנדור מכו׳ דרהמין זעפראן נצף דרהם אפיון ואחד ידק ויעגין במא אל אס ואכראן יזידין חיצץ לולו בכר מכו׳ נצף מתקאל מונרכאב [...] . מעגון אל קרמיז. יוכד לולו בכר גד׳ טבשיר הנדי צנצל אחמר מכו׳ גד׳ צנצל [25] אבייץ דרהם בהמן אבייץ דרהם ונצף זמרד כהרבה מן כול ואחד גד׳ דהב ב׳ קרן ארייאל [sic] א׳ חריר א׳ תפח רטל מא ורד אווק ב׳ סוכר אווק ג׳ ונצף ואחרים אומירים [sic] כד זהב נצף ד׳. מרהם אל אסבידאג נפע ללבוסיר ואל שקאק וילחם אל קוריה יוכד דהן אל חל והוא שירג סיתין דרהם שמע אביץ יד׳ אסבידג אל רצאץ ג׳ דרהם כאפור דרהם [30] ידיכ אל שמע באל דהן תם יגעל אל כאפור ובעד דאלק יסחק אל אסבידג [sic] וידיכ ויחרק ובעד דאלק ינזל ען ען [sic] אל נאר חתא יברד ויגעל ביאץ אל ביץ ותסתעמל מגרד. [f. 2r]

מרהם למאסטריליס ידואי כל קרחה. יוכד אספידאג אל רצאץ מרדסנג מכו׳ דרהם לובן מצטיכי טרמנטינא שמע אביץ מכו׳ דרהם לעאב חלב בזר כתאן מכו׳ נצף דרהם זעפראן שחם תיס ג׳ דרהם זית אווק זפת דרהם יעמל מרהם. [5]

לצועבה אל ולאדה יוכד עצארה ברבינה בניפיד ותילד מסרע. **אכוד** עצרה נענע וכרפס וזעפארן [sic] וקרפה. אכוד כייר שנבר מיניקי אוואק ונצף תשרבה... צמאד לסיקוט אל להאה יוכד זפת לובן מצתיכי חל אל זפת באל נאר ואסחק אל באקי ואכלטהום [sic] וצמיד מוכר אל ראס ללצגאר וללכבר ממריד עלי אל גלד או כרך כתאן דקיק והוא [10] עגיב.

צמאד ינפע לפראניטס. ואלדי לם יקדר ינים ויציח ציאח שדיד פאנה יסכנה ויהדיה גדאה יוכד בזר בשבש בזר כץ בזר רגלה בזר בנג מכו׳ גד׳ ורד בנפסג בזר כזבר טרי מכו׳ גד׳ יסחק ויכלט בדקיק שעיר ועצרתה ענב אל תעלב אלדי יעמל חובוב אסווד ויצמד גבהא ואעלה אל דמאג ומוכרה ויכלט מע דאלק גבריה אל כרבק אל אביץ וידהן גמיע גבהתא בדהן אל יברוח ודהן אל ורד פאנה יסכן ויהדה. [15]

אוקשי קרוצי יועיל לשברי העצמות ולהסיר הכאב משם וכל צמא קשה ירכך והיו הקדמונים מתמידים בזה. יוכד זעפראן זפת קלפוניה מכו׳ ד׳ אואק טרבנטינא מקל ושק מר לובאן מצתיכי מכו׳ אואקיה וג׳ דרהם ועמלה והדה צפת עמלה יוכד מקל ואשק ויסחקהום קליל ויגעלהון פי אל כל ויגטיהון לילה ואחדה תם יגעל עלי אל נאר אלי אן

---

[30] This *pessarium* is not mentioned by Muscio.

[31] .*P. M.*, 5. The end of the *pessaria* taken from Muscio.

ינטוביך תם יצפא וירדא אלי אל נאר אלי אן ינטבך תם יצפא ודלך יעמל אלי אן יפני בעץ אל כלי תם יגעל עליה אל זפת אלי אן ינטבך תם יגעל עליה אל שמע תם טרממנטי' תם אל מסתיכי תם אל לובאן ומור ויחרוק מן אול אלי אל אכר ופי אל אכר יגעלה פי מא אל פאתר וידעבה באל ידין עלה אל רכאם תם יגעל פיה אל זעפרן [sic] ענד תעגינה עלי אל רכאם ואל רכאם מדהון בדהן אל גאר.

יצחק רופא **מעגון** ינפע לסול אל בול אל חר. אכלטה יוכד בלוט גדי' סועד כופי בדי' אמלג בלילג ככלי הנדי גלנאר מצרי רסין ורד גיר צנצל מכוי' די' דרהם וינכל ויעגן בעסל מנזוע אל רגייה מגרב צח עגיב [.]

דרור אלדי עמלנא ליוסף פנירו אל פרנגי והוא מנפיך ליל אכלה ואל קריח אל רטבה יוכד עפץ גלנאר מכוי' גדי' קטר מכי בונוך מכוי' בדי' טלייון רונד ורד[.] תושלבע ספר מסוה ועמו גם ליקוטים אחרים

English translation

To make the menses flow. You should take two ounces each of active sulfur,[32] opoponax, castoreum,[33] rue *mukî* ,[34] butter, trebentine and red natron, ten ounces of wax, one ounce of deer brain, and sufficient old oil, and prepare as a pessary.[35]

To make menses flow. You should take a portion each of butter, trebentine and rose oil, mix and prepare as a pessary.

To make the menses flow. You should take a sufficient portion each of natron's powder and oil, and mix and prepare as a pessary, that brings about a lot of moisture and makes the menses flow.

To make menses flow. You should take a sufficient portions each of black hellebore and myrrh, and pound, then mix with oil and prepare as a pessary in the form of an olive.

To make menses flow. You should take three ounces each of pomegranate flower and wax; eight dirhems each of gander fat and

---

[32] Read: كبريت.

[33] Read: جندبادستر, see *Tuḥfat al-aḥbâb, glossaire de la matière médicale marocaine*, texte publié pour la première fois avec traduction, notes et index par H. P. J. Renaud et G. S Colin, Paris, 1934, no. 103.

[34] There are two species of this plant: سذاب (*Ruta graveolens* L.), and سذاب بري or سذاب جبلي (*Ruta montana* or *Ruta silvestris*, L.). I could not identify the *mukî*, to which the text refers. See *ibid.*, nos. 364, 404; A. Issa, *Dictionnaire des noms des plants en latin, français, anglais et arabe*, Cairo, 1926, p. 159.

[35] On the Arabic term فرزجة see R. Dozy, *Supplément aux dictionnaires arabes*, Leiden, 1881, vol. II, p. 252.

aspergill,[36] two dirhems trebentine; one dirhem each of honey and rose oil, pound and mix in iris juice in order to make a suppository.[37]

To make menses flow. [The woman] should drink pounded pomegranate and honey water in a hot wine; otherwise give her a sufficient portion each of violet seeds, pepper and myrrh, to be pound and drunk with hot wine.[10]

To make menses flow. Jew's mallow, which is *malva visco*,[38] should be cooked in water and then she should sit in it.

A pessary that warms any pain or inflammation of the womb. You should take one ounce each of fenugreek and cotton seed; two ounces of sweet almond oil, cook the seeds pounded in the oil until it [the oil] is consumed, put in it one ounce of wax, take it out of the fire and add it to cotton seed oil or one ounce of fat or deer brain and apply it.

A pessary that warms the womb's pain and eliminates its inflammation. Take ten dirhems each of wax and butter; eight dirhems each of aspergill and bear fat, four dirhems of [15] gander fat, half an ounce of rose oil and apply it.

A pessary for any pain and any ailment in the womb. [You should take] one ounce each of beef fat and burnt centaury;[39] two

---

[36] The medieval Arabic herbalists gave the same name to two distinct plants: *Hyssopus* and *Oesypus*. In order to distinguish between them, the first one is called زوفا رطب and the second زوفا يابس. In many cases, as in the present text, the author does not specify to which plant he is refering. See *Tuḥfat al-aḥbâb*, p. 97, no. 10.

[37] In this case, the author employs the term فتيلة rather than the term فرزجة, which he uses in the remainder of the text. See Dozy, *Supplément aux dictionnaires arabes*, vol. II, p. 240.

[38] This is one of the rare cases in which the author uses a non-Arabic term. We have to underscore the fact that he transliterated the Spanish term perfectly: "Althea en griego quiere dezir propiamente medica al qual nombre por sus virtudes se atribuyó a esta planta la qual también se llama sbiscus y ebiscus como sea especie de malva salvage muy a propósito la llaman *malvavisco* [my emphasis] por toda España", *La 'Materia Médica' de Dioscorides traducida y comentada por D. Andrés de Laguna*, in C. E. Dubler, *La materia médica de Dioscórides*, Barcelona, 1955, vol. III, Lib. I, cap. 157. Cf. M. T. Herrera, *Menor daño de la medicina de Alonso de Chirino*, p. 287.

[39] Read: قنطوريوب . In his glossary, Maimonides refers also to this plant under the name derived from Greek, and he distinguishes between the "little" variety (*Erythraea centaureum* L.) and the "big" (*Centaurea centaurium* L.). See Meyerhof: *L'explication des noms de drogues - un glossaire de matière médicale composé par Maïmonide*, p. 36.

dirhems of gander fat, one ounce of pomegranate juice, and apply [in] a pessary.

A pessary that warms an inflammation of the womb. You should take three ounces each of gander fat, hen fat, fattened pork fat, deer brain, wax, galbanum oil, laudanum[40] oil, cypress oil, nard oil and aspergill juice; and one ounce of trebentine.

A pessary that warms inflammation of the womb. You should take two dirhems each of saffron and aspergill, three dirhems deer brain, two dirhems [20] trebentine, eight dirhems wax, seven dirhems each of green aspergill and butter, three dirhems each of saffron and rose oil, one dirhem each of spikenard oil, pork fat, melilot and fenugreek, two dirhems alecost, eight dirhems each of resin of the mastic tree, deer brain and gander fat.

A pessary that warms an inflammation of the womb. You should take two dirhems each of pheasant[41] fat and butter, three ounces each of deer brain and trebentine, one ounce wax and one ounce gander fat.

A pessary that moistens the hardness of the womb and its closure. You should take three dirhems each of beef fat, deer brain and wax, four dirhems spikenard oil, three dirhems and a half aspergill juice, and apply.

[25] **A pessary** that moistens the hardness of the womb and [brings about] its laxness. You should take one ounce wax, two ounces each of deer brain, butter, fenugreek juice, honey and lily oil, and four ounces spikenard oil.

A pessary that moistens the womb [and softens] its rigidity. You should take deer brain, gander fat, spikenard oil, wax, hens fat and cypress oil.

A pessary that cools the heat of the womb and [is useful] for its pain. You should take cooked Jew's mallow and some calf fat, gander fat and trebentine.

A pessary that cools the womb's heat. You should take ten dirhems each of wax and butter, eight dirhems each of aspergill and deer fat, four dirhems [30] gander fat, sufficient rose oil and apply.

A pessary that cools the womb's heat. You should take ten dirhems of Indian spikenard, two dirhems alum, four dirhems balsam

---

40 On the different Arabic spellings of the term, see Dozy, *Supplément aux dictionnaires arabes*, vol. II, p. 532.

41 The author employs the Spanish term *faisán*, written in Hebrew letters. The Latin text says: "adipes fasiani", Radicchi, *La Gynaecia di Muscione*, p. 326.

wood, six dirhems sweet-flag, three dirhems each of saffron, alecost rob and galbanum, [and] knead into a sufficient portion of honey.

A pessary that cools the womb's inflammation. You should take one ounce saffron, one ounce wax, one ounce each of gander fat, aspergill and deer brain, one dirhem honey, one dirhem egg white and a sufficient portion of rose oil.

A pessary for a woman who does not purify herself of her menses naturally, but rather painfully. You should take one ounce each of opoponax, green rue and myrrh, pound all of them and then mix with a sufficient portion of olive oil and apply.

A pessary for a woman who does not purify [f. 1v] her menses easily. You should take one ounce each of gander fat, old oil, wax, spikenard oil, trebentine, deer brain, aspergill juice, butter and frankincense.

A pessary that postpones the menses period. You should take one portion each of white pepper and fenugreek, pound and mixe with honey, and put into her bath water, which she should enter twice a day.

To abort the foetus. She should take one dirhem opoponax and she will abort quickly. Or let the woman eat green peppermint for seven days on [5] an empty stomach and she will never conceive.

A pessary to dry uterine moisture. You should take two dirhems of the *teliqânis* stone,[42] three dirhems of incense, and mix them with the sap of the plantain and the white of an egg.

A pessary to facilitate conception. You should take four dirhems each of resin, I mean the liquid one,[43] of the storax tree, resin of the mastic tree, cistus, tragacanth, cassia-tree, spikenard, saffron, rabbit's stomach, date and beef fat, and apply a pessary.

A pessary to facilitate conception. You should take one ounce each of wax, theriac, trebentine, gander fat and butter, four ounces each of honey, deer brain, spikenard oil, green [10] aspergill and beef fat; on the eighth day of the month, she should bathe three times

---

[42] The Latin text says: *stibium* (antimony) (*P. M.* 19). It is possible that the word appearing in our text is a deformation of the Arabic term حجر مغناطيس, which does not correspond to the Latin.

[43] Arab medieval pharmacology differentiated between two varieties of this material: الميعة السائلة (the liquid), and الميعة الجامدة (the solid). See Meyerhof: *L'explication des noms de drogues - un glossaire de matière médicale compos par Mïamonide*, p. 27.

with this pessary, and on the ninth, she should lie with her husband, and it has been proven.

A pessary to facilitate conception. You should take four ounces of gander fat, two ounces each of saffron, myrrh, hen fat, resin of the mastic tree, cypress oil, wax, deer brain, aspergill juice, trebentine, bear fat, lioness fat, and apply a pessary.

A pessary to facilitate conception for a [woman's] cold temperament. You should take two dirhems each of spikenard, cistus, sesame oil and myrrh, four dirhems of mummy, eight dirhems each of deer brain and gander fat, three dirhems wax, one ounce spikenard oil, four dirhems rose oil, and apply a pessary.

A pessary to facilitate conception. [You should take] one dirhem each of opium, pistachio[44] and birthwort, three dirhems each of myrrh, deer brain, resin of the mastic tree and gander fat, one dirhem each of opoponax and rose oil. Prepare a pessary and put it in her womb, and the woman should sleep with her husband at night.

A *Miga*,[45] that is a pessary, to dry the cold uterine tumors and to make the menses flow. You should take an equal portion each of the seeds of carrot, celery, resin of behen tree, Armenian borax, mahaleb and nard, and a handful of dates. [It has been] tested and tried.[46]

A pessary, that is a suppository, is useful to purge yellow bile, phlegm and [to cure] dysentery.[47] You should take two dirhems each of pure myrrh and tomato,[48] half a dirhem saffron, one dirhem opium, pound and knead them in myrtle water, and finally add half a miskal each of lycium and unripe marguerite, all mixed.

Kermes electuary.[49] You should take three dirhems of unripe marguerite, three dirhems each of Indian chalk and red bergamot,[50] one dirhem white bergamot, one and a half dirhems white be-

---

44 The text gives the Spanish term *pistacho*, instead of the Arabic فستق.

45 In the text: *miga*, for the Spanish *mecha*. See *Menor daño de la medicina de Alonso de Chirino*, p. 288.

46 Excerpts from the *Pessaria* taken from Muscio's *Gynaecia* end here. The following section, either in its entirety or in segments, was added after the fifteenth century. See footnote 48.

47 Read: زحار.

48 The tomato was not known in Europe nor in the East before the sixteenth century.

49 This name was probably given to the electuary due to the use of kermes, which gave it its special red colour. See Dozy, *Supplément aux dictionnaires arabes*, vol. II, p. 345.

50 Read: صندل.

hen, one dirhem each of emerald and amber, four dirhems kermes, two gold, one deer horn, one silk, one rotl of apples, two ounces rose water, three and a half ounces of sugar, and others say take half a dirhem of gold.

Ceruse[51] **ointment**, [which is] useful [to treat] haemorrhoids and fissures and cures wounds. You should take sixty dirhems of sesame oil, which is *siraj*,[52] ten dirhems white wax, three dirhems lead ceruse, one dirhem camphor; mix the wax in the oil and then add the camphor. After that, pound the ceruse, mix it and burn it. Afterwards, take it off the fire until it is cooled and add the white of an egg, then apply it thinly.

[f. 2r] **Mastarilis' Ointment** [which] cures any wound. You should take one dirhem each of lead ceruse and litharge, one dirhem each of frankincense, resin of the mastic tree, trebentine and white wax, half a dirhem each of mucilage, milk and cotton seed, three dirhems billy goat fat, one ounce oil, one dirhem pitch, and make an ointment.

[5] **For difficult parturition**. [The woman] should take verbena,[53] drunk with wine, to give birth quickly. **Take** peppermint juice, celery, saffron and cinnamon. Take one and a half ounces of purgative [made of] the fruit of cassia tree, and she should drink it.

A bandage for the *suqût al liḥâh.*[54] Pitch, frankincense and resin of the mastic-tree should be taken. Melt the pitch on a fire, pound the remains, mix them, and wrap the back of the head with it. [It is useful] for youths and adults as well, wet with it a piece of leather or a fine piece of cotton, and it is [10] marvelous.

A bandage that is useful for [curing] frenzy[55] and for one who cannot sleep and shouts loudly, and it will warm him and direct him to the right way. Let there be taken a portion each of fennel seeds, lettuce seeds, common purslane seeds and henbane seeds, a portion each of rose, violet and seeds of green coriander, pound and mixed with barley flour and the juice of nightshade, which has black grains,

---

[51] Read: اسفيذاج. See *El libro del 'Amal man ṭabba li-man ḥabba*, p. 40.

[52] The author confused حل, which is sesame oil (see *ibid.*, pp. 19, 49, 67), with سراج, which refers to various plants but not to the sesame (see *Tuḥfat al-aḥbâb*, no. 374; Issa, *Dictionnaire des noms des plants*, pp. 90, 54, 112-115).

[53] Spanish: *verbena*, see Dozy, *Supplément aux dictionnaires arabes*, vol. I. p. 64.

[54] The manuscript states - *sîqût* - but it seems to me that it should be سُقوط (see *ibid.*, vol. I. pp. 661-662), on the other hand, I could not identify the term *al-liḥâh*.

[55] The author employs the term *franitas*.

bandage his forehead, the brain and the back [of the head]. Mix with it the dust of white hellebore and rub it all over his forehead with mandrake oil and rose oil, since they warm and heal. [15]

Uqshi qrusi,[56] which the ancients used constantly and is useful for bone fractures and to remove their pain, [also] mitigates hard thirst.[57] You should take four ounces each of saffron, pitch and solid resin, one ounce and three dirhems each of trebentine, bdellium, gum resin, myrrh and frankincense, and make the preparation as follows: Take the bdellium and the gum resin, pound them a bit and put them in vinegar over night, then put them on a fire until it [the mixture] is cooked and clear, [20] then put it [again] on the fire until it is cooked and clear, do it until it is mixed with the rest of the vinegar. Then put in the pitch, then the solid resin, then the trebentine, then the resin of the mastic tree, then the frankincense and the myrrh, and heat them constantly on the fire, from the first to the last. Finally, put it [the mixture] in mushroom[58] water and spread it by hand on the marble[59], put into it saffron and knead it while the marble is anointed with laurel[60] oil. Yiṣḥaq the Physician.[61] [25]

Electuary useful to relax hot urine. A mixture: there should be taken three dirhems of oak, two dirhems galingale *kufi*,[62] four dirhems each of embelic myrobalan, belleric myrobalan, Indian bean,[63] Egyptian pomegranate Egyptian blossom, rose roots, lime and sandal wood, pound and knead them in honey. It gives hope, and it is tested, true and wonderful.

A medicament we have made for Yusef Faniru the European,[64] useful for a gangrenous sore, ulcers and humidity. You should take three dirhems each of gallnuts and pomegranate blossom, two dirhems each of musk sirup and acacia resin,[65] livelong,[66] laurel and

---

[56] I could not find the meaning of the first word, the second is probably a deformation of قرص or اقراص (pill, pills).

[57] This last sentence is written in Hebrew.

[58] Read: فطر.

[59] Read: رخام.

[60] Read: الغار.

[61] The author does not give any information regarding this physician, nor is it clear whether the previous recipe or the following electuary should be attributed to him.

[62] There are several types of سُعد or سُعدة, but none of them are called *Kufi*. See Issa, *Dictionnaire des noms des plants*, p. 66.

[63] Read: باقلي. See *ibid.*, p. 189.

[64] The text states: *al-franjî*.

[65] Read: بُنك. See Issa, *Dictionnaire des noms des plants*, p.2, no. 10.

rose. Ended and completed, praise God, the Creator of the world. Muscio's[67] Book and other compilations.[68]

[66] Read: طيلافيون (?). See *ibid.*, p. 166, no. 12; Dozy, *Supplément aux dictionnaires arabes*, vol. II. p. 58.

[67] The name is not vocalized in the manuscript, it is written as *mswh.*

[68] The last two sentences are written in Hebrew.

A RECORD OF THE DISEASES OCCURING IN THE GENITAL MEMBERS

Jews' College, London, Ms. Montefiore, 440, ff. 15v-25r.

זכרון החליים ההוים בכלי הריון. מעוט הזרע ובטול התאוה. הסבה אמנם לחולי מיוחד באבר או רוע מזג בו. או בלתי יכולת לאבר או בסבת האשכים השתים וכלי ההולדה. או מרוע מזג קר יבש או בסבת חולשת כח הכליות או חולשת גופם או למיעוט הרוח העשני אשר ישליכהו הלב או לחולשת הכבד או המוח ובכלל האיברים השרים. המקרה יורה על מה שבו בלתי יכולת בהעדר זקיפת השרביט ולא יקווץ במי[1] קרים ומה שהיה מצד האשכים במציאת הזקיפה עם מיעוט הזרע ועוצר צאתו. ואם יהיה מחולשת גוף הכליות במופתי חולשת גופם או יהיה מהכבד בהעדר התאות ובקשת המנוחה ומופתי מיעוט הדם. ואם יהיה הלב חלוש יורה עליהן הדפק.

הרפואה. יתחייב לעשות לכל סבה ההפך. אם תהיה בו בלתי יכולת האבר מרוע מזג קר יתחייב לעשות המשיחות החמות והשמנים החמין כשמן אל כירי דהן אל באק דהן אל נרגס דהן קוסט וירחק החולה מן המאכלים והמשקים הקרים וישים במזונו הבשר המתעכל בנקל באצטו׳ ומכלים[2] מטוגנים במחבת מתובלים בבשמים בבשמים ובכלל יתנהג בקרוב ממנהג רוע מזג בכיס השתן.

ואם יהיה רוע מזג קר באשכים יתחייב השמנים החמים אל האשכים כמו דוהן[3] זינבק ודהן אל כירי יעורב בו מוסך וקשתור ותתן להם זנגביל מרבא[4] ואשקקיל מורבא כפי מה שתראה. ושים מזונו מחזק ומחמם צפרים ובני יונה הקטנים ומח הצפרים ובשר כבש בן שנתו ובשמים קנילא וזנגביל. ויאכלו מזה המעגון לוזים שקדים קלופים פוסתק ואגוז הנדי ובטנים קלופים וגרעיני לנטישקלי מכל אחד י׳ דרכ׳ פלפל ארוך זנגביל מכל [f.16r] אחד דרה׳ יתעצם /יתערב/[5] זה בסוכר קשה ויקח ממנו בכל יום כאגוז.

---

1 Read: במים.
2 Read: ומאכלים.
3 Read: דהן.
4 Read: מרבא .
5 A word added in the margin.

ואם יהיה זה מרוע מזג ישב[6] ומיעוט הזרע הנהיגו במשיחת האשכים בשמן ושעוה ושומן תרנגולת ועשות המזונות המרטבות כבשר הכבשים הקטנים בתבשיל הבצים והתמדת הרחיצה והמנוחה ושתית היין הלבן ואכילת הענבים בלי הקליפה והגרעינים.

ואם יהיה מגיע מזג יבש עם חום יועיל דייב אל בקר עם המנא ומשיחת האיברים בשמן יקטן ודהן לוזים ויאכלו הדגים הלחים הקטנים שלי[7] אש ואבטיח נקי שואין ארמלוץ.

ואם יהיה זה מחולשת הלב ומיעוט התנפחות האבר ממה שיועילם מזה מחנק אל מיסך או אל מתרודיטוס אם ימצא ועשיית תבשיל הבשר והבצים והבצלים והבצים מבושלים בשול בינוני וישתו היין טוב הריח ועשיית הדברים המשמחים.

והדברים הנופחן[8] והמביאין הרוח אל האבר הם לקחת זרעונים שחורים גדולים וישרה אותם במי ארוגא עם התנפחם ואחר ייבשם ואחר ישחקם וילוש אותם עם פניסאו וסוכר קשה ויקח ממנו בקר ובערב כשיעור אגוז. וממה שיועילם זה יקח לב פניוש ואגוז הנדי וזרע אורוגא וזרע אבטיח קלופים מכל אחד חלק ואחר יקח דבש די ספקו. וכמו כן יועילם חלבה שתעשה עם מיץ פשתנגש לחות בדבש וישים בו מנא. אמנם מה שהיה סבתו מן הכליות וחולשת כבד כבר זכרם. ומן הטוב שיעשה להם חוקנא מן הדברים השמנים. ודע כי רפואת המשׂגל על דרך רבות ועברו[9] על דרך הקצור וההעברה במה שיש לנו בו מן העזר.

יתרון התאוה. המים הקודמים ביציאה לזרע זכים או עבים או חדוד הזרע או רובו או חרוך בלי גרב או בגרב בכלי הזרע כמו שיקרה לנשים. או רבוי הרוחות הנופחים. המקרה יורה על מה שסבתו חבור הזרע וצאתו בעת השינה. [16v] והמים הקודמים לזרע יורה על מה שסבתו החכוך שהיה המשגל מרבה בתאות ואותות הנפח רוב זקיפת השרביט.

הרפואה. יתחייב שתדע כי כשיהיה רוב התאוה מבריאות המזג ורב הדם וכוחו לא יאות בכמו זה שתשבור התאוה כי זה ממה [sic] שיזיק בפעולת הטבע אם לא לצורך גדול איך[10] יתחייב בכמו זה לעשות שתשבר החבור בעשיית הדברים המקררים כמו חזרת והלגלוגות וזרעם ואכילת ליינשוש ודלועים הקשואים וישים למדה בחוט השדרה על הכליות נוס[11] עופרת וישים מזונו המאכלים הקרים העשים בחומץ. ומה שהיה סבתו מלוי עם חום רפואתו בהקזה ומיעוט המזון ושיתמיד דברים המְקררים ואכילת העדשים מבושלים במים שניים וזכר גיאלינוס

---

6 Read: יבש.

7 Read: צלי.

8 Read: הנופחין.

9 Read: ועקרו.

10 Read: אך.

11 Read: טס.

כי הנינופאר כאשר יש בה ישבור הזרע ושתית מי אורטיגה במיץ רימונים חמוצים. אמנם הרפואות החמות המיבשות כמו זרע אוקיואש קאשטוש וזרע רודא ומנטשטרא וכמון.

ומן הרפואות המורכבות [15] זרע חזרת וזרע אורטיגא מכל אחד ב׳ דרה׳ זרע רודא דרה׳ ישתה ממנו דרה׳ באישרוב סכנגבין. אמנם רפואות המים הקודמין לזרע יש שהיה מרוב מלוי. ורפואתו ההקזה והכבוס ומיעוט המזון ואכילת פומיש תירה. אמנם מה שהיה סבתו דקיקת הזרע יועיל מזה אכילת האטריפל במרקחת הוורדים ועשיית המזונות המעבים כמו [20] מאכל הקמחים ואם יהיה סבתו בלתי יכלת הכלים חולשת כח המחזיק יועיל מזה האטריפל ועשיית השמנים הקובצים כשמן ההדס עם עמבר וכמו זה תחבושת לבונה עם מי הדס.

רוב זקיפת השרביט בלתי תאות המשגל. הסבה רבוי הרוחות העבות בורידי האבר וחללי העצבים או חלט עבה יוליד הקטורים עבים. המקרה יורה על הרוחות [f. 17r] הבאות אליו בלתי שיתיר לו בו זקיפה בלי רוח. ומופתי מה שהיה סבתו רוח מתילד בו או מחלט עבה התנועעות שבו.

הרפואה. רפואת זה במה שהקדמנו ברפואת רבוי התאוה וזה בדברים השוברים מפרידי הרוחות הממעטים [5] הזרע ויתחייב שתתחיל בהקזה בלי שלשול ואחר תשים על האבר דברים מקררים כמו הצנדל והקלידה והכפור או יולש זה במי חזרת או במי הליסוטיאש וכמו כן ישים מזה על הכליות מלגב וממה שיועיל מזה כאשר אמרנו משקה אשרב עלי הננופר היבש וזרע החזרת וישים על הכליות טסי עופרת ועל העצם [10] השורר ויועילם עשיית הדברים מפרידים לרוחות החמות זרע רודה ואזוב וכמון וכרפס מופרדות או מורכבות מב׳ דרכמש. וכמו כן יאות הכבוס אחר שתדע שיש שם חומר עבה כבסהו הגרעיני[12] הכבד ואל איארג המחוזק ואחר יעשה מה שהקדמנו זכרונו. ויאות לבעלי זה החולי שלא ישמש מטתו כלל [15] ולא יחשוב בו וישים מזונו דברים החמוצים ובכלל הנהגתו הנהגת בעלי רוב התאוה.

המורסה החמה והקרה העבה ההוה באבר גס וחכוך הסבה רוב אחת הליחות הארבעה או מהרכבתם והגרב יתחדש מחומר רע או יתחדש אחר המורסות. המקרה יורה עליהם [20] במה שירגיש בבשר מהחמימות והקרירות והקושי על הגרב הצפראוי בהתפשה אדמימותו ועל היותו מאסודי בנטותו אל השחרות והעכירות והיובש ועל הבלגמיא בהתפשטותא ורכותא.

הרפואה. רפואת המורסה החמה בהקזה מן הגיד הנקרא בסלוקון בכמות רב אם לא ימנעוהו מנוע ואחר יתמיד אכילת[13] מי השעור ושתית סכנגבין ואחר ישים על האבר [f. 17v] נגד[14] טבול בחומץ ומן מי הורדים ויעשה תחבושת בסנדל ומי וורדים וממה שיאות כאשר יהיה החומר חם

---

[12] Read: בגרעיני.
[13] Read: שתית.
[14] Read: בגד.

ויתקבץ מאד באבר שיקח קליפות הרמונים ורדים יבשים ועדשים קלופים יבושל הכל במים עד התרככם מאד חבר עמהם מי [5] שמפרויא ושמן הוורדים. וכמו כן היל הלארמוני בחומץ ואחר כן הדברים נטה אל הדברים המרככים והמלחלחים כמו השעוה והשמן ותחבשת הנעשות מקמח המלוי וקמח פולין עם שעוה והשמן.

ורפואת המורסה הקרה בתחבושות המבשלות כמו חובש קמח תלתן וקמח אמלוי וקמומילא [10] ומוק הוא דילי והתמיד החולה מרבא הורדים עם משקה סכנגבין מהזרעים. ורפואת המורסה הקשה בחכך האבר בשעוה ושמן עם שומן אווז ותרנגלת ואם תצטרך למה שהוא יותר חזק נשים על האבר שעוה עם מוח שוקי הפרות ואמוניאק ושמן אלורד עם שומן אנדי ומונע החולה מהמאכלים העבים [15] אם תצטרך אל הכבוס כבסהו במה שיוציא האסודא.

אמנם רפואת הגרב המתחדש אל האבר החדש יתחייב שתשים עליו אלואן ומרתק ואקלימיא רחוץ במים ומה שיועילם מזה דלועים שרופים אבק או עם שמן ורדים. ואם יהיה הגרב ישן רפאהו בזאת הרפואה ותכונתה פטגי ומרתק ודם דרגון ווראנד [20] שרוף אלום ולבונה ואלואן מכל אחד בשוה ושחוק הכל ותמשח בה הגרב או יקח מהן עם שעוה. ואם יתחדש בהם בשר מת נקהו בחמאה או בקמח העדשים או בחמאה הקשה ויולף ולפעמים תצטרך מרהני אל זריגר[15] ומרהני אל זפאת ואחר זה שים עליו מה שיורה עין הגרב ואם יהיה הגרב בתוך נקב האבר רפאהו ברפואת הגרב המתחדש בבית השתן וזרוק בו הרפואות [f. 18r] ואם נסתם מעבר השתן שים באבר אל ראטטיר עד שיפתח המעבר ואחר הטיף איבו אחר זה חלב הנשים עם שמן ורדים ואשאף אביץ. אמנם רפואת החכוך המתחדש באבר בהקזה ואם לא יספיק זה תביאהו במה שיוציא החום החלט החום השרוף ואחר תחבוש האבר [5] במרחץ בחומץ ודהן אל ורד וממה שיועילם מזה שיחבשו בשאף ממותי ואכסיאה ואלואן וזעפראן ויולש זה בשמן וורדים ויחבוש בו האבר ואם לא יועילם דבר מכל אלו ישים עליו העלוקות כי הם ימוצו החומר הרע ויצא אחר זה הבריאות ברצון השם.

אמנם התנועעות האבר כשיתנועע מעמו במשיחות [10] והשמנים המשיחות כמו שומן תרנגולת ושומן אנד ושעוה והשמנים ושמן נרגיש ואל שירג וירחצה במים פושרין. אל אוראם אל חרבה[16] חד. המורסות החמות המורסות החמות והקרות בפנים ובכיס האשכים. **הסבה** רבוי אחת הליחות הארבעה אל המקרה יורה על כל אחת מהמורסות במה שנאמר לך למופתים ממופת המורסות.

[15] **הרפואה** דע כי רפואת מורסת האשכים דומה למורסת האבר אלא שיתחייב שתחמול על האשכים יותר ובכלל רפואת המורסא החמה ההוה באשכים בהקזת הבסליק מצד האבר אשר בו המורסא ואם יהיה

---

[15] Read: זינגר.

[16] Read: אל חררה.

בשניהם מורסא שים ההקזה תחלה מן היד השמאלי ואחר ביום השני הקיז היד הימני ותוציא הדם כפי מה שתראה מן הכח [20] והשנים ואם לא ימנעהו מונע להנהיג החולה במי השעורים ותן לו אחריו משקה סכרגבין ואחר תחבוש המקום השני בשני מיני הסנדלש ואובא קנילא או ארפא מורסא[17] ומי הדלועין ומי הקנים הלחים אם ימצא מהם ועוד תחבושת יקח קמח השעור וקמח העדשים וילוש אותם במי לייטנש ומי הקנים. ויחבוש אל /בו/[18] המקום וכאשר יעמוד המורסא בעיניה ותצטרך לדברים המתירים התחיל בשעוה ושמן ומי [f. 18v] שמפרויא והוסף עליהם מי השעוה וירחץ המקום במים פושרין.

ואם יהיה המורסא המתחדשת שיש בהם בלגמיא ותראה עם זה רבוי דם הקיזהו ולא תשמר מן ההקזה אלא התמיד החולה במרבה הוורירים[19]. במים חמין במשקה הסכרגבין מהזרעים ואחר כבוס [5] החולה במה שיוציא הבלגם ומשח האבר בשמן יסמין יחבוש אותו בקמח פולין עם מעט כמון ושומן[20] הדליות או בבונג עם מוקל והשעוה והטיף באבר מעט היסמין ודקק המזון ושימהו כמו הזרעונים ואם יחלש הכח עזרהו בתרנגולים השלוקים. אמנם רפואת המורסא הקשה כבס הגוף מן החלק הסאברכי[21] ואחר חבש את המקום בתחבושת תעשה מן בול הכל [10] אצפר ושומן אנד לבלי זות ואמופאק וחבר זה בחמאת הבקר. ועוד תחבושת אחר אמוניאק ומוקל אשתורקש לחה וחבר הכל עם מעט קמח ופולים וירחץ /המקום/[22] במים אשר בושל בהם מורסן ואכליל אל מלך אמנם רפואת המורסות בכיס האשכים תרקב [sic] מזאת הרפואה.

המורסא הממיית. המורסא הממיית ונפח הכיס מסבת הרוח [15] ובקוע הכיס ונפילת המעי בכיס והנפח הבשרי. הסבה סבת המורסא הממיית מהתחדש המים בכיס מהפסד הדם והתחדש הנפח הבשרי מחלט דמיי נוטה אל האסודי והתחדש הנפח הרוחני מבקיעת הספק והוא קרום הבטן. בהתחדש נפילת המעיים מהתרכב שני נקבים אשר אשר לכיס שם ללחות מופסד מאד או לדעקה[23] או למשגל [20] או למלוי או לדלוג או לתנועה מבוהלת וישתתף עם זה הנפח הרוחני.המקרה יורה על הנפח הממיי בגודל הנפח עם להיבות ודקיקת העור וכאשר ימשש עליו ידלג הנפח החצי הנוד. ויורה על נפילת המעי במשוש והרעישה בעת ידחהו או ימרסהו ויורה על כי הבשרי בעובי האבר והתרחצו[24] והתפשטו.

---

[17] Read: ארבה מורא.
[18] A word added in the margin.
[19] Read: הוורדים.
[20] Read: ושמן.
[21] Read: הצפראוי; see f. 17r, line 21.
[22] A word added in the margin.
[23] Read: לצעקה.
[24] Read:והתרחבו .

הרפואה. רפואת הנפח הממי[25] במיעוט המזון ותקון [f. 19r] המזונות וישים אותם נוטים אל היובש. ואחר יחבוש תחבושת מתיר המים בזה של מוניאק בגש פלפל ויעורב זה בשמן ישן ושעוה ויעשה תחבושת. ואם יצטרך למה שהוא יותר חזק תוסף עליו גפרית וזבל העזים וזבל היונים ואם לא תועיל זאת ההנהגה ותצטרך למלאכת היד להוציא המותר לחוץ צוה לחולה שישכב על עורפו וצוה למשרתו שימשוך הגיד לצד הטבור ואחר משוך הכיס והגביה האשכים למעלה ואחר ינקוב המקום בברזל רחב בצד ימין או שמאל לבלתי יגע אשר באמצע הכיס ויגביה הכיס בידו לבלתי יפול על הנקב ויכסנו העור וימרוס יפה עד צאת המותר ההוא ויסמוך ידיו עליו ואחר ישים על המקום הרפואה היבשה כי אין לנו בטחון על הרוב לבלתי ישוב המים ההם ונצטרך לרפואה אחרת ומן הרופאים שיעשו בכויה על זה הדרך שיחממו ברזל דק עקום ויקשרו האשכים רחוק כל מה שיוכלו ואחר יכו בברזל על הכיס במקום שלא ימצאו האשכים ומהם מן הרופאים מי שישבור מעט מהשומן ואחר יעשו הכויה. וירפאהו אחר זה במה שיגדל הבשר ומנע החולה מרוב שתית מים.

אמנם רפואת הנפח בהניח המזונות הנופחים מהגרעינים והפירות ודומיהם ויחכך הכיס בשמן אל קושט ודהן אל יסמין וההתמדה בדברים מפרידים הרוח ועשיית מעגון אל כמון בעת רבוי הרוחות ואכילת מעט רודה ודקק המזון. **אמנם רפואת** הנפח הבשר בכיס במה שהקדמנו מרפואת המורסות הקשות מהחכוך בשומן ומוחות העצמות ויכבס הגוף מן המותר הסודאי.

אמנם סגולות רפואת נפיחת הגידין כאשר תנקה אותו לא יזיק שתפתח אחד מן העורקים הנמצאים בכיס להקל בזה החולי. **אמנם רפואת** השבירה ונפילת המעי שתצוה לחולה בעת שיחזק הכאב ויקרא לו כאב כאב קוליקא ומהרופאים יקראו אותו קליקא משיאון מהבקוע ותאמר אליו שישכב ממול ערפו וימרוס הבקוע בידו וידחהו [f. 19v] למעלה ואם יועיל זה הושב החולה במים חמין וחבש השבר בדברים מרככים ויכסנו בבגדים חמים ואחרי שובו שיקשרהו בקשר מרובע ומהרופאים מי שהקדים על כויתו בכלי כסף או זהב והוא על זה הענין ואם יזדמן החולה מושכב על ערפו שני ימי או שלשת יהיה יותר טוב. ולפעמים יושם על השבר הרפואות המקבצות כמו אלה. יקח אלואן ולבונה ואגוז הנדי אכסיא אנזרות דם דרגון מירא וחצץ וגניברי מכל אחד בשוה ויטיב שחיקתם וילוש אותן באוגדור הדגים או בגמא ארביקא ותשים אותו על המקום ותניחהו ימים רבים סדורים.

זכרון החליים המתחדשים ברחם מהעקרות ועוצר ההריון. הסבה. סבה זה אמנם להפסד זרע האיש או זרע האשה או לרוע מזג ברחם או מורסא קשה או חלי כליי או לקוצר האמה. המקרה יורה על הפסד מזג שזרע האיש יהיה קר או חם כפי שתאמר האשה ואם יהיה

---

[25] Read: המימי.

במיעוטו ואם יהיה לח בדקיקותו ורבויו. ויורה על ענייני הרחם ענייני דם הנדות ובמה שיצא ממנו מן הליחות ויורה על הסתום במיעוט הדם או העדרו מכל וכל ברוב הרפואה אם תהיה הסבה הפסד מזג זרע האיש השיבהו לשווי במה שכנגדו ואם תהיה הסבה חמימות השיבהו לשווי במזונות הקרים ובעשבים הקרים וכבס הליחות החדות. ואם תהיה הסבה רוע מזג ברחם עשה כמו כן מה שכנגדו במה שתדענו מן ההנהגת[26] ואחר הסמוך בטרופיש הקרים והרירים הקרים אם יהיה רוע המזג חם. ואם תהיה הסבה מהקרירות והוא ברוב התמידי הפתילות החמות והשמנים החמין ממה שנזכרהו עוד. ואם תהיה הסבה מסתום פתוח תפתח הסתום ברפואות הפותחות המורידות לדם. ואם תהיה הסבה רוחות ברחם עשה הרפואות המפזרות הרוח כמו הקשטור והרודה וזרעה ואם תהיה שמה לחות וחומר דבק כבס הגוף באל איארג המחוזק או פילולש הסכבינג נעשה אחר זה המעגוניט והפתילות.

עתה נזכור הרפואות [f. 20r] אשר נסיתי ומצאתים שיועילו ברוב זה החולי רוצה לומר שתהיה מקרירות ולחות ומזאת קיבת הארנבת כאשר תשתה ממנה תשאנה האשה עם חמאת בקר בימי הטוהר ומה שיהיה כמו מן הסגולות שתשקה האשה שן הפיל כי הוא מופלא ותעשה זה מהתשמיש ועוד מה שיפול עצמו הפיל כשיגרדו אותן במגרה גם הוא מופלא ועוד בלתי סגולה ההקטרה מועלת ותהיה מעץ בלשמו וגרעיניו ושמנו כמו כן מועיל בהקטרה ובפתילה כמו כן שומן האווזים נתר עם גומא מאילן האל פוסתוק ותחבוש בו האשה הרחם שני ימים.

ומן הפתילות הטובות יקח אשפיק אנדי וזעפראן ומסתק ומירא וקשטור יולש כל זה בשמן הנרדין או בשמן הבאן ושומן האווזה ותעשה מהם פתילות ותשאם בימי הטוהר ותחליפם כל שלשה ימים וממה שיועיל ובסגולה אל הליחות ואל הרוחות תבושל השומים בשירג עד שימחו ותשאם בצמר. ודע כי אם תהר ואחר תפיל ברוב מסבת לחות והקיא אותה בגרענים הסיכנג הנקרא שאקא בינטו ותעשה שמן גירא שוליש ותשתה ממנו בכל יום ב׳ דרכמונים או ג׳ והשמר לך שלא תהיה הסבה חולשה ברחם ותחטא ברפואה. ולא יאות למי שיבקש ההריון שישמש אלא לאחר זמן ארוך ולא ארוך מאד. ולא ישמש אלא בתאות שניהם וישא האיש את ירכותה למעלה מעט מראשה וכזה יאות שמענה ואתה דע לך.

אל רחא והוא החלי תשוב בו האשה כענין ההרות או הנפוחות מהמים הרעים הסבה אמנם מוהרות[27] מודבקות בגלדי הרחם או רוחות עבות ולפעמים יהיה עם זה מורסות קשות או תהיה הסבה תילד בשר בלי צורה על מה שאמרו הראשונים. המקרה יקרה לאלו ענייני ההרות ועוצר דם הנדות ונפלת התאוה ונופח השדים וענייני המים הרעים ויהיה בטנם קשה לא כך כבטני ההרות.

---

[26] Read: ההנהגות or ההנהגה.

[27] Read: מותרות.

הרפואה דע כי זה החולי לפעמים ישאר שנים או ו׳ או יותר מאלו ולפעמים יקרה להרה ענין כחבל [f. 20v] יולדה והמים הנגרים מהם ולפעמים תהיה הסבה התארכות הרחם ודחיית הדבר המכאיבו יצא אחר זה אמנם רוחות עבות עצומות מאד ולפעמים תלד חתכת בשר בלתי צורה ואמרו קצתם כי סבה והולדת זאת החתכה הם שני דברים האחד חומר ישפך ברחם עם חום גדול והשני כי יתילד תכף לתשמיש מזרע האשה כאשר לא נתעכב עמו זרע האיש ולא הגיע אליו יפסד כח המצייר מזרע האיש ואחר יאסוף הרחם אליו המים שהם זרע האשה ותזון אותם ויהיה מזה דבר בלא צורה.

והודיעוני כמה נשים צדקניות וכמה מילדות בלי שקר וכזב כי אשה אחת ילדה שלשה חיות דומות לקראגש והיתה בהם חיות ותנועה. וכמו כן הודיעוני מאשה אחת שילדה עם הנפל חיה דומה לנחש. אמנם רפואת החולי הזה שתנקה גופה בגרעיני איארג ובחזק מאלו גרעינים הנבאשים. ואחר כן תחבושת והרחיצות המתירות לרוח כמו שמן הרודה ושמן הנרגם ושמן הקשט. וצוה עליהן לעשות המעגין והגיארי שנאת המתירות לרוח כגואריש אל עוד אשרב סכריגבין עשוי מי הזרעונים וישתו מי השורשים ויתירו בהם קשתור. ואם ימצאו עובי הנהגתם כהנהגת המורסות הקשות בעשיית השמנים והסיכות והרחצות ומן המעגין המועילות להם מעגין לוגדיה ואם תספיק לך זאת ההנהגה בזאת הרפואה מוטב ואם לא עשה הרפואות המורידות דם הנדות ואשר תפילו הנפלים המתים בטרוסיש אל מנראשיה אל מרו ובשול אל שבינא בלע׳ אל אבהל. כמו זאת הרפואה מר וחבק אל שיוך ואפופוניאק מכא׳ חלק וישתו זה במי הכרפס או במי השומר ושים מזונם תבשיל עשוי מבשר ובצים המבושמים ופרחי יונים ותרנגלים קטנים עשוים במחבת.

עוצר הלידה והוצאת הנפלים המתים. הסבה אמנם מצד האשה כאשר תהיה פחדנית או כחושה או שמנה ביותר או מצד הנפל כאשר יהיה קטן מאד או בפיהו מורסא או חולי אחר או מסבת [f. 21r] אבר השכילו כמו מורסת כיס השתן או במעים או לסבת מחוץ כמו קור. **המקרה**. אמנם מופתי עוצר הלידה על הכללי הוא יטה הכאב לצד הפנים רצוני לומר הבטן ועצם השורר ותהיה לה לידה על כל אחד פרוקי.

הסבות הנועדות הרפואה יתחייב שתתמיד האשה כאשר יקרב עד לידתה המרחץ וטוב שתהיה הרחיצה בבית החיצון לפי שהמרחץ יפיל הכח ומשח הגב ומסה לבטן ועל הכליות בשמן אל כירי ומרח אותן בשעוה ושמן ושומן תרנוגלות נתרים והשקה אותם הרירים כמו ריר חבושים על ריר זרע הפשתן עם גלאב ותן להם בימי הכאב מי אל פנגיריג ומטעמה יהיה תבשיל הבשר והביצים בשומן רב מאד וכאשר יקרב עת לידתה יתחייב שתזמין כל צרכה. והושבה במים שנבשל בהם אל כליל אל מלך וכזבורת אל ביר וסובין ופניגריג והדומה לזה ושים באפה הדברים המעטשין ותפתח פיה למשוך האויר יותר.

ואם תהיה הסבה מן צד השומן יתחייב שתאמר למילדת שתשכיב האשה על בטנה ואחר תשים ארכובתה תחת ירכותה ותשב עליה ואחר תמשח רחמה בדברים המרטבים כמו שומן ושמן ושומן תרנגולת או שומן אנד ועטשה שתשים באפה עץ רך או קראטש פתול וזאת ההנהגה תועיל ואם תהיה הסבה גודל העובר יתחייב אם התחיל לצאת שתמשוך אותו המילדת משיכה רכה אחר שתרחץ המקום במים הפושרין ולפעמים בגדי דק ותמשוך מעט מעט עד שיצא ואם לא יחתוך או יוציא אותו כמו שיוציאו המתים ואם תהיה הסבה מורסא ברחם אין לך לעשות כי אם הסיכות והנהגת השמנות ואם תהיה הסבה חולשת הכח החיה אותו ברחות הטובות ותשקה אותם מי הבשר עם הסמים ואם תהיה הסבה כי האם לא תשבר מרוב עביה יתחייב שתשבור אותה בצפורן או בברזל שיושם בין האצבעות ואם תהיה הסבה קרירות [f. 21v] יתחייב להושיב אותה במרחץ אם יאות או בבית חם מאד ותושיב אותה במים חמים שנתבשל בהם פוליול והאכילה במי הפירולש והזרעונים עם השיכג ושומן התרנגולת וחכך הרחם בשמן חם.

ואם תהיה הסבה חמימות האויר יתחייב שתשב במקומות הקרים ותחבש אותה בדברים הקרים. ואם תהיה הסבה מהפסד תכונת העובר יתחייב למילדת שתשיב אותו בחכמה ואמנם הרפואות המוצאות[28] לעובר המת מהם זאת הרפואה מר וקשטור אשטורקש מכל חד ב׳ דרכמונים קנילא ד׳ דרכמונים גינגברי דרכמונים עלה רודה ג׳ דרכמונים מר דרכמונים והיא שתיה אחת שלמה תשתה אותה בבשול גיגיברי בבקר ובערב. תכונת פתילה תוציא השליה והעובר המת אפופוניאק ומר ולאברום ומררת השור מכל אחד בשוה יודק ויולש ותעשה כמו תמר ותשא אותה ואחר תעשן אותה במר ותעטשנה בכנדס. ואמנם כאשר הפילה או ילדה ולא תנקה מהדם הדרך הנכונה שתעטשה ותעשנה. וחרדל ובכליאום ומר ואם לא יועיל הקז גיד הצפאן או תחת הארכובה ותשקה אותה הדברים המורידים לדם הנדות וכאשר ירבה לצאת הדם ממנה יאות שתשים על בטנה בגדי פשתן טבולים בחומץ ותשא שיאפאת כמו הבלאושטיה והכרבא והורד והלבונה ביין.

במחנק הרחם והוא חולי דומה לצרע שהוא חולי הנפילה ולו עונות. הסבה סבה [sic]. סבת זה החולי אמנם ידע[29] מתאחז ויכבה חמימותו ויהפך לחומר ארסיי אמנם הנדות ומשניהם יעלה קיטור סמי ללב ולמוח המקרה יורה על מה שהיה מהזרע כי הוא יהיה ברוב בקטורים ולא יהיה שמה העדרת דם הנדות והתעלפות גדול או תהיה לאשה אחר זמן ארוך מהתשמיש עם תאוה חזקה. הרפואה אמנם [f. 22r] ההפרש בין זה החולי ובן הצרע כי ידמה לאשה שדבר מתנמל עולה מהרחם לעליון הגוף ואם יהיה חזק יקרה ממנו

---

[28] Read: המוציאות.

[29] Read: זרע.

קונגושטמיט ואם יוסיף עוד הדבר עד אשר תראה האשה כאלו מתה בלי נפשה ולפעמים ימצא לה על הכליות.

ודרך רפואתה זה החולי בהקזת הגיד הנקרא אל צאפן ואם תמצא האשה ברחמה חום דומה לשרפה מדם נאחז וסודא כבס הבטן בבשול מיראבולאנש אינדיש ופוליפודי דלא פיד לאדורי ולפעמים תצטרך אל אפסימו ואחר עשה מה שיוריד ואחר עשה מה שיוריד דם הנדות כמו בשול השרשים עם אשרב סכנגבין הזרעים ואחר צוה אותה שתעשה פתילה עם מעט גליא ומעט אפורבי מופלא מאד להוריד ואחר הושיבוה במים אשר בשל בהם פנגריג וזרע פשתן ומורדוש ועוד פתילה מאשתורקש ופלפל ושומן אניט. ומזונה יהיה המזון הקל כבשר העופות.

והמורידות לדם הנדות כמו פאדילוש ואשפרקש וזרעונים ובסגולה השחורים ושים במזונה קנילה וכמון ומצטכי. ואם תהיה הסבה מזרע הרפואה הנכונה לזה שתזדוג האשה ואם לא יזמן זה יתחייב שתתמיד האשה הדברים המיבשים לזרע כמו מעגון הכמון ויתחייב שתשים המילדת ידה ברחמה ותמשח אצבעותיה בשמן הלור ובשמן אבולוש. ושתמשמש שם משמוש ארוך אולי תוציא בזה זרע קר ותמצא תכף צאתו הנחה או רפואה שלמה וכמו כן שתעשה פתילה מזנגביל ופלפל ורודה ויועיל להן דוא מסך.

ואמנם מה שאות[30] שתנהיג האשה בחולי בחוזק כאשר היא שֹוכבת כאילו מיתה בלא נפישה יתחייב שתשפוך על האשה שומן טוב הריח כמו שמן האדולוש ואחר קשור שוקיה קשר חזק מאד וחזק בגליה וכפות ידיה. ואמור למילדת שתמשמש פי הרחם במה שהזכרנו או תשים בו גאליה עם שמן אבולש ועשן אותה מלמטה עם לאנייה אלובין [f. 22v] ומסך ועטשה בכנדס וצוה עליה שתזעק בקול גדול ותשקה אותה מעט יין לחזק בו הכח ותן לה לה רוטב תרנגולת וכאשר יקרה אי זה החולי להסת די לך בשמנים.

המאמר בשפע דם הנדות. יתכן יציאת דם הנדות וזה החולי נקרא נזף. הסבה אמנם לענין ברחם או לחבורות שבו או לפתיחת עורקיו לחולשתו ומה שיהיה מדם או לרבויו או לדקותו. המקרה אמנם מופתי מה שהיה סבתו מחבורות ואכילת בהמצא הנאב וצאת הונין ושחרות הדם. ומופתי מה שהיה סבתו המלוי באדמימות הלובן הגוף ומלוי הפנים ומופתו מה שסבתו דקיקות הדם שהלובן יהיה ירוק והמצא דקיקות בדם.

הרפואה דע כי ימי ירידת דם הנדות למיעוט הדם הם שלשה ולרוב הם ששה וכאשר ירבה מאד יהיו ימים מכאן ואילך יהיה החולי הנקרא נזק[31]. ואמנם מה שיהיה סבתו חבורות ברחם רפואתו כרפואות המקבצות ואם יהיה סבתו הפתח הגידים בעשית הדברים המקבצים המחזקים כמו זאת הרפואה בחל ובלאו יהיה שהיה יאסף במי ההדס

---

30 Read: שיאות.

31 Read: נזף.

וישימה בצמר ותשאה רוב היום והלילה רוב היום והלילה [sic]. ומה שסבתו חדוד הדם ודקיקותו מן הדברים המועילים לזה מי הפלאנטגי עם שרב החבושים וממה שיועילם עוד מזה שתית החומץ וממה שיחזק פיות הגידים ויקבצם ויועיל מחדוד הדם ודקיקותו שתית ב׳ דרכ׳ מפורסלנש שרופות במי אלסמאק והחבושים וממה שיועיל מחדוד הדם עם חוזק חמימות המזג שתיית הכפנייא עם שרב התפוחים ומה שיועיל תועלת משותפת טרוסיש קוביפש עם רוב החבושים או שרב החבושים ועוד אלו הטרוסיש בולוס של שגלאדום ובולוס ארמניקום ואלום וגאלש ודם התנין מכל אחד רובע דרכמונים כפורא משקל שני גרעינין [f. 23r] מסך שתות דרהם יאסף בשראב ההדס ותתמיד אותן ויועיל מאנזף כאשר ירבה מאד שתעשה לו קלאשטירי מחוי הפלאנטגי עם אקאסיא ודם התנין ומזונם יהיה העדשים בחומץ והתרנגולין במי הסומאק ואם יהיה הסבה מרוב הדם הקיז אותה מגיד הבאסלק וככה לזכות הדם במי הלגלוגולת ושראב הרמונים.

ואם תהיה סבת דקיקות הדם הגברות האל צפרא כבוס הצפרא בדברים המכבסים אותם וכמו כן יועילם הישיבה במים אשר בשל קליפי הרמונים והכרוב ואל בלושטיאש והעפצים בו גאליה עם שמן אבולש ועשן אותה מלמטה עם לאנייה. אלובין ומסך. שמענה ודע לך.

התאחזות דם הנדות ומעוטו. הסבה. סבת זה אמנם כמו רוע מזג קר או יבש או סתום או מורסא קשה או פיות העורקין בשותפות אל האברים אחרים כמו חולשת הכבד או כחשות הגוף או שומן יותר מדאי או לחולי ארוך מעוט הדם בגוף או יובש בחלוני הדם או עובי הדם לרוב מה שיתערב עמו מן החלט העבה.

המקרה יורה על שסבתו הקור ברוב השעה ובלובן מראה הגוף והיציאה תהיה ומיעוט חמימות הגוף על מה שיהיה סבתו נוטה ליובש הרחם והכחשות ועל מה שסבתו חולשת הכבד בהמצא מופתי חולשת הכבד. וכזה מה שסבתו סתום מופתי הסתום. הרפואה דע לך כי יש מהנשים שאין להם דם נדות כל ימיהם כלל או יהיה להם מעט מזער והם אשר ידמו לאנשים מעט [f. 23v] בעובי בשרם ורוב שערה ורוחב גחונם ובזאת יתחייב שלא תתעסק ברפואתם ואמנם מה שיהיה סבתו סתימות בחלוני הרחם רפואתו ברפואות הפותחות לסתום כשראב השרשים עם שמב[32] השקילא והפתילות הפותחות המושכות הדרמן[33] הרפואות הטובות אלא שיתחייב שתשער מעשיכם אם יהיה שמה חמימות מירא ומינטשטרי מכל אחד ד׳ דרכמונים גניברי ח׳ דרכמונים רודה יבשה י׳ דרכמונים ענבים יבשים מנוקין מגרעניהן ד׳ דרכמונים יולש זה במרירת השור ויעשה ממנו פתילה וזה אות לסתום או קור ולא יהיה סבתו רוע מזג קר ברחם ואמנם מה שיהיה סבתו רוע מזג קר והתקבץ פיות הרחם יועיל מזה שתית זאת הרפואה אפפוניאק ודונזור

[32] Read: שמן.
[33] Read: הדם מן.

וקשיה מכל אחד ו׳ דרכמונים ישתה במי בישול מינטשטרי ותעשה כמו תמר מזאת הרפואה ותשים אותה ברחמה וזאת תכונתה מסך וקשטור ומירא בשמן אבולוש.

וממה שיוריד דם הנדות ברוב זאת הרפואה אשנאן היא ארבה דשאוק בלע׳ ופלטרי ואשטז ורובה אנפורבי מכל אחד בשוה יודק ויולש ותשא אותה בצמר ובשמן זנבק. ואם תהיה הסבה מורסא קשה יתחייב שנעשה המרככות והשמנים והשומן והקלישטיריש המתרככות. ואם יהיה הסבה עובי הדם מצד חלק עבה מזה ידמה לי שיקרה ממנו המועטת לא שלא ירד כלל ויתחייב שתתמיד האשה העבה בגרגורוגי ראיאנג דמחזק והתמיד אותה זה הבשול גוגובי ב׳ אוק׳ פאי ד׳ פאידולש ה׳ דרכמונים זרע כרפס דרכמונים רוגה הצבע דרכמונים גרעיני הגינברי ה׳ גרעינים יבושל ויסונן על שראב סכנגבין מהזרעים וכמו זה פתילות מצמר שרוי בשמן אבולש נעשנה בעשון שיעזור להוריד הדם כמו עשון הקולוקונטיר והאמוניאק ואם תהיה [f. 24r] הסבה ממעוט הדם יתחייב שתעזור אליה במזון המוליד לדם ואם תהיה הסבה חולשת הכבד יתחייב שתונין בדברים המחזיקים הכבד. תם ונשלם.

[f. 25v, 21]**מאותות שפעת האם** שפעת האם אנו מבינים תוך חלל ושם שופעות שלשת הליחות. **משפעת הליחה הלבנה שם** יהיו אלה האותות. תהיה האם לחה ולא תתענג במשכב זכר. וכל דבר קר יזיק וכל דבר חם יועיל כמו מרחץ חם ודומיהם ואף אם [f. 25r] הן חפצות במשכב זכר. לזכרים אין חפץ מהם בעבור רב לחותם. וסובלות כאב וכובד תחת הטבור. וקרירות יוצא מעומק. ולחות רב בפי האם. ועם דמי נדתה יתערבו ליחות משפעת הליחה הלבנה. ועב טיט דומה אל יציאת החוטם יתערבו שם. והשתן יוצא מטבעו האדום שהיה כבר ושב להיות שמן או לבן או נוטה ללובן. ולפעמים תהיינה הליחות נתכות ברוח כאשר יעשה באברים הרוחניים במצוקת האם גם חלישות הלב יקרה אליה והוא הנקרא שינקופיט ויכאב ראשה עד שלא תוכל לכופו על ברכיה. ולפעמים יקרה לנשים בסבה הזאת נפח המים הנקרא אגאנוס גם נקי׳ אידרופשיס.

משפעת הליחה השחורה באם והיו אלה האותות. לא יתענגו במשכב זכר. והזרע מעט ומאחורי כאב וכובד והתפשטות נרגש מעומק. ורוח ורעש נרגש באם. ולפעמים יהיה מאותות הליחה השחורה מצוקת האם. ויקרה להיות לה אפיסת כח הלב הוא שינקופיש. וקרירות נרגש סביב האם וסמוך לפיה ובהלה אין הרגש. ודמי נדתה רעים מאד ורעים נוטים לצבע תכלת בסבת ערבוב הליחה השחורה. והשתן דקיק וכבוש. ולפעמים שמן ונוטה לצבע תכלת.

משפעת הליחה האדומה באם יהיו אלה האותות כאב מחודד וחריף ויבשות וקושי. וחום סביבות פי האם וחומצת ומתענגת במשכב הזכר מאד. ואולם בהיות הליחה שופעת מאד ימעט חפץ המשכב ממנה. אך הכאב אינו נפסק. גם הזכרים מתענגים בהם יותר מן האחרות וממהרות

להזריע אך מעט יהיה הזרע. והיו תוצאותיהם מעט ומצבע צהוב. ושפתותיהן יבשות גם כריתות. והנה די במה שזכרנו מאותות שפעת הליחות.

English translation

The paucity of sperm and the disappearance of desire. The cause may be a particular ailment of the member or its bad temperament. It may also be caused by impotency of the member, or by the two testicles and the penis. Or because of a bad cold and a dry temperament, or a feebleness of the kidneys, or [5] bodily faintness, or a paucity of the smoky wind distributed by the heart, or a weakness of the liver or the brain or any of the ruling organs. The case indicates [the causes]: the signs of impotency are the absence of an erection and a failure of the penis to shrink in cold water.

If the cause's source lies in the testicles, the signs are erections with a paucity of sperm which cannot be ejected. If it is caused by weakness of the kidneys, it would be indicated by the weakness of the penis; when the liver is the cause of the ailment, the signs are a lack of [10] appetite, fatigue and [other] symptoms which indicate a paucity of blood. If [it is caused] by heart trouble, it may be evidenced by the pulse.

The treatment must be the opposite of each cause. So, if the impotency is caused by a bad cold temperament, one must employ hot ointments and hot oils, such as gillyflower[34] oil, gillyflower ointment,[35] balm of Gilead[36] ointment, narcissus[37] ointment and kust-root[38] ointment. The patient should be denied cold foods and [15] cold drinks; [instead] he should be prescribed dishes [such as] meat, which is easily digested in the stomach, dishes fried in a pan and

---

[34] The expression combines Hebrew with Arabic: the oil of خيري (*Cheiranthus cheiri*, L.). See *Tuḥfat al-aḥbâb*, no. 422.

[35] For this term, the author exclusively used the Arabic word دهن.

[36] Arabic: البكاء (*Amyris glead*, L.). See Issa, *Dictionnaire des noms des plants*, p. 55, no. 7.

[37] Arabic: نرجس (*Narcissus*, L.). See ابن البيطار, *الجامع لمفردات الادوية والاغذية*, place and date unknown, vol. II, p. 179; cf. Issa, *Dictionnaire des noms des plants*, p. 123.

[38] Arabic: قسط (*Costus speciosus*, L.); see *Tuḥfat al-aḥbâb*, no. 350; Issa, *Dictionnaire des noms des plants*, p. 58, no. 15.

flavoured with spices, and spiced meat and egg dishes. In general, he should follow the diet prescribed [to whomever] suffers from a bad temperament in the urinary bladder.

If the case is of a bad, cold temperament in the testicles, it has to be treated with hot oils such as jasmine[39], or gillyflower ointment mixed with musk[40] and castor. Also give them ginger[41] jam[42] and squill[43] [20] jam, as you see fit. Prescribe him strengthening and warming food, such as birds and young pigeons, birds brains, the meat of a yearling lamb and spices such as cinnamon[44] and ginger. They should [also] eat of the following electuary[45]: ten dirhems each of peeled almonds, pistachio[46], coconut, peeled peanuts and lentil[47] seeds; one dirhem each of long pepper and ginger [f. 16r]. Mix them all with hard sugar and have him eat a nut-size portion every day. If the cause is a bad dry temperament and a paucity of sperm, prescribe him an ointment for the testicles [made] with oil and wax and hen fat. He should eat moistening foods such as lamb meat in egg dishes. He should regularly have a bath, drink white [5] wine, eat peeled and pipless grapes.

If he is afflicted by a dry and hot temperament, it is useful [to apply] a bull penis[48] with its sperm[49], and to anoint the organs with calabash[50] and almond ointments. He should eat little wet fishes, fried on a fire, and clean watermelon, resin of dragon-tree[51] and some beets[52].

---

39 Arabic: زنبق; according to Renaud and Colin, the term signifies "jasmin et huile de jasmin", *Tuḥfat al-aḥbâb*, no. 138.

40 Spanish: *Musgo*, also called *almisce* and *almiscle*, derived from the Arabic مسك. See *Menor daño de la medicina de Alonso de Chirino*, p. 290.

41 Arabic: زنجبيل (*Amonum zingiber*, L.), see *Tuḥfat al-aḥbâb*, no. 143.

42 Arabic: مربى See Dozy, *Supplément aux dictionnaires arabes*, vol. I, p. 506.

43 Arabic: إشقيل (*Scilla maritima*, L.). See *Tuḥfat al-aḥbâb*, no. 31.

44 Spanish: *Canela* (*Cinamonum obtusifolium,* L.). See *Menor daño de la medicina de Alonso de Chirino*, p. 260.

45 Arabic: معجون. See Dozy, *Supplément aux dictionnaires arabes*, vol. II, p. 99.

46 Arabic: فستق (*Pistacia vera*, L.). See *Tuḥfat al-aḥbâb*, no. 321.

47 Spanish: *Lenteja* (*Ervum lens*, L.).

48 Arabic: زُب البقر.

49 Arabic: منى.

50 Arabic: يقطين (*Curcubita lagenaria*, L.). See *Tuḥfat al-aḥbâb*, no. 116.

51 Arabic: شيان. See *ibid.*, no. 118.

52 Arabic: أرمليطة. See Dozy, *Supplément aux dictionnaires arabes*, vol. I, p. 19.

If the cause is feebleness of the heart and the erection is diminished, it is useful to employ musk jam[53] or *al-metroditos*[54], if it is available, and to prepare a dish made of [10] meat, onions and boiled eggs, and to drink perfumed wine and do joyful things.

The following is a prescription for inflating the penis and bringing the wind into it: Take big black grains *[sic]* and immerse them in rocket[55] juice; once they are swollen, dry them, pound and knead them with wild millet[56] and hard sugar. He should eat a nut-size [portion] in the morning and the evening. It is also useful to take, [15] in equal parts, pine-nuts[57], coconut, rocket seed and watermelon seed, all peeled, and then add a sufficient portion of honey. Also useful for them is a confectionary made of fresh galbanum juice and honey, to which sperm is added at the end *[sic]*.

We have already mentioned the treatment in case the problem is caused by the kidneys or a weakness of the liver. You should know that there are many ways to treat a coitus problem; we briefly refered to the most essential of them, and it seems to us adequate to be of help.

[20] **Excess of [sexual] desire** [the signs of which are]: Ejection of water before ejaculation, in which case the liquid may be pure or turbid, and the sperm itself, all or part of it, may be thin, or scorched. Sometimes the genital organs may be affected by an itch, as occurs with women, or an excess of inflating winds. According to the symptoms, it is possible to determine if the cause is hot sperm and nocturnal pollution. [f. 16r] Ejaculation of water before the sperm indicates that the cause is an excess of desire during coitus, and finally, prolonged erection means that he suffers from inflating winds.

---

[53] Arabic: مخنق المسك.

[54] A deformation of *mithridaticum*, an antidote prepared by Mithridates VI Eupator, used until the 19th century. See *Hippocrates Pseudepigraphic Writings*, ed. and trans. with an Introduction by W. D. Smith, Leiden, 1990, p. 71; Platearius, *Le livre des simples médecines*, translated and adaptated by G. Malandin *et al.* Paris, 1986, p. 357.

[55] Spanish: *Oruga* (*Eruca sativa*, L.). See *Menor daño de la medicina de Alonso de Chirino*, p. 292.

[56] Spanish: "Se cuenta entre las especies de grano, es semejante al mijo y en la mesma forma se masa; *latine panicum. Dioscoridem*, lib. 2, cap. 89.", S. de Cobarruvias, *Tesoro de la lengua castellana o Española*, Madrid, 1611, fasc. edition, Madrid, 1977, p. 849.

[57] Spanish: *piñiones*. See *ibid.*, p. 871.

The treatment. You must take into consideration that if the excess of desire results from a healthy temperament and the quantity of the blood and its power, you should not, in this case, diminish that desire, since such a treatment contradicts nature's work, unless it is of urgent necessity. In this last case, the recommended treatment is blood-letting.

If the reason is hot sperm, you should treat it with cooling materials, such as horseradish, purslane and its seeds, and serve lentils and marrow. It is recommended to place a piece of lead on his back and on the kidneys, and to keep his meals cold in nature, and made with vinegar. When [10] the cause is an excess of blood and fever, the remedy is blood-letting and a small quantity of food. He should continue to apply cooling treatments and eat lentils boiled in water and vinegar. According to Galen, nuphar[58] applied [on the member] weakens the sperm, and the patient should drink nettle liquid with juice of a sour pomegranate. Regarding the hot and drying medicaments, they are chaste-tree[59] seed, rue seed, mint[60] and cumin. Of the compound medicaments, take two dirhems each of horseradish seed and nettle seed, and one dirhem of rue seed; he should drink one dirhem of it [the compound] with a beverage[61] made from oximel.[62]

Concerning the treatment of water ejected before ejaculation, when it originates from an excess of blood, the treatment is a combination of blood-letting, purification [of the body], a small quantity of food, and eating fumitory.[63]

If the cause is thin sperm, it is useful to eat atriplex in a rose confection and to be nourished by thickening foods, such as [20] dishes made of [different kinds of] flour.

If the cause is impotency of the organs and a feebleness of the erecting power, it would be useful to apply atriplex and a preparation of constrictive oils poured into myrtle oil [mixed] with ambergris.

---

[58] Spanish: *nenufar*. See *Menor daño de la medicina de Alonso de Chirino*, p. 290.

[59] The Hebrew text states: *aquivas qastus*, which is the corruption of the Latin term: *agnus castus=Vitex agnus castus*. See Issa, *Dictionnaire des noms des plants*, p. 190, no. 1.

[60] The Hebrew text states: *mentastra*.

[61] Arabic: شراب ; and Spanish: *asarab* or *xarope*. See *Menor daño de la medicina de Alonso de Chirino*, p. 313-314.

[62] Arabic: سكنجبين; see *Tuḥfat al-aḥbâb*, nos. 372, 400.

[63] Spanish: *Fumusterra* (*Fumaria oficinalis*, L.). See *Menor daño de la medicina de Alonso de Chirino*, p. 277.

Likewise, [he may be treated] with a frankincense bandage [doused] with myrtle liquid.

A prolonged erection without sexual desire. The causes are an increase of thick winds in the veins of the penis and in the cavities of the nerves, or a thick humour[64] which causes thick vapors. In case the problem is caused by the winds, [f. 17r] the erection would be impossible without these winds. The proof that it is caused by wind in the organ or by a thick humour is its swaying.

The treatment. The treatment of this case is similar to what we have described in the case of an excess of desire. Which means using materials that break and dissipate the winds and reduce [5] the sperm. You should begin with blood-letting, but avoid diarrhoea, and apply cooling materials to the organ, such as sandal wood[65], *qaleda*[66], and camphor, or anoint it with horseradish juice or with lettuce juice. He should also put some of these materials on the kidneys, on the back. As we have mentioned, it is also useful [to drink] a beverage made of dry nymphaea leaves and horseradish seed, and to place pieces of lead on the kidneys and on the spinal column. It would be useful for them to apply materials which dissipate the hot winds: rue seed, asparagus, cumin and celery; these may be applied as separate medicaments or in a compound, in which case take two dirhems of each.

In case you discover that he suffers from thick matter, it would be proper to purify him. The purification has to be done with heavy grains and a strengthened purgative[67], and followed by the treatment mentioned above. It would be appropriate for someone who suffers from this illness not to have any sexual relations [15] and not even to think about them. Generally, he should conduct himself as one who suffers from an excess of [sexual] appetite.

[On a] hot abscess and a cold and thick one, which afflict the organ and cause friction. The cause may be one of the four humours or a combination of them. The scabies may be caused by malign matter or may occur after the abscesses. The diagnosis should be made [20] according to the warmth, coldness and hardness which the patient

---

64 Arabic: خلط.

65 Arabic: صندل (*Santalum album*, L.). See *Tuḥfat al-aḥbâb*, no. 297.

66 I could not identify this term.

67 Arabic: الايارج . The origin of the term is Greek. For the various species of the plant, see *El libro del 'Amal man ṭabba li-man ḥabba*, p. 12.

feels in his flesh. If the scabies is caused by biliousness[68], the sign is reddishness; if it is caused by black bile[69] it is blackish, turbid and dry; if the cause is phlegmatic[70], it is whitish and soft.

The treatment. The hot abscess should be treated by letting of a significant quantity of blood from the vein called basilikon, if there is no impediment. Afterwards, he should continuously drink barley liquid and oximel[71], and place on the organ [f. 17v] a cloth immersed in vinegar and rose juice, and make a bandage of sandal-wood[72] and rose juice.

When the matter [of the abscess] is hot and concentrated, it would be proper to apply the following: Take pomegranate peels, dried roses and peeled lentils, cook them all in water until they are very soft, then add [5] house-leek tree[73] sap and rose oil. Then apply Armenian cardamom[74] in vinegar; afterwards, softening and wetting materials, such as wax, oil and a bandage made of mallow[75] flour and broad bean flour mixed with the wax and the oil.

The treatment of the cold abscess is carried out with bandages which cause it to ripen, such as clover flour, mallow flour, camomile[76] and [10] *muql*[77], which is bdellium[78]. The patient has to continuously drink rose jam and oximel[79] with seeds. The medicament for a hard abscess is to rub the organ with wax and oil and fat from a gander and a hen. In case something stronger is needed, place wax

---

68 Arabic: صفراوي .

69 Arabic: سويداء.

70 Arabic: بلغمي.

71 Arabic: سكنجبين ; see note 62.

72 Arabic: صندل ; see note 65.

73 Spanish: *Siempereviva* (*Sempervivum*, L.).

74 Arabic:هيل (*Elettaria cardamomum*, L.).

75 Spanish: *Malva* (*Malva sylvestris*, L.); see *Menor daño de la medicina de Alonso de Chirino*, p. 287.

76 Spanish: *Camomilla* (*Anthemis nobilis*, L.); see *ibid.*, p. 260.

77 Arabic: مقل . Note that the scribe omitted the *lam*.

78 The form which appears in the Hebrew text is a deformation of the Romance *bedelio* or *bedelion*. The Spanish physician Alonso Chirino states: "Bedelion que llaman en arauigo mocal...", *Menor daño de la medicina de Alonso de Chirino*, p. 112. Cf. *L'explication des noms de drogues - un glossaire de matière médicale composé par Maïmonide*, no. 230; *Tuḥfat al-aḥbâb*, nos. 61, 257, 426, 439.

79 The author employs the Arabic term but adds: "[made of] the seeds", without any specification. The oximel is, in fact, a mixture of vinegar and honey, so that it is plausible that he means "to add" some kind of seeds.

with marrow taken from a cow leg, amoniac, rose[80] oil and goose fat[81] oil, on the organ, and prevent the patient from eating thick food. [15] If it is necessary, purify him with materials that draw out the black bile.

Regarding the treatment of scabies which recently afflicted the organ, you should apply saltwort[82], litharge[83] and cadmium[84] cleaned with water on the area. It is also useful for them [to take] pumpkins burned to ashes or [mixed] with rose oil. In case the scabies are old, treat them with the following medicine: An equal quantity each of pottage[85], litharge, dragon-tree, burned [20] laurel[86], aloe, frankincense and saltwort are pounded together to anoint the scabies, or apply them with wax. In case there is dead flesh, clean it with butter or lentil flour or hard butter, and it will disappear. Sometimes you may be obliged to apply verdigris liniment[87] and pitch liniment[88] [first], and then put a proper medicament for scabies on the organ. In case the scabies afflict the orifice of the organ, treat them with the medicament used for the scabies which occur in the urinary bladder, and apply them inside.

[f. 18r] If the urinary passage is blocked, put zygophyllum[89] on the organ until it opens, then sprinkle in women's milk with rose oil and white collyrium[90]. The proper treatment for the friction that afflicts the organ is blood-letting. If this is insufficient, apply materials which take out the burned brown humour, and then bandage it [5] in

---

[80] Arabic: الورد.

[81] Arabic: هندي ; see Dozy, *Supplément aux dictionnaires arabes*, vol. II, p. 774.

[82] Spanish: *Alumbre*; see *Menor daño de la medicina de Alonso de Chirino*, p. 249.

[83] Arabic: مرتق; see *Tuḥfat al-aḥbâb*, no. 256.

[84] Arabic: إقليميا ; see Dozy, *Supplément aux dictionnaires arabes*, vol. I, p. 30.

[85] Spanish: *Potaje*; see *Menor daño de la medicina de Alonso de Chirino*, p. 295.

[86] Arabic: رند, (*Laurus nobilis*, L.); see *Tuḥfat al-aḥbâb*, nos. 173, 437.

[87] Arabic: مرهم الزنجار.

[88] Arabic: مرهم الزفت.

[89] The form that appears in the text is probably a distortion of the Arabic الطرطير or الرطريط (*Zygophyllum coccineum*, L). See Issa, *Dictionnaire des noms des plants*, p. 193, nos. 3,4.

[90] Arabic: اشياف ابيض . The Arabic term شياف is used both for a suppository and an eyewash; in the present context, the author refers to the second. Ibn al-Khatîb, in the chapter on illnesses of the eye, mentions the cure with different types of eyewashes. These compound medicamets are divided according to their colour, including a white one, but he is not precise about their components. See *El libro del 'Amal man ṭabba li-man ḥabba*, p. 45.

a bath with vinegar and rose oil[91]. It is also useful to bandage it with red-horned poppy[92] oil, acacia, and saltwort and saffron[93], knead it with rose oil and bandage the organ. In case all these treatments are in vain, you should apply leeches, since they suck out the malign material; afterwards, he will be cured, God willing.

Regarding the treatment of the organ's movement, when it moves unwillingly *[sic]*, it should be carried on with ointments [10] and oils. The ointments are hen fat, goose fat oil and wax. The oils are narcissus[94] oil and hyacinth[95]. Afterwards wash it with lukewarm liquid.

On very hot tumors.[96] On hot and cold tumors which appear on the inside and the outside of the scrotum. **The cause** is an excess of one of the four humours. According to each case of tumor, it is possible to define the cause, based on what we have said about the diagnosis of tumors. [15]

The treatment. You should know that the treatment of a tumor of the testicles is similar to that of an organ tumor, but you must treat the testicles more carefully. Generally, the treatment of the hot tumor which afflicts the testicles is blood-letting from the basilikon vein, on the side where the tumor appears. If the tumors afflict both sides, let blood first from the left-hand side and on the second day, let blood from the right-hand side. Regarding the quantity of the blood, take into consideration the physical condition and the age of the patient, [and examine] whether these two factors permit blood-letting. I recommend giving the patient barley liquid, and afterwards give him oximel to drink. Then bandage the [afflicted] place with the two species of sandal[97], white stonecrop[98] or black-nightshade[99], and the sap of pumpkin or green cane, if they are available. Another ban-

---

[91] Arabic: دهن الورد.

[92] Arabic: ماميثا (*Glaucium corniculatum*, L.); see *Tuḥfat al-aḥbâb*, no. 264.

[93] Arabic: زعفران (*Corcus sativus*, L.); *ibid.*, no. 151.

[94] Arabic: نرجس (*Narcisus*, L.).

[95] Arabic: سراج (*Hyacinthus orientalis*, L.); see *Tuḥfat al-aḥbâb*, no. 374; Issa, *Dictionnaire des noms des plants*, p. 95, no. 18.

[96] Arabic: الاورام الحرارة.

[97] Spanish: *Sandalos*. In fact, during the Middle Ages, three kinds of sandal were known: white (*Santalum album*, L.), bright red (*Petrocarpus indicus*, L.), and citric (*Santalum freycinetianum*, L.). See *Menor daño de la medicina de Alonso de Chirino*, p. 299.

[98] Spanish: *Uva canilla* or *Uva cana*, "dog grape", which is called also *uva de gato*, "cat grape". See *ibid.*, p. 310.

[99] Spanish: *Yerua mora* (*Solanum nigrum*, L.). *Ibid.*, p. 315.

dage may be made of barley flour and lentil flour; kneaded in liquid of waybread and cane. In case the tumor persists after the bandage [is applied], you need to employ [other] things which dissolve it. Begin with wax, oil and extract of [f. 18v] the house-leek tree[100], add liquid wax and wash the place with lukewarm water. In case the tumor is caused by phlegm[101] and a great quantity of blood is diagnosed, you should let blood even if his general condition is feeble, but give him rose jam, hot water, oximel and seeds. Afterwards you must purify [5] the patient with medicaments which take out the phlegm, and anoint the organ with jasmine oil and bandage it with bean flour with a small quantity of cumin, goose fat or camomile[102], bdellium and wax. Drip a small amount of jasmine on the organ and give the patient thin food, such as grains and oil; if he is feeble, give him roasted cocks.

Concerning the treatment of a hard tumor, purify the body from the yellow bile[103] and then cover the place with a bandage made from yellow [10] urine[104] and goose fat, tragacanth[105] and opopanax[106], and mix them all in cow butter. Another bandage [is composed of] ammoniac, bdellium and storax[107], all of them mixed with a small quantity of bean flour. You also have to wash the place with water in which myrtle[108] and melilot[109] have been boiled. Indeed, the treatment of the tumors in the scrotum is based on this one.

The dropsical tumor. On the dropsical tumor and the inflation of scrotum caused by the wind, [15] the separation of the scrotum, the scrotal hernia and flesh inflation. The cause: the dropsical tumor is caused by dropsy in the scrotum and the corruption of the blood; the inflation in the flesh is caused by a sanguine humour tending to blackishness[110]; and the windy tumor is caused by the break of peri-

---

[100] Spanish: *Siempreviva*; see note 73.

[101] Arabic: بلغمي.

[102] Arabic:بابونج (*Matricaria aurea*, L.). See *Tuḥfat al-aḥbâb*, no. 86.

[103] Arabic: صفراوي.

[104] Arabic: بول اصفر.

[105] The word was distorted by the scribe, read: انزروت. See *Tuḥfat al-aḥbâb*, no. 35.

[106] Spanish: *Opoponac*. See *Menor daño de la medicina de Alonso de Chirino*, p. 291.

[107] Spanish: *estoraque*. See *ibid.*, p. 246.

[108] Arabic: مرسين (*Myrtus communis*, L.). See *Tuḥfat al-aḥbâb*, no.272.

[109] Arabic: إكليل الملك ; see *ibid.*, no. 4.

[110] Arabic: اسودي.

toneum, which is the abdomen membrane. The scrotal hernia is caused by the accumulation of very corrupted humours in the two cavities of the scrotum, or by an exceedingly great cry, or by coitus, or by [20] an excess of material, or by a jump, or by a sudden movement, as in the case of the windy tumor.

The signs of a dropsical tumor are its size, fever and thin skin; when you touch it the tumor moves. When the tumor is windy the signs are a separation and a noise; sometimes it moves and at other times it is motionless. The scrotal hernia may be diagnosed by touch, and is noisy when pushed or pressed. If the tumor is in the flesh, it can be seen by the thickness of the organ and by its expansion.

The treatment. The treatment of a dropsical tumor has to be carried out by limiting food and by prescribing a diet [f. 19r] of dry foods. Then prepare for him a bandage which disperses the water: It is composed of ammoniac and pepper grains; mix it with old oil and wax and prepare a bandage. If he needs something stronger, add sulphate, goat dung and pigeon dung. If even this preparation is not sufficient, you should take out the excess matter by surgical intervention. Order the [5] patient to lie on his back, and order his servant to pull his penis towards the umbilicus. Then, pull the scrotum, lift the testicles and in this position make a hole in the right or the left side with a wide scalpel, being careful not to touch them in the middle of the scrotum. He should lift the scrotum with his hand in order to prevent it from falling, so that the skin will not cover the hole. [Holding this position] press properly until the surplus [matter] comes out, and then apply the drying medicament to the place because in most cases we are not certain that the water will not reappear, [10] which obliges us to turn to another treatment.

There are some physicians who treat [the tumor] by scorching; that means they heat a thin and curved scalpel, they tie back the testicles as far possible and treat the scrotum in the afflicted place, not touching the testicles. Some other physicians first cut a small part of the fat and then they scorch it. The post-surgical treatment involves using crusting medicaments and preventing the patient from drinking too much water. The treatment of the inflation is to abstain from inflating foods, such as grains, [15] fruits and similar things, and to rub the scrotum with kust[111] oil and jasmine oil[112], and to keep treating it with medicaments which scatter the winds. In case there is

111 Arabic: القسط. See *Tuḥfat al-aḥbâb*, no. 350.

112 Arabic: دهن الياسمين. *Ibid.*, nos. 138, 205.

an excess of winds, apply a cumin electuary[113], [and] give him a small amount of rue and thin foods to eat.

The treatment of the swollen flesh in the scrotum is similar to what we have mentioned regarding the treatment of the hard tumors. Rub it with fat, marrow and oils, and purify the body from the surplus black bile.[114]

The virtues of the swollen scrutum treatment is that when you clean it, it causes no harm to open one of the veins which are in the scrotum in order to ease the illness.

The treatment for a hernia and a collapse of the intestine [in cases where] the patient suffers from great pain similar to colic[115], called *colica masion* by some physicians. Order him to lie on his back, to press the hernia with his hand, and to pull it [19v] upwards. If this treatment proves to be useful, seat the patient in hot water and bandage the hernia with softening materials and cover him with hot clothing. When the hernia reappears, tie it with a square knot. Some physicians anticipate this treatment by scorching [the hernia] with a silver or golden instrument. It is recommended that the patient lie on his back for two or three days.

Sometimes we apply [5] combined medicaments to the hernia, such as the following: Take sulfuric acid, frankincense, coconut, acacia, tragacanth[116], common dragon, myrrh, box-thorn and ginger, in equal amounts, and knead them with fish liver[117] or with gum-arabic[118]. Apply this on the place for many successive days.

A record of the diseases occurring in the womb. On sterility and [10] the impediments to pregnancy. The cause might be a corruption of the man's sperm or the woman's sperm, or a malign temperament in the womb, or a hard tumor, or an ailment in the organ or a short penis. According to the case it may be possible to determine the reason, [whether it is] a corrupted temperament, or if the man's sperm is cold or hot, as the woman feels it, whether the sperm is in a small quantity, or whether it is [too] wet or thin or [according] to its quantity.

---

113 Arabic: معجون الكمون. *Ibid.*, no. 229.

114 Arabic: سوداء.

115 Spanish: *Colica.* See *Menor daño de la medicina de Alonso de Chirino*, p. 264.

116 Arabic: عنزروت. See *Tuḥfat al-aḥbâb*, no. 35.

117 A distortion of the Spanish: *higado.*

118 Spanish: *Goma arabica.*

If the cause is a uterine problem the signs may be found [by examining] the menstrual blood and the humours which exude from it. If the womb is blocked, the indication is a small quantity of blood, or even its complete [15] absence despite medical treatment. If the cause is a corrupted temperament of the man's sperm, you should equilibrate it with its contrary. If the cause is [an excess of] warmth, equilibrate it with cold foods and cold herbs, and purify the acute humours. If the cause is a malign temperament in the womb, counteract it as you learned before, and apply cold truffles[119] and cold liquids if the cause is a hot malign temperament. If the [20] cause is coldness you should continuously apply warm suppositories and warm oil, as we mentioned before. If the cause is blockage, you should open it with medicaments which open the blockage and cause the blood to flow. If the reason is winds in the womb, prepare medicaments which disperse the wind, such as castor, rue and its seed. If you find humidity and sticky matter there, purify the body with a strengthened purgative[120] or ginger[121] pills[122], and then prepare electuaries[123] and suppositories.

At this point I will record the medicaments [f. 20r] with which I [have] experimented and found useful in most cases of this illness, by this I mean [those] caused by coldness and humidity. Of these, it is recommended that the woman drinks from a rabbit's stomach and to apply it [the stomach] with butter during her menses days [in her womb]. Some remedies are also useful, such as giving the women ivory to drink, because it is really wonderful, and the woman should take it a short time before having sexual relations. Drinking scraps of [5] elephant skin is also excellent. Another useful treatment, which does not function by virtue, is to apply a fumigation of balsam[124], its seeds and its oil. It is useful to apply it both as a fumigation and as a suppository. Also, take gander fat, natron and a gum[125] taken from the mastic tree[126], and bandage the woman's womb with it for two days.

---

[119] Arabic: ترفاس . See *Tuḥfat al-aḥbâb*, no. 220.
[120] Arabic: إيارج . See note 67.
[121] Arabic: سكنجبير . See *Tuḥfat al-aḥbâb*, no. 143.
[122] Spanish: *Pildoras*. See *Menor daño de la medicina de Alonso de Chirino*, p. 294.
[123] Arabic: معجون.
[124] Spanish: *Balsamo*.
[125] Spanish: *Goma*.
[126] Arabic: الفستق (*Pistacia vera*, L.). See *Tuḥfat al-aḥbâb*, no. 321.

Of the good suppositories. Take spikenard[127], saffron, mastic, myrrh and castor, [10] knead them all in nard[128] oil or in oil of the ben-oil tree[129] and goose fat, and make them into suppositories. She has to carry it during her purification period, and to change it every three days. A useful virtue to treat humours and winds is to boil garlic with sesame oil[130] until it becomes a mush, which she has to carry in a piece of wool.

You should know that if a pregnant woman aborts, in most cases it is because of moisture, so you have to provoke vomiting by giving her the resin of fennel[131], also known as *sacauiento*[132]. Also prepare oil of sunflower[133], and [have her] drink two or [15] three dirhems of it every day, but be careful, since if the reason [for the abortion] is feebleness of the womb, caused by a malign temperament, you may be giving the wrong medicine. If she wants to be pregnant again she should wait a long time, but not too long. The man should have sexual relations with her only if both of them desire it, and the proper position is to lift her legs above her head, listen and know [all these things].

On the swelling of the womb[134], which is an illness that causes a woman to resemble one pregnant or swollen with malign water. [20] The causes are malign matter sticking to the womb's skin, or thick winds, which sometimes appear with hard tumors. The reason may also be, as the ancients said, the creation of a formless piece of flesh. The signs resemble those of pregnant women: they do not menstruate, desire [for intercourse] declines, and the breasts inflate. If the cause is dropsy, the abdomen would not be as hard as in pregnancy.

The treatment. You should know that this illness may last for six years or even more. Sometimes it may happen that the woman suf-

---

127 Spanish: *Espicanardi* (*Nardus stricta*, L.). See *Menor daño de la medicina de Alonso de Chirino*, p. 273.

128 Arabic: ناردين (*Valeriana*, L.). *El libro del 'Amal man ṭabba li-man ḥabba*, p. 81.

129 Arabic: بان (*Moringa aptera*, L.). *Ibid.*, p. 13.

130 Arabic: سيرج. *Ibid.*, p. 49.

131 Arabic: سكبينج (*Ferula scowiziana*, L.). *Ibid.*, p. 46.

132 Spanish: *Sacauiento*. See *Menor daño de la medicina de Alonso de Chirino*, p. 299. The same identification is given by Maimonides: سكبينج هو معلوم اسمه بعجمية الاندلس سكا بينة. *L'explication des noms de drogues - un glossaire de matière médicale composé par Maïmonide*, no. 280.

133 Spanish: *Girasol*. See Cobarruvias, *Tesoro de la lengua castellana o española*, p. 641.

134 Arabic: الرحى . See *El libro del 'Amal man ṭabba li-man ḥabba*, pp. 7, 167.

fers the same phenomenon [f. 20v] as in giving birth, accompanied by a fall of water. At times she may give birth to a formless piece of flesh. Some physicians give two reasons for the birth of that piece [of flesh]: the first is that the matter [of the sperm] is poured into the womb with great heat; the second is that it is formed immediately after coitus by the [5] woman's sperm. The woman's sperm does not mix with the man's sperm, and therefore the man's sperm loses its formative power. The woman's sperm enters into the womb, it is nourished there and develops a formless thing. I have been informed by some just women and some midwives, without any lies and falsehoods, that one woman gave birth to three animals resembling quadrupeds[135]; they were alive and they moved. They also informed me of a woman who gave birth, with the aborted foetus, to an animal [10] resembling a snake.[136]

The treatment of this illness must be carried out by purifying her body of the humours with purgative grains and even those stronger than these, the stinking grains. Afterwards use bandages and baths, such as rue oil, narcissus[137] oil and Arabian costus oil, which dissolve the wind. Order them to apply an electuary,[138] which dissolves the wind, such as Indian aloe-tree[139], and a beverage made of fennel[140] seeds, and to drink root water in which castor is melted. If you find thickness, [15] treat it in the same way you would treat hard tumors, with oils, ointments and baths.

Of the electuaries[141], a useful one is the laxative pastille[142]. It would be best if these treatments are sufficient but if not, apply the medicaments which cause menstrual blood to flow and those which abort the dead foetus, such as a compress[143] of Egyptian marjoram[144], [also called] maru[145], and boiled savin[146], which is called *al*

---

[135] Arabic: كرج. See Dozy, *Supplément aux dictionnaires arabes*, vol. II, p. 461.

[136] On Talmudic tradition regarding an abortion of a formless piece of flesh or animals, see *Babylonian Talmud*, Nidda, 21a-24b.

[137] Arabic: نرجس. See note 37.

[138] Arabic: معجون.

[139] Arabic: جواريش العود. See *Tuḥfat al-aḥbâb*, no. 308.

[140] Arabic: شرب سكبينج. *Ibid.*, no. 372.

[141] Arabic: معاجين.

[142] Arabic: معجون لوغاذيا. See *El libro del 'Amal man ṭabba li-man ḥabba*, pp. 13, 167, 170.

[143] See Radicchi, *La Gynaecia di Muscione*, p. 485.

[144] Spanish: *Mentastro* (*Origanum maru*, L.). See *L'explication des noms de drogues - un glossaire de matèire médicale composé par Maïmonide*, no. 235.

abhal [147] in the foreign language. Another medicament is composed of a portion each of [20] myrrh[148], Egyptian marjoram[149] and opopanax[150], to be drunk in celery water or in fennel juice. Order them [the women] to eat food made of meat and perfumed eggs, young pigeons and young cocks fried in a frying pan.

On retention of the foetus and on removing a dead foetus. The cause might be the woman herself, if she is frightened, or too thin or too fat; or the foetus itself, if he is too little, or has a tumor in his mouth, or another ailment, or because [f. 21r] of an organ afflicted by an illness, such as a tumor in the urinary bladder or in the intestine, or for external reasons such as [excessive] cold.

The symptoms. In general, the symptoms of the retention of the foetus are internal pains, by this I mean in the abdomen and in the navel.

The cases which deserve treatment: The woman [5] has to bathe herself when the time of birth is approaching. It is desirable for her to wash her external parts, because the bath weakens [her] force. Anoint the back, and rub the abdomen and the kidneys with wallflower[151] oil, then anoint them with wax and hen fat, and give them [the women] liquids to drink, such as cydonia liquid and linen seed liquid mixed with julep[152]. During the days of her labour, give the woman fenugreek juice to drink and she should eat [10] foods made of meat and eggs with a lot of fat, and when the time of birth approaches, you should satisfy all her needs. Order her to be seated in water in which common melilot[153], maidenhair[154], bran, fenugreek and similar herbs have been boiled. Put sneezing materials in her nose and she must keep her mouth open so as to breath as much air as possible.

---

145 Arabic: المرو. See *ibid*; cf. Issa, *Dictionnaire des noms des plants*, p. 130, no. 4.

146 Spanish: *Sabina* (*Juniperus sabina*, L). See Cobarruvias, *Tesoro de la lengua castellana o Española*, p. 918; *Tuḥfat al-aḥbâb*, no. 26.

147 Arabic: الابهل. *Ibid.*

148 Arabic: مر. See *Tuḥfat al-aḥbâb*, no. 265.

149 Arabic: حبق الشيوخ. See Issa, *Dictionnaire des noms des plants*, p. 130, no. 4.

150 Spanish: *Opoponac*. See note 106.

151 Arabic: الخيري. See note 34.

152 Arabic: جلاب. Issa, *Dictionnaire des noms des plants*, p. 81, no. 14.

153 Arabic: إكليل الملك. See note 109.

154 Arabic: كزبرة البير (*Adiantum capillus veneris*, L.). See *Tuḥfat al-aḥbâb*, no. 65.

If the cause is fatness, you should order the midwife [15] to lay the woman on her back, and put her knees under the woman's hips, to sit on her and to anoint her womb with moistening things such as fat and oil, hen fat or goose fat oil, and to make her sneeze by putting soft wood or twisted papyrus in her nose; this treatment is very useful. If the reason is the size of the foetus, when he begins to emerge the midwife must pull him out gently after washing the area with lukewarm [20] water, and at times with pounded saffron[155]. She has to pull him little by little, until he is outside. If that is impossible, you should cut him [to pieces] or get him out in the way we do with a dead [foetus]. If the cause is a tumor in the womb, the only thing to do is to apply ointments and to treat her the same way as with fat women. If the reason is her feebleness, strengthen her with pleasing smells, and give the woman perfumed boiled meat broth to drink.

If the reason is too thick a placenta[156], which does not break, cut it with your nail or with a scalpel placed between the fingers. If the reason is coldness, [f. 21v] you should bathe her or put her in a very warm house, and seat her in hot water in which penny royal[157] was boiled, and give her the water of the pills[158] to eat with its grains, sesame oil[159] and hen fat, and rub the uterus with warm oil. If the reason is warm air, she should be seated in cold places, and bandaged with cold [5] things. If the reason is the bad presentation of the foetus, the midwife must remove it according to her wisdom.

The medicaments which force out the dead foetus are the following: two dirhems each of myrrh[160], castor and storax[161] , four dirhems cinnamon[162] , [...] dirhems ginger[163]. Another drink: four dirhems the soft part of bread, three dirhems rue leaves, two dir-

---

[155] Arabic: جادي. See Dozy, *Supplément aux dictionnaires arabes*, vol. I, p. 177.

[156] The text states *ém*, i. e., womb.

[157] Arabic: فوليون, originally from the Greek. See *L'explication des noms de drogues - un glossaire de matière médicale composé par Maïmonide*, no. 72.

[158] Spanish: *Pilloras*. See *Menor daño de la medicina de Alonso de Chirino*, p. 294.

[159] Arabic: سيرج. The scribe replaced the Hebrew letter *resh* by a *kaf*. See *El libro del 'Amal man ṭabba li-man ḥabba*, pp. 47, 48, 50.

[160] Arabic: مر. See note 148.

[161] Spanish: *Estoraque*. See note 107.

[162] Spanish: *Canela*. See note 44.

[163] Spanish: *Gingibre* (*Amonum-zingiber*, L.). See *Menor daño de la medicina de Alonso de Chirino*, p. 279. The text does not indicate the quantity to be taken of this plant.

hems[164] myrrh; drink them all with boiled ginger morning and evening.

Description of [10] a suppository which removes the placenta and the dead foetus: equal amounts each of opoponax[165], myrrh[166], black-chameleon[167] and bull's gall, pounded and kneaded; then shape it in the form of a date. She should carry it; then fumigate her with myrrh and make her sneeze with soap root[168].

In case the woman has given birth or aborted, and has not been cleaned of the blood, the proper treatment is to provoke sneezing and to fumigate her with mustard, *bakaleum* [169] and myrrh. If this treatment does not help her, let blood from the saphena[170] vein, or from under the knee, and give her to drink those things [20] which provoke menstrual blood. When a considerable quantity of blood has flown, it would be proper to place upon her clothes made of linen immersed in vinegar. She should also carry suppositories[171] made of pomegranate[172], caper[173], rose and frankincense mixed with wine.

On suffocation of the uterus, which is an illness similar to *sar'*[174], that is epilepsy, [except that] it is periodic. The cause. The cause of this [20] illness is the remains of sperm which have lost its warmth and become poisonous, or menstrual blood from both, [causing a] poisonous vapour to ascend to the heart and the brain. The case itself indicates whether the cause is the sperm, in which case there is a great deal of vapour, but not a lack of menstrual blood. [In this case the woman also suffers] from intense fainting, which occurs long after coitus, and great sexual desire.

---

[164] The scribe omitted the quantity.

[165] Spanish: *Opoponaco*. See note 101.

[166] Arabic: مر.

[167] *Labrun* (*Cameleunta nigra*, L.). See *Platéarius, Le livre des simples médecines*, pp. 333, 320.

[168] Arabic: كندس (*Gypsophilla struthium*, L.). See *Tuḥfat al-aḥbâb*, no. 225; Issa, *Dictionnaire des noms des plants*, p. 90, no. 14.

[169] I could not identify this term.

[170] Arabic: الصافن.

[171] Arabic: شيافات pl. form of شياف. On the different varieties of this type of suppository, see *El libro del 'Amal man ṭabba li-man ḥabba*, pp. 52-53.

[172] Spanish: *Balaustia*. See *Menor daño de la medicina de Alonso de Chirino*, p. 257.

[173] Arabic: كاربا, called usually كهربا, it is the resin of *Populis nigra*, L. See *L'explication des noms de drogues - un glossaire de matière médicale composé par Maïmonide*, no. 199.

[174] Arabic: صرع.

The treatment. [22r] The difference between this illness and epilepsy is that in this case the woman feels as if ants are moving from her uterus to the upper part of her body; if this sensation is strong, she may lose consciousness, and if it endures, the woman may appear to be dead and without breath, and at times she might experience this sensation [of ants moving] in the kidneys.

The method of curing this illness is to let blood from the saphena vein. [5] If the woman feels heat as if a fire were in her womb, caused by the remaining blood and a black humour[175], you should purify the abdomen with boiled embelic myrobalan[176], polypody[177] and an electuary[178] of lepidium. At times you should use absinthe[179] and then apply a treatment that provokes menstrual blood, such as boiled roots with oximel[180] and seeds, and then order her to put in a suppository with a small quantity of galia[181] and spourge[182], which are wonderful for provoking [menstruation]. Then seat her in water in which there were boiled [10] pennyroyal[183], linen seed and sweet-marjoram[184]. [Have her insert] another suppository made of storax, pepper and anise[185] oil, and prescribe light food such as fowl.

And those which provoke menstrual blood, such as pills[186], asparagus[187] and black grains, which have a [magical] virtue, and put cinnamon[188], cumin and mastic[189] in her food. If the cause is the

---

175 Arabic: سوداء.

176 Spanish: *Mirabolano* (*Phyllanthus emblica*, L.). See *Menor daño de la medicina de Alonso de Chirino*, p. 289.

177 Spanish: *Polipodio* (*Polypodium vulgare*, L.). *Ibid.*, p. 295.

178 Spanish: *Letuario* = Electuarium. *Ibid.*, pp. 282-283.

179 Arabic: افسنتين (*Arthemysia absinthium*, L.). See *L'explication des noms de drogues - un glossaire de matière médicale composé par Maïmonide*, no. 3.

180 Arabic: شرب سكنجبين. See note 62.

181 Arabic: غالية. See *El libro del 'Amal man ṭabba li-man ḥabba*, p. 60.

182 Arabic: افربيون, is the resin of *Euphorbiae resinifera*, L. See *L'explication des noms de drogues - un glossaire de matière médicale composé par Maïmonide*, no. 25.

183 Arabic: فودنج (*Mentha pulegium*, L.). See *Tuḥfat al-aḥbâb*, no. 325.

184 Arabic: مرددوش (*Origanum majorana*, L.). *Ibid.*, no. 253.

185 Spanish: *Anís* (*Pimpinela anisum*, L.).

186 The term that appears in the Hebrew text is probably a distortion of the Spanish: *Pildoras*, See note 122.

187 Spanish: *Esparragera* and *esparrago*. See *Menor daño de la medicina de Alonso de Chirino*, p. 273.

188 Spanish: *Canela*. See note 44.

189 Arabic: مصطكى, the gum made of *Pistacia lentiscus*, L. See *Tuḥfat al-aḥbâb*, no. 251.

sperm, the proper treatment for [15] her is to have sexual relations. If this is not possible for her, she should apply drying things such as a cumin electuary[190], and the midwife should place it in her womb after anointing her fingers with laurel oil and ebony[191] oil. The midwife should massage here and there for a long time, hoping that the woman will, as a result, emit cold sperm and immediately feel better, or make a complete recovery. Also prepare for her a suppository made of ginger[192], pepper and rue; it would also be useful to apply a compound [20] medicament[193].

Indeed, a proper way to treat the woman, when the illness is grave and she is lying down as one dead and breathless, is to pour a good smelling oil on her such as ebony[194] oil, and to tightly tie her knees and her hands, and strengthen her with galia[195]. Then order the midwife to massage the orifice of her womb with the materials mentioned above, or to use galia with ebony[196] oil and to fumigate her from below with *laniya*[197], cowpea[198] and [f. 22v] musk. Make her sneeze with soap-root[199], order her to cry loudly and give her some wine to drink in order to strengthen her, and give her hen soup to eat. In case the illness is not difficult, treat her only with oils.

A chapter on a surplus of menstruation. The menstrual blood may flow [abundantly], and [5] this ailment is called loss of blood[200]. The cause may be the uterus itself or bruises found within it, or because its veins are open or because it is weak. Another reason is the blood, if it is in abundance or because it is too thin. If bruises and consumption are the cause, the signs are paroxysm[201], extraction of venomous matter and a blackness of the blood. The signs of surplus blood are redness of the white parts of the body and her face

---

190 Arabic: معجون الكمون.

191 Arabic: ابنوس (*Ebenus*, L.). Issa, *Dictionnaire des noms des plants*, p.73, no. 2.

192 Arabic: زنجبيل. See note 41.

193 Arabic: دواء مسك. On this medicament, see *El libro del 'Amal man ṭabba li-man ḥabba*, pp. 100, 102, 106.

194 Arabic. See note 191.

195 Arabic: غالية. See note 181.

196 Arabic. See note 191.

197 I could not identify the term.

198 Arabic: اللوبيا (*Dolichos lubiya*, L.). See *Tuḥfat al-aḥbâb*, no.16.

199 Arabic: كندس. See note 168.

200 Arabic: نزف.

201 Arabic: نوب.

red. If the cause is diluted blood, the signs are [10] a greenness of that [which normally is] white and watery blood.

The treatment. You should know that the period of menstruation is in some cases three days and at most six days. When its duration is more than this period of time, it is considered an illness called "loss of blood"[202]. The remedy for bruises of the uterus are constraining medicaments; if the cause is open veins, treat them with [15] constraining and strengthening things such as the following remedy: [Take] antimony and the remains found in myrtle water, put them in wool and order her to carry it almost constantly, day and night. The useful things to treat sharpness of the blood and its dilution are waybread water with a beverage made of cydonia; it is also useful to drink vinegar.

[A remedy] to strengthen and constrain the openings of the veins, also useful for treating the warmth of [20] the blood and its dilution: [Give her to] drink two dirhems of burnt porcelain[203] [mixed] in sumach[204] and cydonia water. It is useful to treat hot blood accompanied by a very hot temperament by drinking pine resin[205] with an apple beverage. It would be useful in both cases to make a compress[206] with curdled cydonia[207] or a cydonia beverage[208]. Also [apply] the following compresses: a quarter dirhem each of "sealed bole"[209], Armenian bole[210], aloe, resin of gall-oak[211], and resin of dragon-tree, the weight of two grains of camphor[212] and [23r] one

---

[202] Arabic: نزف.

[203] Spanish: *Porcelanas*. See Cobarruvias, *Tesoro de la lengua castellana o Española*, p. 877.

[204] Arabic: سماك (*Rhus coriaria*, L.). See *Tuḥfat al-aḥbâb*, no. 368.

[205] Spanish: *Calafonia*. See *Menor daño de la medicina de Alonso de Chirino*, p. 259.

[206] Latin: *Trochiscus*. In Muscio's *Gynaecia*, *trocisci* were also used to cure genital bruises and bleeding. See Radicchi, *La Gynaecia di Muscione*, pp. 110, 134.

[207] Arabic: روب.

[208] Arabic: شراب.

[209] Latin: *Bolus sigillatus*. "Terre sigillée. Elle doit son nom ce que ... on la marquait d'un secau pour l'exporter. La terre scellée est une de ces terres argileuses appelées 'bols' dont usait l'ancienne pharmacie. Connue plus tard sous le nom de 'terre de Lemnos' ou 'terre sigillée', c'est du carbonate d'alumine." *Platéarius, Le livre des simples médecines*, p. 349-350.

[210] Latin: *Bolus armenicus*. Also called: *Bolus orientalis*. See *ibid.*, p. 319.

[211] Latin: *Galla*. See Radicchi, *La Gynaecia di Muscione*, p. 373.

[212] Arabic: كافور. The resin of *Laurus camphora*, L. See *Tuḥfat al-aḥbâb*, no.212.

dirhem of liquid musk. Put all these into myrtle beverage[213], give her this mixture to drink continuously, and it will help.

If the haemorrhage[214] is very serious, you must treat it with a clyster made of waybread grains[215] with acacia and resin of dragon-tree. The woman should eat lentils with vinegar and hens in sumach[216] water. If the cause is a surplus of blood, you have to let blood from the basilicon[217] vein, and to purify the blood with the water of purslane seed and a pomegranate beverage[218].

If the reason is thinness of blood resulting from an increase in yellow bile[219], you have to purify the yellow bile with the proper means; it is useful to sit in water, in which pomegranate peels, carob and flowers of the male pomegranate[220] have been boiled; [you may also add] galia[221] and ebony[222] oil, and fumigate her from below with *laniya*, cowpea[223] and musk.

Listen and know **on the retention of menstrual blood and its diminution**. The cause: The cause may be in the uterus, such as a cold or a dry bad temperament, or if it is closed, or if a tumor is found in it, or if the orifices of the veins [are closed], or because of other organs, such as a feebleness of the liver, or if the body is too lean or too fat, or because of a chronic illness, or a scantiness of blood in the body, or a dryness of the veins, or a thickness of the blood, usually because it is mixed with a thick humour[224].

In case the reason is coldness, its signs are a whiteness of the body and a small quantity of menses. Coldness of the body demonstrates that the cause is dryness of the uterus and leanness; if the cause is a weakness of the liver, the signs would be appropriate to [a condition of] weakness of the liver. And in the same manner, when the cause is a blockage, the signs would be of a blockage.

---

213 Arabic: شراب.
214 Arabic: النزف.
215 Arabic: حب [?].
216 Arabic: سماك, see note 204.
217 Arabic: الباسليق.
218 Arabic: شراب.
219 Arabic: الصفراء.
220 Spanish: *Balustias* or *Balostias*. See *Menor daño de la medicina de Alonso de Chirino*, p. 257.
221 Arabic: غالية. See note 181.
222 Arabic: ابنوس. See note 191.
223 Arabic: اللوبيا. See note 198.
224 Arabic: خلط.

On the treatment. You should know that some women, by their nature, never have any menstrual blood all their lives, or they have only very little. Those women resemble men by the thickness of their flesh, the abundance of their hair and the width of their belly. You should not treat this kind of woman in any way. When the cause is a blockage of the uterus' openings, the remedy is in the medicaments which open the closure, such as a root beverage or a squill[225] beverage. It is also beneficial to apply suppositories which draw the blood, but act cautiously, since the area might become [too] warm. [Take] four dirhems each of myrrh[226] and horse mint, eight dirhems of ginger, ten dirhems of dried rue and four dirhems of dried and seedless grapes. Knead them all in bull gall and make a suppository.

This is the treatment you should use in cases of blockage or coldness, but not in the case of a bad cold temperament in the uterus. To treat a bad cold temperament and the contraction of the uterus' orifices, it is useful to drink the following medicament: six dirhems each of opopanax[227], drosera[228] and cassia, drunk in boiled horsemint juice. Also prepare [a medicament] in the form of a date from the following materials: musk, castor, and myrrh, mixed in ebony oil; [then] place it in the womb.

To provoke menstrual blood, use the following medicament: an equal quantity each of kali[229], which is called soap-herb[230] in the foreign language, pellitory[231], astragal[232], rue and euphorbia, pound and knead them [together]; she should carry it in wool, immersed in jasmine[233] oil. If the reason is a hard tumor, we must pre-

---

225 Arabic: إشقيل (*Scilla maritima*, L.). See *Tuḥfat al-aḥbâb*, no.31.

226 Spanish: *Mirra*. See *Menor daño de la medicina de Alonso de Chirino*, p. 289.

227 Spanish: *Opoponaco*. See note 106.

228 The scribe probably distorted the term. It should read *Droseras*, also called *Herba sole* (*Drosera rotundifolia*, L.). See *Platarius, Le livre des simples médecines*, pp. 325-326.

229 Arabic: اشنان. See *Tuḥfat al-aḥbâb*, no. 38.

230 Spanish: *Yerva xabonera*. See Cobarruvias, *Tesoro de la lengua castellana o Española*, p. 1014. The Spanish term refers to a plant; the Hebrew author, however, was referring to a mineral.

231 Spanish: *Palitaria*. See *Menor daño de la medicina de Alonso de Chirino*, p. 292.

232 Arabic: إشخيص (*Atractylis gummifera*, L.). See *Tuḥfat al-aḥbâb*, no. 52.

233 Arabic: زنبق. The Arabic term was used for both the plant (*Jasminum officinale*, L.) and the oil produced from it. See. *ibid*, no. 138.

pare emollient oils and fat, and softening clysters[234]. If the reason is thick blood, caused by fatness [of the woman], it seems to me that in this case she would nevertheless have little [menstrual flow] [20], so the woman has to be continuously treated with thick [materials] like rocket[235] and fennel[236], which [provide] strength. Also treat her continuously with the following boiled preparation: two ounces of jujube[237], four rush[238], five pills[239], two dirhems celery seed, two dirhems red[240] colour[241] and five ginger grains. Boil and filter them and mix with an oximel beverage[242] made of seeds. It is also useful to prepare suppositories of wool immersed in ebony[243] oil, and to fumigate her with materials which help to discharge blood, like a fumigation made of vitriol[244] and ammoniac.

If [f. 24r] the cause is a small amount of blood, you should help her by giving her food that generates blood. If the cause is weakness of the liver, she has to be nourished by things which strengthen the [5] liver. Finished and completed.[245]

[f. 24v, line 21] **The signs of uterine surplus**. Uterine surplus means that there is an excess of three humours in the cavity. **In case of an excess of white humour**[246], the signs are: a wet womb and the woman does not enjoy sexual relations. Everything cold is harmful and everything warm is useful, such as a hot bath and the like. Even if [f. 25r] they desire sexual relations, men do not desire these

---

234 Latin: *Clysteris*.

235 Arabic: جرجير (*Eruca sativa*, L.). See *Tuḥfat al-aḥbâb*, no. 95.

236 Arabic: رازيانج. The scribe has omited the letter *zayin*; the plant is *Foeniculum vulgare*, L. See *ibid.*, no. 358.

237 Spanish: *Jujubas*. See *Menor daño de la medicina de Alonso de Chirino*, p. 281-282.

238 French: *Paille*. On its medical uses in the Middle Ages, see *Platéarius, Le livre des simples médecines*, pp. 331, 340; *Tuḥfat al-aḥbâb*, no. 34.

239 Spanish: *Pildoras*. The author does not specify the kind of pills.

240 Spanish: *Roja*.

241 The scribe omitted the name of the ingredient.

242 Arabic: شراب سكنجبين.

243 Arabic: ابنوس. See note 191.

244 Arabic: القلقطار. There are several *atramenta* divided according to their colour, see *Tuḥfat al-aḥbâb*, no. 144.

245 The original treatise ends at this point. The compilator of the codex added some additional prescriptions (f. 24r-24v) and a chapter on uterine surplus (f. 24v-25r). This last part is of interest because of the medical treatments it includes; I have attached it as a continuation of the original text.

246 In contrast to the previous treatise, in the present text all medical terms appear in Hebrew, although the author occasionally also adds their Greek synonyms.

women because they are excessively wet. They suffer from pain and difficulty under the navel; and coldness emerges from inside, and the orifice of her womb is very wet. Also, her menstrual blood is mixed with other humours because of an excess of white humour, and it is also mixed with dirty matter similar to mucus. Her urine loses its red colour *[sic]* and becomes fat or white [5] or tends to whiteness.

At times those humours are mixed with breath, as happens in the case of uterine suffocation. She suffers from a weakness of the heart, which is called *syncopis*, and headache, so that she cannot bend her head to her knees. At times it causes women to inflate with water, an illness which is called *aganos* and *hydropsis*.

On an excess of black humour. Its signs are the following: the women do not enjoy sexual relations, nor do men enjoy having relations with them. The women have small amounts of sperm and after [coitus] they feel pain, difficulty and a spreading sensation coming from their depths. At times, the signs of the black humour are similar to those of uterine suffocation, and she may feel heart exhaustion, called *syncopis*. Coldness is felt about the womb and near to its orifice, and [at times] panic and senselessness as well. Her menstrual blood is of a small quantity and malign; it tends to blue [15] because it is mixed with the black humour. Her urine is thin and acidic, at times it is fat, and its colour tends toward blue.

On an excess of red humour in the womb. These are the signs: acute and sharp pain, dryness and hardness, warmth around the womb's orifice; she desires and very much enjoys sexual relations. But when the humour is of a great quantity, her sexual desire diminishes although the pain [20] continues. In addition, the men enjoy being with them more than with other women [because] these women are quick to ejaculate, but in small quantities. Their excrement is small in quantity and its colour is yellow. They [the women] feel bites around the uterus' orifice, their urine is red or reddish or yellow, and their lips are dry and cracked. We have mentioned sufficient signs of the excess of humours.

GALEN'S BOOK ON THE WOMB, WHICH IS CALLED GENICIAS[1]

Jews' College, Ms. Montefiore, 440, fol. 53v-59v.

ספר האם אל גאלינוס הוא הנקרא גניסיאש[2]. הקדמתי אני לראות דבר מועיל לכתוב לכם מרב התחלואים המשתנים אשר יקרו תמיד באם ויש מהם קשים אשר לא יוכלו [5] להרפא בעבור שהן מתבישות לגלותם. ויש מהם אשר יתרפאו בהיותם קלים להרפא. על כן באתי להורות עזר לכלם בהקדמת האותות[3] לפני כל אשר מהם לפתוח [P. 5] דרך ולגלות מה שהצניעות והבושת מכסה[4] ומעלים בהם[5] בעזרת[6] האל.

מתנועת האם. בהיות האם נעה יחול שם כאב ומקרים [10] קשים ורעים. ואם מהר לא יעזר להם יעשו[7] נגעים שם. ואם היא מונחת תחת הצלעות יולד שם מצוק. גם יולד שם כאב גדול ללב. גם אסטניסות. ולפעמים יעשה רוקה כמו חומץ ופיה מלא מים. ושוקיה קרים וראשה ולשונה יופרפו אליה הוא כרופמי גולד[8]. [15] ואפס קולה בסבת כל המקרים האלה. העזר יאות להניח תחת האם צמר כרוך בבגד[9] לבן וטבול בַשֲמִי. או בשמן טוב וערב. ולהריח לאפיה נשים אֲשפַלטוֹס. ובהיותו רך הוא [P.10] טוב יותר. ותעורר אליה אסטניסות[10] עם קרן עזה שחורה. או עם שוקי האיל או עם נוצה טבולה בחומץ. ותשים להריח

---

[1] As indicated above, this is the Hebrew translation of the Latin text *De passionibus mulierum*. For comparison, I used Monica Green's draft edition. It is possible that once the Latin edition, with all variants, is completed, we will be able to determine which Latin version was used by the Hebrew translator. I am indebted to Monica Green, not only for being the first to identify the Hebrew text with the DPM B, but also for permitting me to use her draft edition.

[2] Parma manuscrit (P): אופיסיאס

[3] P: אותות

[4] P: שהצנועות ומבויישות מכסות

[5] P: ומועילים

[6] P: בעזר

[7] P: מהר יעזר להם ועשו

[8] P: פרומיגולא

[9] P: +לבן וטבול

[10] P: אסטנסות

לאפיה דבר המעטיש. וכאשר תוכל לדבר[11] תתן לה לשתות קשתור[12] עם יין חם. ותשים לאפיה האצבעות טבולים בשמן. והצמר[13] הנזכר יהיה שם לבל תסירהו[14] עד שתתרפא[15]. כי אם תסירהו[16] ישוב החולי שם. על כן נכון להניחו פעמים רבות.

[f. 54r] **ממצוקת האם** או תהיה[17] לה השתטות[18] כאב בצידי הערוה הם אְנגֶש[19]. אז יכאב אליה בתוך המקוה גם יעצר השתן וירפרפו שוקיה [P. 15] גם יכאבו. העזר תשים לאפיה כל דבר אשר ריחו טוב כמו מירא. ולאם כל דבר אשר ריחו רע שתקטירה[20] בם עד שתתרפא. מן האם הליחה[21]. בהיות רב ליחות האם יכאבו עיניה וראשה נוטה לחום וחלש כאלו הולך אליה[22] בגלגל. העזר לזאת תעשה מוך בענין זה תקח שמן אווז חמאה אניש כתוש לאבק[23]. ותניחהו לה[24] בצמר או בבגד פשתים וזה יטהר כל תחלואי האם.

מנפח האם ואם[25] יכאבו מקומות סתריה או תרגיש [P. 20] נשיכות ברחם בהתחברה עם זכר אז תדע כי האם נפוחה ויותר בפנים. והאות על זה הוא[26] כי יכאבו אליה קצות[27] העינים ופניה מאדמים יותר ממכורכמים. ומזה החולי מתבישות[28] לרופאים. העזר תקח חלב אשה אשר ילדה זכר ותערב אותו עם שמן ורד בד בבד ותחמם אותו ותעשה מוך מצמר רך ותטבול אותו שם ותשימה עד[29] ראש הרחם. עזר אחר תכתוש מעט גַלבְנום ותערב אותו עם שמן וורד ותועיל[30]. מן [P. 25] התולעים הם הנקראים לוֹמְבְריקש[31]. הם[32] יכאבו אליה צידי הרחם אז תתבונן כי יש אליה תולעים עגולים רצים תמיד במעים וברחם על כן

---

11 P: וכאשר אין יכולה
12 P: קשטורו
13 P: והנצמר
14 P: תסרירם
15 P: שתרפא
16 P: תסירמו
17 P: יהיה
18 P: השטטחות
19 P: אנגיס
20 P: שתקטיר
21 P: הלחה
22 P: -
23 P: + דק
24 P: -
25 P: אם
26 P: היא
27 P: קצוות
28 P: + להגיד
29 P: ותשימהו על
30 P: ורד ויועיל
31 P: לומריצי
32 P: אם

מתאוות להתגרד[33] מאד הבטן והגוף וליחת הגוף תזל עד שתדמה[34] כמו מֶרַבְּמַס[35] היא הזלת הקרירות. העזר תקח שרש אִירִיס[36] כתושה היטב ותערב שם מיץ אַגִילֶנְט. ומיץ רמון ומזה תעשה אליה מוך. וכאשר יהיו התולעים[37] העגולים באם והם מתקרבים אליה דרך מעי אחד[38] אז יחול [P. 30] אליה עיות הבטן רב וזיעה[39] עבה עד שהזיעה ההיא [f. 54v] תתקשה אליה מאד. והנה תעזור אליה עם אותו[40] המיץ עצמו כאשר נעשה לה[41] טבול נמוך[42].

מנפח האם. אם נפח או זה חולי יחל לעשות[43] באם אז[44] יעלה נפח בדדיה ויתקשו[45] מאד. ושב מראה פניה כעין תכלת. [5] וסובלת כאב כל זמן עד כלות החולי מן האם ואז יתרפא הבא[46] מעט מעט. ועל כן יש מהן אשר לא[47] תזרענה ומגען קשה מאד. גם קודם אכילה נדחה רוח חמוץ דרך גרונם [P. 35] כבד וקשה מאד לסבול ואבד מהם חפץ כל אוכל ותדמו[48] בנפשם כאלו[49] הם מלאות. העזר תקשיר[50] ותטבול האם עם טבול שמן[51] ומים ומעט דבש ואחר [5] כן תקח יין עם [P. 46v] מירטיל בשומן אווז ותרחץ שם רגליה תמיד.

עוד מנפח האם. הנשים לאשר ירד לחות האם אל הרחם יהיו גופיהם[52] קר ואין להם חפץ ממשכבי זכר כי גופיהם קר בפנים עד החלקים האחרונים. העזר תקח קלפת עץ פין גטלש בשוה ותכתוש[53] הכל יחד ויטבלו גופם בזה בפנים וזה ראוי לעשות [15] יום אחד ולדלג יום אחד אחר כן תבשל לנטישקלי והדס[54] עם יין אדום ותטבול[55] ממנו בערב

33 P: + תמיד
34 P: - תזל עד ש...
35 P: + כל כך תיזול
36 P: איריס
37 P: עגולים
38 P: + עגול
39 P: זיעה
40 P: זה
41 P: -
42 P: במוך
43 P: לעלות
44 P: או
45 P: ויתקשרו
46 P: הכאב
47 P: מהן שלא
48 P: ותידמו
49 P: כאילו
50 P: תקטיר
51 P: + וכאת
52 P: גופם
53 P: ותיכתוש
54 P: + ותערב
55 P: ותייחל

עד שתתחמם[56] ויכסו אותה היטב במקומה משם. [P. 5] ואם רוצה[57] להזדוג עם איש לא תחזיק[58] הרפואה הזאת ממנה לבלתי התמידה.

עזר אחר אל הלחות היורדות מן האם והבטן. תקח סיבי[59] הברזל הוא הנקרא קַאקַאפר ותכתוש [20] אותו לאבק ותערבהו עם חומץ ותעסיהו לו כמוך[60].

מן קרנק האם. אם יולד קרנק לאחת מן הנשים באם אז ידמה אליה כאלו יש לה עץ או קוץ בגוף. ולפעמים יצא משם דם בכאב רב מאין[61] שיעור. העזר תקח רודא[62] מדברית. אלום קרוע. ניטרי[63] ותכתוש הכל ותשים לה [P. 10] תחבושת. וזה טוב לכל חולי ולכל נגע קרנק באם ובשאר מקומות הגוף. אחר [f. 55r] כן תשים אליה מיץ שוֹלַטְרֵי[64] עם שומן אווז בשוה ותרגיל ממנו במוך. גם לכל כאב הנשים תקח מיץ פוֹרְ[65] ותערב אותו בשוה עם שמן גיליאַני ותרגיל בו. גם אל קרנק תכתוש רַפֵּא הוא המחודד[66] ותערבנו עם דבש ותליחנו[67] לה ויועיל מאד.

מן פלקמון[68] זה החולי הנקרא [5] כן נולד באם. ובסבתו יולדו קדחות חדות לנשים ונפח הבטן וקשיו וכאב הכליות. גם חולי [P. 15]אחר מן האצטו' הנקרא אְנַאטְרוֹפַּא[69].

ומצוק הבא מליחה חמוצה[70] או מן האדומה היא[71] קוֹלֵירָא[72] ועצור השתן גם הבטן. וקיא וצמאון ונחור הלשון וצבעה כצבע אַרַמֵנְט[73] וכאב הצואר גם העינים יכאבו. וקצוי האצבעות והצפרנים. ואם האצבע מונח [10] בערותה תרגיש כאב גדול שם ויובש וקושי ועצור וסתימה בפי האם.

העזר תמזוג חמאה ומוח[74] איל בשקל שוה ביין ותרגיל בו. גם הנפוחות ואשר אין יכולת להשתין תמזוג בשוה. שומן אווז [P. 20] וְאַרְדוּרַא גִינִיש[75] ותכרוך שם הצמר[76] ותניח אליה.

---

[56] P: שיתחמם
[57] P: -
[58] P: תרחיק
[59] P: סיגי
[60] P: ותכניסהו לה במוך
[61] P: באין
[62] P: רוטא
[63] P: -
[64] P: סולאטרי
[65] P: עורו
[66] P: + מאד
[67] P: ותניחנו
[68] P: פליקמון
[69] P: אנא טרופא
[70] P: -
[71] P: הנקרא
[72] P: קולרא
[73] P: איריאנט
[74] P: עם מוח

מוך אחר לתנועת האם ולנפח ולמוקד[77] הנקרא אִנְגְנִס שַׁקְרוֹס[78]. ואל הקדחות הפשוטות ואל אִיפוֹפְטֶשְׂיס[79] ולמחשך העינים ולנשיכות[80] הגוף עוזר[81] להפלא. תקח דונג מוח איל[82] דרכמו׳ טרבנטינא[83] מוח אווז ד׳ דרכמו׳ אופי אובוליש ב׳ דרכמו׳. ועם שמן שיפריש תעשו ותתקנו המוך. מוך אחר זה[84] טוב לכל מחלת[85] האם. תקח שומן חזירה שלא ילדה ותמסוך אותו עם דבש [P. 25]ותעשה המוך ותרגיל בו אחרי צאתה מן המרחץ ויועיל מאד.

ממצוקת האם. זה יקרה להן מהתמדתן להפיל או מצער לידה או ברב עציקת[86] דם נדתה[87] או בנפח האם. וכל פעם שתעלה האם עד כנגד החזה יציק להן עד אשר תשכבון נטויות למות. והיו אלה אותותיו בעלות האם עד החזה והם נופלות ושלא מדעת ובאין[88] הרגש ותתאלמנה שפתותיהן וחורקות שיניהן[89] ולפעמים ידיהן[90] ורגליהם לא ינועו ולפעמים [P. 30] שוכבות ישרות שהקרבים[91] נפוחות[92]. גם הקרב העליון הנקרא [f. 55v] טוֹרק וכבד[93] מאד. ומקורות מצחם נפוחים וזיעה קרה תזל מן המצח והפנים ולא נמצא להם שום דפק כי אם מזער וקצר מאד. ולפעמים שבות מאד[94] ומתאמצות ויודעות מה שעבר עליהן[95]. ולפעמים אינם יודעות מאומה וסובלות כאב הראש והצואר מאד. העזר בנפול האשה בחולי הזה[96] יתכן להשכיבה במטה מוצעת בחמה ולא[97] בבית אפל אך שיזרח האור שם. ולהגביה מראשותיה וידיה ורגליה [P. 47r] שטוחים. ולהניע תמיד פניה גם לחמם פניה במים חמים לאט בבגד דק

75 P: ואנדרגינש
76 P: צמר
77 P: ולנח ולדוס
78 P: אנגאנא שקרוס
79 P: איפושטשיס
80 P: ולינשכות
81 P: עזר אחר
82 P: + ד
83 P: טרמינטינא
84 P: הוא
85 P: מחלות
86 P: ברוב עצירת
87 P: נידותה
88 P: ואין
89 P: ותאלמנה שפתותיהם והורקות שיניהם
90 P: ידיהם
91 P: והקרבים
92 P: נפוחים
93 P: טוראק כבד
94 P: -
95 P: עליהם
96 P: זה
97 P: וחמה ואל

ואם תבארך[98] שלא תדבר תמהר לשום כוסות המציצה על גב הערוה ובצדי[99] הם אנגש ותטיף מים חמים [10] בפיה לאט ותמזוג בהם מולשא. גם תניעה תנועת נחת במטת התינוקות היא בריץ[100]. וכאשר תשוב רוח אליה והיא עיפה מאד באין שהות תקנוה[101]. וביום השלישי תעזור אליה במשיחות [P. 5] שמן ומיצים ואחרי המשיחה תאכילה מאכל דק ודקיק ותאמצה היום ומחרתו ואולם היום ומחרתו[102].

ואולם בכל יום תרגיל אליה מיני תחבושת וחמום [15] ורכוכים רכים[103] ופשוטים. גם רחיצות ושינוי מאכלים ערבים ויין דק וטוב. ואם ישוב החולי להיות קרוניקא[104] ואשר יתמידה תמיד ירגיל[105] אליה העזר הנזכר ולהניעה תנועת נחת ויושר ולגרד קצותיה בידים לאט. ולהרגיל אליה סִינָא פִּישְׁמִי[106]. ואם כל אלה זה לא יועיל אליה יאות להוליכה בים וביבשה כמו בגרות[107] ולרחוץ במים חמים תמיד. [20] והרופאים[108] צוו להריח לאפיהן כל דבר בלוי וכל דבר נבאש. והיו עושים הקטרה למצוקת האם להשיב להן[109] [P. 10] הדבור ולעורר אותן[110]. גם את זה תעשה פִּיוסֶדָנִי[111] ו׳ דרכמי׳ גַלְבְנוֹס[112] קשתור[113] יב׳ אישְׁקרוֹפולש[114] ויא׳ גרגרים פלפל. ומעט אוֹפוֹ בָלשַׁמוֹס[115] ותשים גלבנום בחומץ טוב[116]. ושאר הדברים תכתוש ותערב היטב שילחלח. ובעת הצורך תקח מזה שעור לוז ותניח על גחלים מהבהבים ותריח [f. 56r] לאפיה.

מהשטחות[117] **האם והנפח**. זה יקרה תחת הטבור[118] מעט גם כאב הבטן והכליות ומחוש הראש והאסטוי׳ ועצור השתן גם תעורה [P. 15] ונשיכות. ואינן יכולות להטהר מנדתן[119] ובשום האצבע שם נמצאת [5]

---

[98] P: תתארך השתיקה
[99] P: הסתר
[100] P: ברץ ובלשון קלבריאה נאך
[101] P: הקזה
[102] P: - ואולם היום ומחרתו
[103] P: רבים
[104] P: קורוניקא
[105] P: נרגיל
[106] P: סילא פשימי
[107] P: בנירות
[108] P: + הקדמוני׳
[109] P: להם
[110] P: אתהן
[111] P: פיאטרוני
[112] P: גלאבנום
[113] P: קשטורו
[114] P: אשקרופולי
[115] P: אופן בלסמוש
[116] P: -
[117] P: מהשטטחות
[118] P: טיבור
[119] P: מנידותן

האם נפוחה. והעזר הנכון על זה ככל הכתוב על חמום האם באין תוספות ומגרעת. מנפח[120] האם והבטן. זה יקרה בסבת קרירות או שהפילה או נשאר שם הדם מקובץ ועל כן שבה נפוחה עד שנתמלא הבטן. והיה הנפח אשר בנעוץ[121] עליו האצבעות יניח מקום ומיד ישוב לאחור גם בהכות עליו האצבעות[122] ירים קול כמו תוף. ולפעמים ירוץ הקבוץ[123] [10] [P. 20] ולא ינוע. גם לפעמים יניח מקום. ובראותך האותות האלה תעזור[124] כן. העזר. תעשה כל הנזכר על עצור וחמום האם גם המילדת או האשה החכמה תשתדל להוציא לחוץ כל אותו קבוץ הדם בלא היזק. וכאשר יקרה הנפח להיות קרוֹנִיקָא אז נרגיל לה[125] הדברים הנזכרים במצוקת הרחם הם הנקראים מֶטַשִׁין קְרֶיטִיקָאש אז[126] נניח [P. 25] שם מיני תחבושות [15] אשר האחד נקרא אַשְׁטֵיאָה והאחר נקרא פוֹלְיאַרְגֶיאוֹן והאחר דִיאשפֵירמַטוֹן[127] וזה נעשה עם המים באשר נתבשל פוליג[128] מרובי ואגודת אזוב ועלי לַבְרֵיר ואחרי הבשול הזה[129] נעשה לה טבול הוא אֵנַקאטִישְׁמֵי[130]. ומוך העשוי כן רודא ניטרי פוליג[131] מרת הפר ובהתחבר כל אלה יושם אליה במוך. מוך אחר תקח תאנים כתושים היטב עד שלא [20] יתראה בהן[132] כמון ב' דרכמו' אפרוניט דרכמי' וזכור כי כל מוך שהוא חמוץ[133] כאשר [P. 30] יהיה כרוך בצמר יתכן להעבירו[134] בשמן או בחלב. גם נניח בחלקים ההם כוסות המציצה הם מֵיטַאשִׁין קריטיקאש[135]. ונמשוך בחוזקה[136] הנה והנה ונביא אתהן בכח. ונרגילה במים חמים ובסוף[137] קרים.

מן הנפח הנקרא טומור בהיות החולי הזה באם יהיה הקושי תחת הטבור[138] עם נפח. [f. 56v] וכאשר תנעוץ[139] אצבעה על הנפח יפול

120 P: מנגע
121 P: בניעוץ
122 P: ידים
123 P: + הנה והנה גם נשיכות ועוות הבטן ולפעמים יעמוד הקיבוץ
124 P: + לה
125 P: -
126 P: או
127 P: דיאשפרמאטן
128 P: נבשל פולייו
129 P: -
130 P: אנקטימש
131 P: P: פולגי
132 P: בהם
133 P: חומץ
134 P: להעביר
135 P: מטאשין קרישקש
136 P: בהקזת
137 P: ובחרך
138 P: הטיבור
139 P: תעוץ

ובשהות מועט ישוב. ועור הבטן אינו[140] בצבע הראוי לו. ובנעוץ האצבעות בעור יצא אחריהם. ובעזר [P. 47v] הנזכר[141] על נפח האם תעזור לזה. ואחרי העזר הנקרא אֶשְקוֹפִישְׂיאוֹשׂ[142] תקח שמן שיפריש ותכניסהו בפנים ובהפרד החום [5] מן האם נשאר שם הקושי ולפעמים יתקשו כל חלקי האם ולפעמים החלקים האחרים. ואלה אותותיו[143] קושי גדול נמצא בחוץ במשוש וכאשר יגדל הקושי תרגיש הכאב בכליות ובבית הסתרים. וכובד על גב הערוה. ואם יהיה הקושי בצואר האם יהיה גם הקושי בחוץ בפי האם[144]. ונמצאת פי האם פתוחה עד [P. 5] שמרגישה כאב ונשיכות סמוך [10] לשכבה עם איש. ומרגישה[145] שם עומס רב עד שאין המקום ההוא מרגיש מאומה. והעזר על זה ככל הכתוב על עצור האם וקשיה לא תוסיף עליו ולא תגרע ממנו.

מן הכאב הבא אליה אחרי לדתה. בבוא[146] הכאב אחרי הלידה[147] יהיו אלה אותותיו. בהתקרב הכאב אל האצטו׳ אז יהיה הכאב חזק מאד. ויהיה הגוף עצור[148] [15] ולפעמים עומדת נטויה למות בהיו[149] החולי דומה אל הנקרא כומיציאל[150] אך יש ביניהם חלוק כי [P. 10] בזה לא תתהפך העינים[151] ואין לה שפעת רוק גם לא נכבשו הגידים. אך השינה קרובה אליה מאד. העזר. אם הכאב גדול מאין יכולת אליה לסבול תעזור אליה מאד יציאת הדם. ואם הכאב מזער[152] אז יאות לשום כוסות המציצה בבתי הסתר הם [20] אנגש[153]. ואם[154] לשכב ותרגיל השתיקה לבוא אליה[155] אז יאות להריח לאפיה דבר שרוף ונבאש ולהזות מים קרים על פניה או להניח על הערוה רודא כתושא[156] בדבש או בשמן שיפריש[157]. ולגרד אליה הגוף והירכים ולהניח על בטנה סֵינא פִּישְׁמִי. וביום השלישי או הרביעי יתאדם הגוף. ואם ישאר [P. 15] ויתארך

---

140 P: איננו
141 P: + אחורי
142 P: אשקפולי
143 P: אותות
144 P: - יהיה גם קושי בחוץ בפי האם
145 P: ומרגיש
146 P: בבא
147 P: הלדה
148 P: עכור
149 P: בהיות
150 P: חמציל
151 P: העטים
152 P: הכא מצער
153 P: אנגיש
154 P: + תאריך
155 P: -
156 P: כתושה
157 P: ציפריס

הקושי תבשל שוֹלַטרֵי[158] בחלב ותכתשנו עם דונג לבן ומוח איל עם טרינו ושמן [f. 57r] סֵדְרי. חלב פר או חלב תיש מעורב[159] עם שמן ורד ותתן אליה במשקה או אניט. ואם הרחם נגוע בנגעים אז תקח וורדים[160] עם שומן חזיר חדדש ותתערב עם לובן ביצים וחוץ[161] ויתערב שם אבק ורדים כתוש היטב גם יקטירו האם עם גפרית.

ואם לא תטהר מדמי נדתה[162] תניח כוסות המציצה בבתי הסתר הם אנגש. או תחת הדדים. ואם יצא הדם בשפע יאות לשום לה קוֹשְׂט[163] פוליג[164] ויאולה לבנה[165] [P. 20] שדריה אישופו[166] והאכילה מאכלים הנאותים לה. כמו פור[167] רודא חרדל כמון בצל ואם הדם שהיה[168] רגיל[169] לצאת למטה ישוב[170] לצאת בנחירים יאות לשום כוסות המציצה למטה בעגבות ואם תרגיל לעשות כן בשלשה או בארבעה חדשים מחדש לחדש תדע כי נתרפא החולי באמת. ואם לא יצא הדם תדע באמת כי אז יחול כאב הראש ואז יאות להקזה[171] מן הזרוע ותתרפא.

מקושי האם. זה החולי נקרא מוֹלַא הוא קושי האם ונעשה מן החמום שהיה לה[172] בתחלה[173] ועל כן נשתטח[174] הבטן מהכל עד שנראית [P. 25] כמעוברת. ולפעמים יגדל בשר רע יוצא מן הנגע אשר באם. ואם המילדת תכניס אצבעה לפנים תמצא שם כמו[175] צואר ונקרא מולא בעבור שינוע בכבדות. ויש חלוק והפרדה בין הסובלת[176] מולא ובין המעוברת[177] כי המעוברת סובלת[178] אסטניסות וכובד בכליות והבטן הולך וגדל תמיד. **והסובלת**[179] מולא תרגיש בכל יום נשיכות וכאב[180]

[158] P: קולטרי
[159] P: ויעורב
[160] P: ורד
[161] P: וחומץ
[162] P: נידתה
[163] P: -
[164] P: פלייג
[165] P: לבונה + נפיטא
[166] P: שרויה אישפו
[167] P: פורו
[168] P: -
[169] P: הרגיל
[170] P: ושוב
[171] P: להקיזה
[172] P: -
[173] P: לתחילה
[174] P: נשטטח
[175] P: כמן
[176] P: הסובלות
[177] P: המעוברות
[178] P: המעוברות סובלות
[179] P: והסובלות
[180] P: הנשיכות כאב

ובהתארך העת לא תרגיש עובר חי ולא מת. והמעוברת תתחיל[181] להרגיש מארבעה חדשִׁים והלאה. והאחרת בעבור עשרה חדשים יכלה הגוף וידל והבטן והירכים יעלו ויגדלו. אך שניהם [P. 30] שוות שאינם נטהרות מדמי נדתם.

וזה החולי[182] דומה לחולי המים הרעים. אך זה נפרד ממנו בזה כי בהכות הבטן ביד לא ירים קול. העזר. רבים אומרים כי החולי הזה אין לו עזר. ורבים אומרים כי יש לו עזר בתחלתו. ואנו אומרים כי כאשר[183] ישוב זה החולי להיות קְרוֹנִיקַא[184] נעזור אליו עם הרפואות [f. 57v] הנקראות פֵּירַאגוֹרִיקֵש ועם מיני תחבושות וטבולים[185] כמו דִיַאקִילוֹן[186] או מְנַאשֵׂס. גם נחבר שם מִיטַאשִׁין קְרֵיטִיקַש ומַלְקְמַא כמו דִיַאשְׁפֵּרְמֵטוֹן או פוֹלִיַארְגִיאוּן[187]. גם טבול באשר יבושלו בַּאגש דְלַבְרִיר[188]. אגודת אזוב. מינטה[189] מרובי ויועיל מאד ויעשו לה מוך העשוי כן[190]. חמאה [P. 48r] מיץ אישופו שומן אווז מוח איל מן העצמות וממוח הראש דבש תאנים יבשים שמן זית ישן שמן שיפריש[191] שמן איריש ואחר כן נכניס אותה במים חמים ונצוה להשיטה בים[192]. ואם בכל זה יתארך החולי נתן אליה לֵיבוֹר.

מדם האם. דם האם יקרה כאשר מתקשה מאד ללדת או כאשר הפילה או מנגעי האם או בסבת שפעת דם יוצא למטה שנכרתו המקורות. ויקרה בזה עיפות הגוף וחולשה [P. 5] ורזון. ומראה פניה רע ואסטניסות וזה החולי יתיבש ויעצר בכבדות רב. ואולם לפעמים לא יזל מן האם כי אם מחיק הערוה. העזר יאות להשכיבה במטה קצרה ובבית אפל ובמקום שלא ינוע ואשר יגביהו רגליה. גם במנוחה והשקט. ואשר לא ישמע בבית דבר וקול אדם כי הזלת הדם תנוע בסבת כל תנוע[193]. ותשכב בענין כאלו רגליה עקומים וסדין אחד טבול במים קרים או תוך[194] פושקא הוא[195] מים בדבש יניחו על הערוה והכליות ובתי[196] הסתר ובקיץ [P. 10] ישיבו אותו שם תמיד בעבור שהחום לא יחמם אותה גם

181 P: והמעוברות תחל
182 P: -
183 P: -
184 P: קורוניקא
185 P: תחבושת וטיבולים
186 P: דיאקלון
187 P: פילי ארגיאון
188 P: דלאורו
189 P: מנטא
190 P: מן
191 P: שיפריס
192 P: במים
193 P: קול תנועה
194 P: -
195 P: או
196 P: ובבתי

יטבלו אותה במי[197] קרים וכל הגוף יתנשב במנשבי הרוח. גם נמשח כל גופה בשמר[198] קר.ולפעמים נשקה אותה חומץ[199] ונעשה לה טבול מן [20] פושקא קרה ובמים[200] אשר נתבשלו[201] מירטא לינטישקלי סלתיקא[202] מדברית קלפת רמון או ענפי העץ אשר[203] אחר שיתבשל ויתקררו ויושיבו[204] האשה עליהם. ואם לא תוכל לשבת בסבת ההזלה יכניסו אלה המים אליה עם תשומת כלי הוא קלישתרי[205] או מיץ פלאנטאגי[206] או מיץ אִינִיטאַברוֹס[207] או מֵאוֹבא[208] [P. 15] לוּפִינא או[209] פוֹלִיקאַרִיא כל זה יניחו[210] לה במוך. ואם יתארך החולי תקח אִיפוֹקִישִׁיטִידוֹש[211] אֶכאסִיא[212] אופי מזוג [f. 58r] בחומץ וכתוש היטב ותניח בצמר לבן כמו מוך. ותערב שם שמן אוֹנְפַסִי[213]. ותשים מעט צמר גפן[214] בפי האם לקבל הדם הנזול[215] משם ותחליפהו תמיד שלא יקפא הדם שם. וכן כוסות המציצה באש רב תניח על החלקים החצונים ותסירם בערבות[216] ובנחת ויעילו[217].

[5] תחבושת לזה. תקח תמרים חבושים אלום קרוע גטלאש אִיפִּקִישָׁטִירוֹש אכאסיא[218] שמן אונפסי [P. 20] שמן ורד או מירטי או לִינְטִיסִי ויחובש עליה גם את זה תקח בורטוליגא קֵנִילַאַרַה נִיקְטִילַא[219] פוֹלִיקַרִיא אובַא לופִינא פְלַאנְטאגִי[220] אִינְטִיבַא[221] כל אלה יכתשו היטב

197 P: פניה במים

198 P: בשמן

199 P: בחומץ

200 P: וממים

201 P:+ שם

202 P: סיליטקא

203 P: -

204 P: שיתבשלו יתקררו וישיבו

205 P: קלישטורי

206 P: פלאנטאגיני

207 P: אינטפרוס

208 P: מובא

209 P: -

210 P: יניח

211 P: אפוקישטירוס

212 P: אכסיאה

213 P: אינפאסי

214 P: -

215 P: הניזול

216 P: ותסיר בשבות

217 P: ויועילו

218 P: גטלש אפקשטי רוס אכציאה

219 P: ברטוליגא קאנילאדא ניקאליטש

220 P: פלאנטאגיני

221 P: אינדיביאה

ויתערבו עם קמח חטים ועם חומץ. מוך טוב לזה תקח גטאלא[222] מנא לבונה ועם מיץ [10] העשבים הנזכרים למעלה יתערב[223] אבק אלה גם פוליאוס או דשן ספוג שרוף כן תטבול הספוג החדש בשומן חדש נזול ותשומנו בכלי חדש[224] עד שיתקשה ויבש. ותוכל לעשות ממנו אבק ותערב עם המיץ [P. 25] הנזכר ועם לובן ביצים. ואם לא[225] תתרפא[226] ההזלה בזה תרגיל לעזור אליה הרפואות באשר נעזרים סובלי דישנטיריאה[227]. גם האכילה קמח חטים [15] מבושל היטב ותערב שם מעט חומץ ספרדי. ותתן לה אִינְטִיבָה[228]. גם ליטוגה רכה. וביצים רכים במחבת ויונים מדברים פרדיץ מבושלים עם פושקא ועם באגש דלברר[229] מירטא שמן ספרדי. ובאחרונה ניתן אליה יין טוב וערב ומזוג ויועיל[230] בעזרת האל.

מהזלת דם האם. הזלת דם הנשים יקרה בשפע רוב[231] ליחות ויוציא תמיד[232] מן האם עד ישתנה[233] מראיה ופניה רעים. ויחול[234] עליה רזון[235] אסטניסות ובלכתה יעלה נפח ברגליה.[P. 30] והיו האותות[236] החולי בענין זה. פעמים תבוא ההזלה[237] בכאב ופעמים בלא כאב. ופעמים בנגע ופעמים בלא נגע ופעמים ההזלה מגואלת ופעמים זכה. ההזלה שהוא[238] בלא נגע ובלא כאב יתכן לעזור בכל העזר שהזכרנו על דם האם. וכפי הראוי אל הרופא [f. 58v] עזר אחד טוב. תיקח קיבת[239] ארנבת או[240] [P. 48v] מעגל או מטלה או מאיל גטלאש קליפת רמון קליפת פין. ותכתוש כל אלה לאבק ותערב במים חמים באשר יבושלו חדושים ותתן לה[241] תמיד[242]. בהיות ההזלה בכאב תעזור אליה עם מיץ אַלִיסִי או טִיבְשֵׁאנָה [5] ובמאכל טוב וערב. גם בזה נעזר חמום[243] האם אם הנגע

[222] P: גטולא
[223] P: ותערב
[224] P: חרס
[225] P: -
[226] P: תתרפא
[227] P: דיסנטריא
[228] P: אנדיביאה
[229] P: ראגש דלאבר
[230] P: ויטיל
[231] P: ברוב שפע
[232] P: דם
[233] P: שישתנו
[234] P: יחול
[235] P: רזות
[236] P: אותות
[237] P: תבא הזלה
[238] P: שהיא
[239] P: תקח קבת
[240] P: ארנבת או -
[241] P: חבושים ותן
[242] P: -
[243] P: חימום

מגואל אחרי צאת הדם [...] [...] זכה או מגואלת נעזור אליה בעזר סובל דושנטריא[244] או הנג[ע זך] ונאמר כל העזר הזה שלם על נגעי האם. אם החולי יהיה קרוניקא או אַפִּימְרָא[245] נעזור בכל דבר מֵאְטֵשִׁין קרֶיטיקַאש[246] ויועילו בעזרת האל.

מן העקור. זה החולי[247] לזכר ולנקבה ויקרה בסבות רבות. או שהאשה לא תקבל בפנים[248] ולא תהר. או שלא תוכל לצאת עד עת נכון הוא עד[249] שיגמר העובר שלם. וזה העקור יקרה כאשר הזכר או הנקבה יהיה להם חולי בגופם או שהחלקים הנאותים אל ההריון יהיו מבולבלים. ובסבת הזכר לא יגמר ההריון כאשר יהיה לו[250] חולי קרוניקא[251]. וזרעו יהיה דקיק או מומי[252] או קר או חם יותר מן הראוי. או נשחת הזרע או שיתמיד לצאת בהיותו שטוף בזמה וכשישתבר ויהיה חלש באין אומץ. גם ימנענו בהיות לו מקור בצדו באשר ישפך הזרע ולא יכנס במקומו.

וכן נמצא העקור בנשים בהיות[253] רזות ודקות[254] ודלות בשר[255] וכל גופן יבש. או שהן טְשִׁיקְש[256] או שמנות יותר מדאי[257] או כעסניות או משוגעות. וכן כאשר אינם[258] יכולות להטהר בנדתם[259] או אשר כי האם נשמט או עקום או הכלי הנקרא מִימראנו̇ס סגור[260] או דומה כמו צואר הוא קול[261]. או שיש להן קושי ועל כן אינם מקבלות הזרע ונעשו עקרות. העזר. כל אחד מן האנשים נעזר בעזר[262] נכון הראוי לעשות לה[263]. או שיחליפו כח [f. 39r] מן העמל והיגיעה אשר עברו עליהם או בשינוי מאכלים ומשיחות. וכן הנשים אם[264] פי האם סגור מאיזו סבה

244 P: דיציאנטיריא
245 P: אפימי
246 P: קריטיקש
247 P: + שוה
248 P: -
249 P: + עת
250 P: + בימים
251 P: קורוניקא
252 P: ממיי
253 P: בהיותם
254 P: ורקות בשר
255 P: -
256 P: טשקש
257 P: מדי
258 P: אינן
259 P: להיטהר בנדתן
260 P: ממארוניס סוגר
261 P: קולי
262 P: עיזור העזר
263 P: לו
264 P: או

יאות לפתחו. ואם הנגע אשר באם זך או מגואל יאות לטהרו. וכן הצוא[265] והקושי יתכן [לרכך כראוי. צואר הא]ם הוא קול[266] יק[רא זה] בארבעה ענינים פעמים[267] תהיה [האם נמוכה ועקומה] ופעמ[ים[268] תעלה] למעלה וזה נקל להכיר [P. 20] באצבע[269] [הגדולה ואם נשמטת] לאחד מן הצדדים הרגל[270] שהיא מן הצד הה[וא הכאב והיא תר]גיש קרירות בגוף[271] ולא תוכל ללכת. ואם נשמטת [לאחור] אז יצאו התוצאות ברוח גדול והיא יושבת בכובד רב ו[אם נשמ]טת מצד הנקב התחתון אז יהיה הכאב על גב ה[ערו]ה.

והעזר[272] לאלה העזר הנזכר למעלה. מן פַּרְלֶשִׁין [הבא א]ל האם כל פעם שתסבול האם זה החולי יהיה פיה חזק ומלא כאלו מלא[273] [בגר]ס ועם קרירות רב אשר לא תרגיש אצבע המילדת ובורחת [P. 25] ומואסת הנהגת הבטן כמו מן[274] התוצאות והשתן. ואולם אחרי שהיא[275] יגעה מאד מן העמל הזה יקרה אליה הריון[276] בסוף. גם יכאבו עליה[277] ולא תוכל ללכת ועת נדתה נעצר או יקרה אליה שלא כסדר. וזאת נעזרת בעזרת הסובלות עצור האם. או בעזרת הנטהרות בכאב.

מהשמטת האם. השמטת האם תקרה לנשים תמיד ואז יהיה להן שפעת דם נדתן ויקרה[278] להן אסטניסות תמיד ואין חפץ אוכל ומגרשות[279] הזרע משם וזאת סבה להן להפיל. ולא [P. 30] ינקבו ויפתחו מקורות דדיה בעת נכון והאם אשר לא ילדה מעולם מגרשת הזרע לחוץ בשנה הראשונה או בשנייה[280] או בשלישית ומפלת בחדש השני או השלישי לעבורה[281]. ותכונת הנפל דקה ותגרשהו בטרם היותו חי. והלידה היא אין[282] מבושלת כל זמן שהנפל יגורש לפני זמנו או לפני היום הקרוב לזמנו. [f. 59v]

---

[265] P: הצואר
[266] P: קולי
[267] P: פעם
[268] P: ופעם
[269] P: באצבעו
[270] P: הרגש
[271] P: גוף
[272] P: ותעזור
[273] P: -
[274] P: -
[275] P: אשר היא
[276] P: אל ההריון
[277] P: רגליה
[278] P: נידתן ויקלה
[279] P: ומגרשת
[280] P: בשניה
[281] P: לעיבורה
[282] P: אינה

[העזר]. העזר על הזלת האם ודמיה. ואל הנשים אשר תזל [חלביהן יותר מן הראוי] יאות להרגילן[283] בעמל ובנגינה [למעט כמות] החלב. ואם החלב עבה יאוּת [P. 49v] להרגילן במאכלים [...] [ולש]תות] מים ול[...] [מכובד הלידה. בסיבת כובד הלידה יקרה [...] מיאוס והוא [יעלה בפי האם. העזר. אם יהיה החולי חדש בלא חמום נמשחנו [...] [קלטיאה נקש [...] [ואם] יעשה החולי שם [מן צואר יאות לרכך אותו] [...] הסירו בברזל ויתרפא מהר.

[מן] התחתוניות [ה]ם מוֹרוֹאִינֶשׁ[284] ונמצאות מזער[285] [בנשים] ולפע[מים] [P. 5][...] בפי האם והיו האותות האלה שם ש[פעת] דם רב ושלא [כסדר] וכרכמות פניה ויגיעה וחולשה בכ[ל] הגוף. ולפע[מים] [הש]תטחות[286] וכובד. ואולם התחתוניות מ[תחלפות] בעצמן פעמים יש[287] שהן[288] פשוטות ולחות ורכות וחלקות ויש מהן קשות מאד כגודל הקדרות וכאב גדול שם לכל האברים הקרובים מן המקום ההוא. והם גדולות ונחורות ונעזרות[289] בקושי גדול בסבת רב[290] המקרים אשר הקרו[291] שם וכן בעבור [P. 10] היותם בפנים במקום גבוה.

העזר. אם יהיה מזער ובתחילת[292] החולי נעזור אליה במה שהזכרנו בחמום האם. ואחר עבור הכאב אם ישאר שם שפע רב[293] מדם[294] נחבר שם הדברים[295] העוצרים ונפזר עליהם אבק קלפת רמון וענפים ויעצור אותן[296] להפליא.

מן הקבוצים כאשר יקרה חמום רב באם והיה כן מתחלה. יולידו[297] שם הקבוצים[298] והזלת מים רעים ועם הענין ההוא נעשות נשיכות בפנים. ולפעמים בסבה הזאת יקשו התוצאות ודרכי השתן. ורגליה וכל הגוף ינועו בכבדות. ולפעמים בשפעת הקבוץ יעלה נפח על גב[299] הערוה. וכאשר יעשה ראש דרך חוץ או[300] ימצא בראש האצבעות[301]

283 P: להרגילם
284 P: מורידאש
285 P: מצער
286 P: השטטחות
287 P: -
288 P: P: מהן
289 P: ונעדרות
290 P: רוב
291 P: יקרו
292 P: מצער בתחילת
293 P: -
294 P: דם
295 P: דברים
296 P: אותם
297 P: יולדו
298 P: קיבוצים
299 P: -
300 P: אז

[P. 15] המילדת אך הקבוץ הגבוה לא יתפש ואז תעלה[302] הזיעה במצח ובראש.

העזר כל הקיבוצים הנמצאים בגוף ירוככו ואותם שהיו בפי האם יהיו נטהרי׳ ברוב הקזה וכאשר תיבוש הליחה פתיחת המקורות יאותו נטבלים תוך פושקא גם ספוג רך יאות להניח שם בתוך הערוה וביום השלישי יאות להסיר הכל ואם יהיה הנגע מגואל תקח דבש זך שהוסר קצפו ותערב עמו טיטרא פרמאקא ויטהרו היטב מאד ואם יהיה הקובץ בתוך האם בגובה מעלותיה שלא יוכל האצבע להשיג [P. 20] שם גם כאשר יפתח הפתח הנקרא אורגאנום שלא תוכל העין לראות שם ואין יכולת לחתוך שם דבר יאות להסר במיני תחבושת חזקים ובחימום ספוג ובריכוכים ממיני מוך קלאשטינקאש גם בריכוכים פשוטים כמו דיאקולון עד אשר ירוככו וישחתו הקבוצים ויפרדו כל הלילה.

עזר אחר אם לא תרגיש התמדת הרפואות הנזכרות גם הכאב לא יחסר אז נרגיל מיני תחבושת העשויים מגרעינים תקח פוליגנו הוא קמח שעורים גם אורבי וכמון ותאנים מבושלים וכתושים עם טרמיינטינא ותחבוש עליה ותצליח בעזרת האל.

טיבול טוב לזה תקח ליבורייו פלייג׳ מרובי ארצימסא אשקופאריגיאה סינטוריאה מינטא ותבשל במים ותטבול המקום תמיד וזה יאות למהר בעבור שלא ישאר שם הקיבוץ באריכות פן יזיק לאם וישחית ברעתו.

מוך תקח חמאה מיץ אישופו שומן תרנגולת ניטרי צמוקים קלויים ותכתוש הכל ותעשו מזה מוך ותניח שם אלה הקיבוצים שהזכרתי היו רגילים לבוא בפתע פתאום ובמרוצה עד שהליחות [P.30] נגרש חוץ בשאר החלקים כי לפעמים נבקע לפעם ויוצא הליחות נשמד בחלק הנזכר בוקע לפעמי׳ עור הבטן ויוצא וכל פעם שנבקע באם נטהר דרך האם ואם יעשה ראש לחוץ יאות לשום שם תחבושת לרכך ואח׳ להוציאו משרשו בכלי הברז.

אחר להריון[303] מופלא תקח מרת פר ותכרוך בו הצמר ותניח על פי האם סמוך לוסתה ותסיר בלילה ותשכב עם בעלה ותהר בה׳. **להריון** אופו בלסמו ב׳ דרה׳ פראזראני ב׳ דרה׳ שומן אווז דרה׳ מיר כוכוע דר׳ מוח [P. 35] איל אופופוניו דרה׳ ותכתוש הכל עם שמן ורד ותניח שם ב׳ שעות רצופות ותוציאנו ותשכ׳ עם בעלה ותהר רק תתמיד אותו. **אחר להריון** תקח מרת תישית כמון ותרקח בשמן ורד [P. 59v] פינצויט ותניח כמשפט. **אחר להריון** תכתוש [...]

---

301 P: אצבעות

302 The London text of the treatise breaks off at this point due to the loss of several leaves. The remaining passages are based on Parma Ms. only.

303 The following three prescriptions to facilitate pregnancy were added by the translator or by a copist of the original *DPM B* text.

מנגעי האם[304] לפעמים היא חרוכה ונגועה כחומץ [...] הראש גם מקום הנגעים שב והליחה יוצאת בכאב [...] ופעמים במעוט ואם הנגע במקומות השפלים יהיה הכאב רב מאד [P. 5] בצואר יקרה מזה חימום והשטטחות רב ודפק גבוה והליחה מועטת [...] בנגע אז יחסר הנגע ומראה הליחה כניצן תכלת וכמו [...] קרנק או לצאת הבלויה גם נבאשת עד אין יכולת לסבול ותמיד נזול הדם [...] ויחול כאב הראש והצואר והענים ושורשיהם.

העזר געול הנגע [...] טיבשאנא העשויה בשפעת דבש ועם טיטרא פראקו הנתך בשמן [...] [P. 10] יבושל פייניגרייג וסובין חטין גם לינטישקולא ובזה תרחץ הנגע היטב ואם [...] שם מרובי פולינאש אורובי אירשימיליקא תשים שם ותעשה תחבושת מחוץ [...] שעורים ושמן אונפאצי ואם יולד קרנק בנגע תעשה כל הרפואות הראויות אל קרנק [...] קרוב ואם יהיה בפנים אז הוא חולי כבד מסוכן בעבור שלא נוכל להניח שם הרפואות ניתן להרגיל בפנים רפואות קלות מיני טיבולים פושרים ברוב דבש ומעט שמן ועם פיניגרייק [P. 15] מבולל במים וכפות תמרים כל זה יכתש היטב ותשים שם מעט יין טוב או חומץ גם אם יגדל הקרנק נבשל ביין קליפת רימון עלי ורדים ענפי זית חבושים אלום קרוע אכאסייא לוציאוס ונטה להכניס בפנים בפעם וכאשר יהיה הנגע זך נתן אליה מאכלים ערבים ויין טוב.

English translation

[f. 53v] It seems to me useful to write to you about the various ailments which occur frequently within the womb. Some of them are difficult and [5] incurable, since women are ashamed of them. Some others are curable, since they are easy to treat. Therefore, I will teach the treatment for all of them, in the first giving the signs of each ailment, so as to open [P. 5] the path and uncover that which modesty and shyness shroud and conceal[305], with God's help.

On the movement of the womb[306]. When the womb moves it produces pain, and [10] hard and malign effects. If it is not treated quickly, it provokes ailments[307] there. If it lies under the ribs, it pro-

---

[304] The last chapter of the *DPM B.*

[305] P: shy and modest women cover, and what is useful for them.

[306] DPM B: "De motu matricis".

[307] DPM B: "uulnera". The Hebrew translation employs the Biblical term *nega'im* (see Ex. 11,1; Lev. 13, 9.), which generally signifies leprosy.

duces distress[308], and it provokes a hard pain in the heart[309], and nausea. At times the woman's spittle becomes like vinegar, and her mouth fills with water; her thighs become cold and her tongue and head flutter[310]; her colour turns yellow; these phenomena cause her to lose her [15] voice[311].

The treatment. It would be proper to place wool under the womb, bound in a white piece of cloth immersed in balsam[312], or in a good and pleasant oil. Give her asphalt to smell, which is better [P. 10] when soft. Cause her to vomit by using a horn of a black she-goat, or deer legs, or a feather immersed in vinegar. Make her to smell something that causes [20] sneezing. When she is able to speak, give her castor with warm wine to drink, and put anointed fingers in her nose. The above-mentioned wool has to remain there until she is cured, since if you remove it the area will become afflicted by the illness again; therefore, it is proper to repeat the treatment many times.

[f. 54r] **On the distress of the uterus**[313]. In this case, she will suffer from pain on the sides of the pubes, which are called *Inges*[314]. She will also feel pain in the urinary bladder, suffer from retention of urine, and a flutter [P. 15] and pain in the legs.[315]

The treatment. Put in her nose everything that smells good, like myrrh, and put in her womb [5] everything that smells bad, and fumigate her with these until she is cured.

On the humid womb[316]. When there are too many humours in the womb, the woman suffers from pain in the eyes, and the head is hot and feeble as if it were spinning.

---

308 The Hebrew translation employs the term *mazoq* for the Latin *suffocatio*, which generally is translated in Hebrew texts by the more precise term *maḥnaq*. As we will see in the continuation, the term *mazoq* is also used for other pathologies.

309 DPM B:" ad os", but does not mention the heart at all.

310 The translator used the word *yerafref* (flutter) for the term "formicatur" in the Latin text. However, he was aware of his problematic translation, and therefore also gave the Latin verb, which has been distorted in both manuscripts, L: *krofimi gold*; P: *fromigola*.

311 The Latin text states nothing about a change in colour.

312 The Latin text says "in white balsam", while the Hebrew translator added the colour to the cloth.

313 DPM B: " De infusione matricis". In this case, the Hebrew translator again used the term *mazoq*. See note 308.

314 DPM B: "in inguine".

315 DPM B: "et formicatio tibiarum"

316 DPM B: "De humorosa matrice".

The treatment. Prepare the following suppository: Take gander fat, butter, pounded anise, and put this [in her womb] in a piece of wool or in a cloth made of linen. This purifies all the ailments of the womb.

[10] **On the inflation[317] of the womb[318]**. If she has pains in her hidden places[319] or if she feels [P. 20] biting sensations in her womb during sexual relations, you should know that the womb is inflated, especially in the inner part.

The symptoms are pains at the corners of her eyes and her face becomes more red than yellow. They [women] feel ashamed to reveal this ailment to the physicians.

The treatment. Take the milk of a woman who has given birth to a male infant, [15] mix it gradually with rose oil, and warm it. Make a suppository of soft wool, immerse it and place it at the head of the womb. Another treatment: pound a small amount of galbanum, mix it with rose oil and it will be useful[320].

On [P. 25] worms called *lombriqis*[321]. When she suffers pains on both sides of the womb, you may find that she has ring-worms [20] running continuously in her intestines and womb. Therefore, she has a great desire to scratch her belly and her body, and the body's humour flows down until it seems like *merabemas*[322], which is the chilling humour[323].

The treatment: Take well-pounded iris, mix it with the juice of pimpernel[324] and pomegranate, and make a suppository.[325] When the ring-worms approach the womb through the intestine, [P. 30] she will suffer a spasm of the belly and she will break out in a thick

---

317 The Hebrew text states *nefaḥ*, which means inflation, and not tumor, as it appears in the Latin text.

318 DPM B: "De tumore uulue". The translator used the term *em* (literally = mother), which was the standard medieval Hebrew translation for the Latin *matrix*. The word is vague and in the present case fails to provide a precise anatomical indication.

319 DPM B: "mulieris loca".

320 DPM B: "pessum inice".

321 DPM B: "De lumbricis".

322 Both Hebrew manuscripts use a distortion of the Latin: "reumatica".

323 DPM B: "Et humor sepe ducurrit de corpore, ita ut putet se reumaticam factam".

324 Both Hebrew manuscripts say *aguilent*, a distortion of "anagallis" (*Anagallis arvensis*, L.). DPM B: "et rubi et maligranati succum commisce".

325 The Hebrew text omits the following sentence: "Sed antea fomentet se, et sic subiciatur".

sweat, [f. 54v] which will be very difficult for her[326]. The treatment is the same as we mentioned before, with an immersed suppository[327].

On the inflation of the womb[328]. When an inflation begins to afflict the womb, her breasts will also become inflated and very hard. The colour of her face will turn blue and she will [5] suffer constant pain until this ailment of the womb ends, and the pain is gradually cured[329]. Therefore, some of the women do not ejaculate sperm[330] and they feel very hard when touched. Before they eat[331], acid, heavy and hard smells are emitted through their throats, [P. 35] which is very hard to bear[332]. They lose their appetites and feel as if they are full.

The treatment: Fumigate and bathe the womb with oil[333], water and a small amount of honey, then [10] take wine [P. 46v] and myrtle mixed with gander fat and frequently wash her legs with it.

More on the inflation of the womb[334]. When the humour of the vulva descends into the womb[335], the women's bodies become cold and they do not desire to have sexual relations since the interiors of their bodies are cold up to the extreme parts.

The treatment: Take an equal quantity of bark from the pine tree and of galbanum, pound them together, and sprinkle the woman's inner parts with the [blend]. The treatment has to be given [15] intermittently, every two days. Then boil lentils and myrtle with red wine and sprinkle [her] with that until she becomes warm, while covering the area well. [P. 5] But if she would have sexual relations [during the treatment], the medicament will not cure her, because of the interruption. Another treatment for the humour descending from the womb and the belly. Take base iron, which is called *Qaqafer*[336],

---

[326] DPM B: "et sudor spissus ut putent se ab humore molestari".

[327] DPM B: "Hec postquam urinam fecerint, de succo edere, fomententur".

[328] DPM B: "De uicio matricis".

[329] DPM B: "...et fiat decursus foras. Deinde sic sedatur paulatim dolor...".

[330] DPM B: "unde sine filiis quedam earum fiunt".

[331] DPM B: "Preterea quando sine cibo sunt".

[332] DPM B: "putantes se plenas esse medicinas".

[333] The Hebrew text omits the use of cypress.

[334] DPM B: "De humorosa matrice".

[335] In this case, the translator used the term *em* to designate the vulva, while the appropriate Hebrew word *reḥem* for the womb. Cf. note 318.

[336] DPM B: "Ferri eruginem".

pound it [20] to a powder, mix it with vinegar and make a suppository[337].

On cancer of the womb[338]. If a cancer is produced in the womb of a woman, then she feels as if she has a piece of wood in her womb or a thorn in her body; at times it bleeds with immeasurable pain.

The treatment: Take rue, alum and nitre, pound them all [together] and [P. 10] bandage her. It is useful for every illness and all kinds of cancer which afflict the womb and other parts of the body. Afterwards, [f. 55r] place in her [womb] a suppository of the following materials: winter cherry juice mixed with the same amount of gander fat.

Also, for all the pains which occur to women, take the juice of leeks and mix it with an equal quantity of iris oil, and apply. Also for cancer, pound radish, which is sharp, mix it with honey, put it in her [womb] and it will be very useful. On the ailment called *flegmon*[339], which [5] inflicts the womb and causes women [to experience] acute fevers, pain and hardness of the belly and pains in the urine bladder. It also causes a stomach illness [P. 15] called *anatropa*[340], and nausea caused by an acid humour or by a red one, which is *colera*[341]. In addition [it provokes] urinary retention and [rigidity] of the belly, vomiting, thirst, and dryness of the tongue. Her colour becomes black[342], she suffers pains in the neck, in the temples, in the eyes, in the extremes of her fingers and in the nails. If a finger touches [10] her pubes[343] she feels a great pain there, dryness, hardness and a restriction of the womb's orifice.

The treatment. Put butter and deer brain of equal weights into wine and apply it. Also, for those who have tumours and cannot urinate, take an equal quantity of gander fat [P. 20] and green purslane, put them in wool and apply. Another suppository to cure womb movement, its inflation and heat, called *sacer ignis*, for simple fevers

---

337 P: "and put it in with a suppository".

338 DPM B: "De cancro matricis". The term for cancer used in both Hebrew manuscripts, and which was common in most Hebrew medical treatises in the Middle Ages, is *qarnaq*.

339 DPM B: "De flegmone matricis". L: *fleqmon*; P: *fliqmon*. The fact that the translator did not even attempt to translate this and the words following demonstrates that he did not understand them.

340 DPM B: "stomachi anatropa"; L: *enatropa*; P: *ana tropa*.

341 DPM B: "flegma aceti uel colera".

342 DPM B: "atramento"; L: *arament*; P: *iriant*.

343 DPM B: "in natura ipsius".

and pustule[344], for darkened eyes and bitings in the body[345], which is wonderfully helpful. Take [seven] dirhems each of[346] wax and deer brain, four dirhems gander brain, two dirhems odorous opium with cypress oil, and apply in a suppository.

Another suppository useful for every sickness of the womb. Take the fat of a sow that has not given birth, mix with honey [P. 25] and make a suppository. Apply it when she comes out of a bath, and it will be very useful.

On suffocation of the womb. It happens because of repeated abortions, or hard labour, or a retention of menstrual blood over a long period, or a tumour in the womb. Whenever the womb ascends to the chest, they suffocate and lie down as if dead. These are the symptoms: when the womb ascends to the chest they fall down and lose consciousness. They lie senseless, their lips are dumb and they grind their teeth. At times their hands and legs rest motionless, and at times [P. 30] they lie straight and their entrails are swollen. The upper entrail, which is called [f. 55v] *torax*, also becomes very heavy[347]. The veins of their forehead swell, and cold sweat runs from their forehead and their face. They do not have a pulse, except perhaps a feeble and very short one. When they recover, [they] sometimes know what happened to them, but other times they know nothing, and suffer from headaches and hard pains in the neck.

The treatment. When the woman is afflicted with this sickness, it is proper to put her in a warm bed, not in a dark room but rather in a lighted one; to lift her head and to keep her hands and legs [P. 47r] flat. You should move her face constantly and warm it with hot water, lightly with a soft cloth. If you see that she is unable to speak, you should quickly put cupping glasses on the back of her pubes and on their sides, which are called *inguinis*[348], and drop into her mouth warm water mixed with wine sweetened with honey. You should also rock her easily in a cradle, which is called *breṣ*[349]. When she recovers, but is still very tired, phlebotomize her immediately. On the third day treat her with ointments [P. 5] and juices, and

344 DPM B: "apostasin"; L: *ipopetasis*; P: *ipostasis*.

345 DPM B: "punctiones doloris".

346 Both Hebrew manuscripts omit the quantity.

347 DPM B: "torax grauior fit"; L and P: *toraq*.

348 DPM B: "et inguinibus appositis"; L and P: *ingas*.

349 DPM B: "et in pensili lecto eam"; L and P give the Occitan term: *breç* (see Barkaï, *Les infortunes de Dinah*, p. 169, n. 8), but P adds: "and it is called *nakh* in the Calabrian language".

after the ointments give her lean and fine food to eat. Order her to take exercise on the same day and the following one. And every day apply various bandages to her, warming [things], [15] and softening [things], [which are] soft and simple[350]. She should also have baths and eat varied and tasty foods, and drink fine and good wine.

If the ailment becomes chronic, constantly recurring, treat her as mentioned above, move her gently and correctly, scrape her extremities slowly with your hand and apply sinapism[351] to her. If all this does not help her, you should make her walk by the sea and on the land as if in a boat[352], and always wash her face with warm water. [20]

The [ancient] physicians[353] ordered them to smell everything tattered and stinking. They also used to fumigate[354] the women in order to cure uterine suffocation, in order to restore their speech [P. 10] and to revive them.

Also use the following [recipe]: [take] six dirhems of hog fennel, twelve *escrupules*[355] of galbanum and castor, eleven grains of pepper, and a small quantity of balsam resin. Put the galbanum in good vinegar[356], pound all the others, and then mix them until the mixture becomes wet. When necessary take the amount of a nut, put it on burning coal and give her this to smell.

[f. 56r] **On the stretching of the womb and its inflation**[357]. This occurs under the navel, with pain in the belly and in the kidneys,

---

350 DPM B: "cataplasmatibus et fomento curata cum appositione cerotarii, et malagmatis simplicis utantur".

351 L: *sina pisimi;* P: *silapsimi;* DPM B: "sinapismo". It is doubtful whether the translator knew the meaning of the term. For its composition and uses in medieval medicine, see Radicchi, *La Gynaecia di Muscione*, p. 471.

352 The Latin text states: "... deinde peregrinari eas iubemus terra et maris". The two Hebrew manuscripts add two different words, L: *be-guirot*; P: *benirot*. Both make no sense in Hebrew; therefore, it seems that they are distortions of *be-sirot* = "in boats", a form which also appears in the Hebrew adaptation of Muscio's *Gynaecia*. See Barkaï, *Les infortunes de Dinah*, p. 169.

353 DPM B: "Veteres autem medici..."; the reference to the "past" physicians is retained only in manuscript P.

354 DPM B: "Fumigium ad prefocationem matricis". While the term is used as a heading to introduce the subsequent recipe in the Latin text, the Hebrew translator employs it in the sense of its medical function.

355 The Hebrew translator employs an Occitan term, while the Latin text states: "xii dirhems".

356 DPM B: "in aceto optime".

357 DPM B: "De tensione seu inflacione matricis".

headache and pain in the stomach. She also suffers from retention of urine, insomnia [P. 15] and [feels] pricks [there]. They are not purified [by expelling the] menstrual blood, and if you place a finger there you find [5] the womb open.

The correct treatment for this is the same as that written for the heat of the womb, without any addition or deletion.

On the inflation of the womb and the belly[358]. This happens because of coldness, or because she aborted or because the remaining thick blood collected there. In consequence, she becomes inflated and her belly becomes feeble. If you press the inflation with your fingers, it withdraws and immediately returns, and if you hit the place it sounds like a drum. At times the inflation moves and at times [10] [P. 20] it is steady; also, at times it moves from its place. When you observe all these symptoms you have to treat her in same way we mentioned[359] concerning the retention and the heat of the womb. The midwife or the wise woman[360] should try to remove all the blood that has collected without causing any harm.

When the inflation becomes chronic, we apply all those things mentioned concerning womb suffocation to her, which are called *metasincritica*[361]. We would also place various bandages there, [15] one of which is called *postea*[362], the other *poliarchion*[363], and another *diaspermaton*[364]. We should do it with water in which pennyroyal, horehound, hyssop and laurel leaves were boiled. We should

[358] DPM B: "De inflatione matricis".

[359] DPM B: "dicemus".

[360] The Latin text states only: "obstetrix".

[361] Latin text: "metasin creticis"; L: *metasin creticas*; P: *metasin criscas*.The translator evidently did not understand the meaning of the *metasyncrisis*, "cyclic cure", which is of fundamental importance in Soranus' Methodical system of medical treatment. The *metasyncritica* is "a general course of therapy" for restitution of health by evacuation of humours. The translator treated these concepts as if they were names of medicaments, as he also did in his translation to Muscio's *Gynaecia* (see Barkaï, *Les infortunes de Dinah*, p. 172). Cf. Hanson and Green, "Soranus of Ephesus: *Methodicorum Princeps*", pp. 1055, 1060; Burguire *et alia.*, *Soranos d'Épheèse*, pp. XIV-XVI; Radicchi, *La Gynaecia di Muscione*, pp. 406-407.

[362] L and P: *astea*. The translator understood the Latin word "postea" (thereafter) as a name of one of the "epithima" which are mentioned in the Latin text. Yet, it is also possible that the Latin version he was translating indeed indicates *astea.*

[363] L and P: *poliargueon*. See Radicchi, *La Gynaecia di Muscione*, p. 441.

[364] L: *diaspermaton*; P: *diaspermatan*. See *ibid.*, pp. 343-344.

then prepare a bath for her, called *encatisma*[365], and a suppository made of rue, nitron, pennyroyal and bull gall. Mix them all and apply them to her in a suppository.

Another suppository: Take figs and crush them completely, [20] two dirhems cumin and [half a] dirhem[366] of African nitron. You should remember that every acid suppository, when [P. 30] it is bound up with wool, may be[367] immersed in oil or in milk.

We should also put cupping glasses, which are called *mitasincritica*[368], in these places. We should strongly push them and forcefully pull them. We should also bathe her [first] with warm water and lastly with cold water.

On inflation called tumour[369]. When this ailment afflicts the womb, there is hardness and inflation under the navel. [f. 56v] When you press your finger on the inflation it disappears, but after a little while it reappears. The skin of the belly does not have its proper colour and if you drive your fingers into the skin, it follows the fingers.

The treatment [P. 47v] for this ailment is the same as for womb inflation. After that, employ the treatment called *encolpismum*[370]. Take cypress oil and insert it. When the heat [5] of the womb disappears, it remains hard. At times, all parts of the womb are hard, but sometimes only some sections.

These are the symptoms: when you touch the womb from the outside, you feel a great hardness; when the hardness becomes larger, she will feel pain in the kidneys and in her hidden place[371], and heaviness on her pubes. If the hardness is found in the womb's cervix, it would be [felt] outside as well, in the womb's orifice. The womb's orifice will be open [P. 5] and she will feel pain and pricks immediately after [10] having sexual relations. She feels such a burden that the place will become senseless.

---

[365] L: *encatismi*; P: *encatimas*; Latin text: "encatisma". The *encathisma* is a rinse of the interior members of the body containing water in which medicinal herbs have been immersed.

[366] The Hebrew manuscript does not give the exact quantity. DPM B: "half a dirhem".

[367] According to the Latin text, it "ought to be".

[368] DPM B: "Curcurbite etiam metas critice partibus ipsis bene imponimus". The translator mistakenly identified the "curcurbite" (cupping glasses) with the "metasincretica".

[369] DPM B: "De tumore matricis".

[370] L: *escopisios*; P: *escapoli*. See Radicchi, *La Gynaecia di Muscione*, p. 354.

[371] DPM B: "inguina".

The treatment for this ailment should be the same as prescribed for womb rigidity and hardness; do not add or omit anything.

On the pain afflicting her after birth[372]. When the pain appears after she gives birth, these are the signs: When the pain approaches the stomach it is very hard, the body is rigid, [15] and at times she seems to be near death because this ailment resembles one called *comicial*[373]. But they differ [P.10] since in this one her eyes do not turn over, she has no surplus saliva, and her nerves are not strained, but she feels a great desire to sleep.

The treatment. If the pain is unbearable, bloodletting would be very helpful; if the pain is minor, it would be proper to put cupping glasses on her secret places, called [20] *inguine*. If she lies down speechless for long time[374], it would be proper to give her something burnt and stinking to smell, to sprinkle cold water on her face, or to place pounded rue mixed with honey or with cypress oil on her pubes. Also massage her body and her legs and put a sinapism on her belly. On the third or fourth day the body will be reddish[375]. If the hardness remains, [P.15] you should boil nightshade with milk and pound it with white wax and deer marrow, iris oil and [f. 57r] the fat of a bull or a goat. Mix them all with rose oil and give it to her in a drink or in anise[376].

If the uterus is afflicted with ulcers[377], take roses with new pork fat and mix [them] with egg whites and apply it to her. You may also use egg whites with vinegar, mixed with well-pounded rose powder, and fumigate[378] the womb with sulphur.

If she is not [5] purged of her menstrual blood, put cupping glasses on her secret places, called *inguine*, or under her breasts. If the blood flows abundantly, put cost, pennyroyal, white violet, [P. 20] savory and hyssop on her, and give her proper foods, such as leek, rue, sinap, cumin and onion.

---

[372] DPM B: "De dolore matricis post partum".

[373] DPM B: "ut in commiciali morbo uideatur esse"; L: *comicial*; P: *hamicil*. The translator did not understand that the Latin refers to epilepsy.

[374] L omits "for a long time".

[375] DPM B: "sinapismum super uenterem impone tertio die vel quatro intermissio ne corpus rubeat".

[376] DPM B: "In potione dandum est castoreum uel aneteum".

[377] Here again the translator employs the vague Hebrew term *nega'im* (see note 307), while the Latin text is very precise: "Si uero uulua ulcerata est".

[378] DPM B: "et subfumentum matricis fiat"

If the blood, which usually flows from below, comes from the nostrils, it would be proper to put cupping glasses below, on her buttocks. If you persist with this treatment every month, for three or four months, you can be sure that the ailment will be cured. If the blood does not flow, you will recognize it because she will suffer from headache. In this case, you should let blood from her arm, and she will be cured.

On the hardness of the womb[379]. This ailment is called *mola.* It is a hardness of the womb and is caused by the heat she suffered before, and for this reason her belly is expanded and she seems [P. 25] pregnant. At times, malign flesh grows out of the womb's lesion. [15] If the midwife puts her finger inside, she will feel something like the cervix there, which is called *mola*[380]. It is so called because it moves heavily. There is a difference between one who suffers from mola and one who is pregnant. The pregnant woman feels sick, heaviness on the kidneys and her belly constantly enlarges. One who suffers from mola feels pricks and pains every day, and after a while she does not feel the foetus[381], either alive or dead. The pregnant woman begins to feel [the foetus] from [20] four months. After ten months, the other woman's body becomes thin, but her belly and legs become more and more fat. On the other hand, both [P. 30] of them are not purified by menstrual blood[382]. This ailment resembles hydropsy but differs from it because, if we knock on the belly, it does not make a sound.

The treatment. Many people say that this ailment is incurable. Many others say that it is curable only at the onset. We say that when this sickness becomes chronic, we can treat it with medicaments called *peragoriqes*[383] [f. 57v] and with various bandages and baths, such as *diaquilon* or *manasen*[384]. We would also put there [in

[379] DPM B: "De duricia matricis".

[380] DPM B: "si obstetrix mittit digitum in orificium uelud callum inuenit".

[381] DPM B: "et accedente tempore motum infantis non habet"

[382] In the Latin text, this remark appears at the beginning of the comparison between pregnant women and those who suffer from mola.

[383] DPM B: "paragoricis"; L and P: *peragoriqes*. It is evident that the translator was not familiar with these tranquillizing medicaments. See Radicchi, *La Gynaecia di Muscione*, pp. 425-426.

[384] DPM B: "manasen"; L and P: *menases*.

the womb] *mitasin critica*, and *malqama*[385] such as *diaspermaton*[386] or *poliarchion*[387], and prepare a bath in which were boiled grains of laurel, hyssop, mint and horehound, which is very useful. Make her a suppository of the following: butter, [P. 48r] juice of [5] hyssop, gander fat, deer's marrow and brain, honey, fig-cake, old olive oil, cypress oil and iris oil. Then bathe her in warm water and order her to swim in the sea. If after all these treatments the ailment persists, we will give her hellebore.

On a bleeding womb[388]. Bleeding from the womb may occur because of hard labour, or abortion, or lesions of the womb, or a surplus of blood flowing from below because [10] the veins were cut. It causes fatigue of the body, feebleness [P. 5] and leanness; her face looks ill and she feels disgust. In fact, it is very difficult to dry and to restrain this ailment. At times the source of bleeding is not the womb but, rather, the vagina[389].

The treatment. Put her in a short bed in a dark room, in a place in which she will not be able to move, and lift her legs. She has to lie down peacefully and quietly, so there must be no noise or human voice in the room, because bleeding [15] is provoked by any movement. She should lie down and cross her legs, and [you must] put a sheet, immersed in cold water or in *pusca*, which means water mixed in honey[390], on her pubes, kidneys and hidden places. In summertime, [P.10] she always has to rest, in order to avoid the heat. And to bathe in cold water, and to expose her body to gusts of wind. We should anoint all her body[391] with cold oil, and from time to time give her vinegar to drink.

We should also prepare her a bath of [20] cold oximel and water, in which were boiled myrtle, lentils, mulberry, peel of pomegranate or its branches. After it has boiled and cooled, you may sit her in it, but if she cannot be seated because of the bleeding, insert the water

---

385 DPM B: "malgama"; L and P: *malqama*. The translator correctly transcribed the Latin term but did not know that it means emollients. See Radicchi, *La Gynaecia di Muscione*, pp. 395-396.

386 DPM B: "diaspermaton"; L and P: *diaspermeton*. See *ibid.*, pp. 343-344.

387 DPM B: "poli archion"; L: *poliarguion*; P: *piliarguion*. See *ibid.*, p. 441.

388 DPM B: "De sanguine matricis".

389 The translator employed the Hebrew term *ḥeiq ha-'ervah* , which means vagina, for the Latin "sinus mulierum".

390 Explanation added by the Hebrew translator.

391 DPM B: "caput eius".

by means of an instrument, which is a *clyster*[392]. Or apply by means of a suppository [made with the] juice of waybread, or of endive, or of nightshade, [P.15] or of flea-wort. If the ailment persists, take dogrose, acacia and opium mixed with [f. 58r] vinegar, pound these well, and administer them to her with a suppository made of white wool. Also mix some green olive oil with a piece of cotton and place it in the opening of the womb[393] in order to absorb the blood flow, and change it constantly to prevent its clotting. Also place cupping glasses with a lot of fire on the exterior parts, and remove them gently and tenderly. [5] A bandage for this [ailment]: Take dates, cydonia, aloe, tamarisk, dogrose, acacia, green olive oil, [P. 20] rose oil or myrtle oil, or lentil oil and bandage her with it. Also take purslane, *caniglara*[394], nightshade, waybread and endive, pound all these well and mix with wheat flour and vinegar. Another good suppository for this [condition]: Take tamarisk, frankincense and the fluid made of the [10] above-mentioned herbs, mix it with the powder[395] or the ashes of burnt sponge. Also, immerse a new sponge in new liquid fat, and place it in a new vessel until it is hard and dry. Then you will be able to make a powder of it, and mix it with the above-mentioned [P. 25] fluid and with egg whites.

If the flow is not cured by all these, then treat her with the medicaments designated for those who suffer from dysentery, and feed her with [15] well-cooked wheat flour mixed with a small amount of Spanish vinegar[396]. Give her endive, lettuce, soft eggs cooked in a frying pan, desert birds [called] partridges boiled with oximel, laurel grains, myrtle and Spanish oil. Finally, we will give her good and perfumed wine; it should be beneficial with God's help[397].

On the flow of blood from the womb. The flow of women's blood occurs because of a surplus of humours. It flows constantly from the womb, until she looks different, and her face looks bad. She become lean, disgusted, and when she walks, she suffers from swollen legs.

---

392 DPM B: "clistere"; L: *clisteri*; P: *clistori*. See Radicchi, *La Gynaecia di Muscione*, pp. 325-326.

393 DPM B: "et penicellum aceto plenum orificia matricis apponatur".

394 L: *qenilara niqtila*; P: *qanilada niqalites*.

395 Hebrew text: *pulius*.

396 DPM B: "oleo yspano".

397 The last sentennce was added by the Hebrew translator. On the other hand, he omitted the following sentece: "Sane si simplices potiones datur iuuat".

[P. 30] The signs of the sickness are the following: At times it occurs with pain, at times without pain. At times lesions also occur, at times they do not. Sometimes the flow is unpure, sometimes it is pure. The flow without bruising and pain is to be treated in the same way we mentioned on the bleeding of the womb, and according to the physician's ability[398].

[f. 58v] One more useful treatment: Take the stomach[399] of a rabbit, or [P. 48v] a calf, or a lamb, or a deer, tamarisk, pomegranate peel and pine bark, pound them all[400] and mix them in hot water, in which cydonia was boiled, and apply this to her consistently. If the flow is painful, give her a drink made of spelt or of crushed barley [5] and good and pleasant food. We would also treat the womb's heat with this. If the lesion is dirty, you may recognize it by examining the blood flow [to see] if it is dirty or pure; we should cure her with the treatment designated for those who suffer from dysentery or lesions[401]. Thus far we have completed the description the treatments for the ailments of the womb.

[P. 5] If the sickness is chronic, we should treat her with all kinds of *metasin creticas*, which will be beneficial with God's help[402]. [10] On sterility[403]. This ailment occurs to the male and to the female as well, and it has many causes: either the woman is not receptive inside, or she can not complete the period of pregnancy, which means [she cannot sustain the pregnancy] until the foetus is completed. Sterility occurs when the male or the female has an ailment in the body, or the reproductive organs are confused[404].

In the case of the male, the pregnancy can not be completed when he has [15] a chronic disease, or because his sperm is too thin or watery, or too hot or too cold. [P. 10] Or because the sperm is corrupted, or because he is lascivious and ejaculates too much, or if he has a vein at the side, through which the sperm pours out rather than entering the proper place.

---

398 The last sentence does not exist in the Latin text.

399 DPM B: "coagulum".

400 The Hebrew text does not give any amount. DPM B: "two dirhems".

401 The Latin text refers to the cure as being given later: "Dicemus etiam plenam curam de his omnibus ubi tractabimus de uulneribus matricis".

402 Addition of the Hebrew translator.

403 DPM B: "De sterilitate matricis".

404 *Sic* the Hebrew translation! DPM B: "aut partes ille conceptui necessarie impediuntur".

Women are sterile if they are lean and thin, they have meagre flesh and all their body is [20] dry. Or they suffer from phthisis[405], or they are too fat, or irascible, or insane. Also when they do not purify [themselves] properly, or they suffer from womb prolapse, or the womb is distorted, or the organ called the membrane is closed, or it resembles a neck, called *col*[406]. Or they have [P. 15] a hardness which prevents them from receiving the sperm, and they become sterile.

The treatment. Each has its proper treatment, according to the cause. They have to recover from the fatigue, [f. 59r] the labour and the exhaustion they have endured[407]. They also have to eat varied foods and to apply ointments. For the women who have a closed womb orifice for any reason, it should be opened. If the lesion in the womb is dirty, you should purify it. The cervix and the hardness have to be softened.

On the womb's cervix, called *col*[408]. It happens [5] because of four different causes. At times it declines and at times it ascends; it is easy for the midwife to verify [P. 20] this with her longest finger. If it inclines to one of the sides, the leg of that side will be painful and she will feel cold in her body and will be unable to walk. If the womb s, then she defecates with strong wind, and she sits with great difficulty[409]. If the womb prolapses [10] towards the anus[410], then she will have a pain on the pubes. The treatment should be as mentioned above.

On the paralysis of the womb[411]. Every time the womb suffers from this sickness, its opening is full with matter and is hard and it will be very cold, so she will not feel the midwife's finger. She avoids [P. 25] and dislikes her relieving nature, such as feces and

[405] DPM B: "ptisice"; L and P: *tisices*. See Radicchi, *La Gynaecia di Muscione*, pp. 447-448.
[406] DPM B: "Aut certe callositatem".
[407] DPM B: "singule res predicte conpetentibus diligentis ita ut fatigatio exerciciis".
[408] DPM B: "De matricis collo".
[409] DPM B: "cum ingenti difficultate mulier sedet, maxime si ad anum fuerit inclinatio".
[410] DPM B: "Si uero in priorem partem facta fuerit inclinatio".
[411] DPM B: "De paralisi matricis". L and P: *parlesin*.

urine[412]. But once she [15] recovers from this labour, she can finally conceive. If she has pain, she is unable to walk and the time *[sic]* of her menstrual blood stops, or becomes irregular.

The treatment for this case is the same as for rigidity of the womb or for the retention of menstruation.

On the prolapse of the womb[413]. Uterine prolapse frequently occurs to women. It provokes a surplus of menstrual blood, they are always [20] disgusted and have no appetite to eat[414], they expel sperm from there and this causes them to abort. Their [P. 30] nipples do not open at the proper time[415], and the womb which never gave birth expels sperm during the first, the second and the third years[416], and she aborts in the second or third month, while the foetus is still very thin yet alive. Premature birth occurs when the foetus is expelled before its proper time or its approximate day. [f. 59v] The treatment of this sickness is the same as prescribed for the feebleness of the womb and its bleeding.

On an abundance of milk[417]. For women who have an abundance of milk, it is proper to order them to work and to play music[418] in order to diminish their milk. If the milk is thick, give [P.49v] them appropriate food and water to drink and [a bath every day][419].

[5] On a difficult birth.[420] The difficult birth provokes [...][421] a lesion in the orifice. If this ailment occurs without fever, we should anoint her [with] *caltea niqis*[422] [...][423], and if the ailment is in the

---

412 The Latin text refers to intercourse: "usum veneris odit et fugit". It seems that the translator confused the word "veneris" with "venter", which is correctly translated into Hebrew as *beten.*

413 DPM B: "De lapsa matrice".

414 DPM B: "occurrit cum fastidio uiri".

415 This sentence has nothing in common with the Latin: "et ad legitimum tempus pecus [foetus] non perferat".

416 DPM B: "primo aut secundo aut .iii. die foras excludat". It is difficult to explain how the translator confused a "day" with a "year".

417 DPM B: "De lactis copia".

418 DPM B: "forcioribus excerciciis uti debent...", but there is no mention of playing music.

419 DPM B: "et cotidiano lauacro utantur".

420 DPM B: "De difficili partu".

421 A lacuna of one word in the Hebrew text. DPM B: "Ex difficili partu uel ex nimio labore".

422 DPM B: "calasticis"; The translator transcribed the Latin term, but it seems that he did not knew that it refers to an "emollient preparation". See Radicchi, *La Gynaecia di Muscione*, p. 309.

cervix you should soften the place [and then][424] remove it with an iron [scalpel], and it will be quickly cured.

On haemorrhoids called *emorroidis*[425]. It occurs rarely to women and at times [P. 5] it [appears][426] in the womb's orifice. The signs are an abundance of [10] blood, her face becomes pale, she feels fatigue and feebleness in all her body[427], and at times also rigidity and heaviness as well. There are different kinds of haemorrhoids: sometimes they are simple and humid, soft and smooth; others are very hard and as big as a pot[428]. She feels great pain in all the parts close to them. They are very big and pierced, and are very difficult [15] to cure, due to all the circumstances [of their symptoms] and especially because they are [P.10] inside, in a higher place.

The treatment:[429] If the sickness is minor and has just commenced, we should treat her in the same way we treat uterine fever. We will then treat the pain, and if she still has an abundance of blood, we will put medicaments there which will stop it, and pulverize [the haemorrhoids] with the powder of pomegranate peel and its branches[430], which will stop it wonderfully.

On collections[431]. When a great fever occurs in the womb[432], it causes collections and the flow of bad water[433]; as a result, she feels pinprincks inside. At times it also causes her difficulties in defecating and urinating, and her legs and her body move heavily. At times, because of the abundant collections, her pubes becomes swollen. The midwife can feel, with her fingers, [P.15] the collections which are in the exterior part, but she cannot feel the higher ones; in that case

---

423 A lacuna of one word in the Hebrew text.

424 A lacuna of one word in the Hebrew text.

425 DPM B: "De emorroidis". The Hebrew text gives both the Talmudic *(taḥtoniyot)* and the Latin (L: *moroines*; P: *moridas*) names of the ailment.

426 A lacuna of one word in the Hebrew text.

427 DPM B: "et pallor cum lastitudine corporis".

428 DPM B: "durissime et dolore...".

429 The Hebrew text omits the following passage: "Antiquis uero tolerare eas placebat, aut uasa eorum scarificantes puluerum ibi apponebat, ut paulatim mortui caderent, que omnia reprobamus. Nos ergo...".

430 DPM B: "corrio maligranati et galla"

431 DPM B: "De nimio feruore precedente". The Hebrew translator gives another heading to this chapter. He refers to the Latin term "collectiones" (tumefactions), which he renders into Hebrew literally by the word *quibuzim* (collections).

432 DPM B: "in sinu mulierum".

433 DPM B: "et foris orror occurrit et orrore".

there appears[434] a cold sweat on the forehead and the head [of the woman].

The treatment. All the collections which are found in the body have to be softened[435]; those which are in the womb orifice should be treated by a considerable quantity of bloodletting. When the humour is dry, immerse the openings of the veins in oximel; it is proper to place a soft sponge in her vulva, and to remove all these on the third day[436]. If the lesion is dirty, take honey, of which the foam has been removed, and mix it with tetrapharmacum[437] and it will purify the lesions very well. In case the collections are inside the womb, in its higher part, so that it is impossible to reach them [P. 20] with the finger, and you cannot see them even when the orifice, which is called organum[438], is open, so that you are not able to operate, you should treat her with strong bandages and a hot sponge. You should also apply emollients, such as calasticum[439], by mean of suppositories and simple emollients, such as diaquilon, until the collections are softened and destroyed, and [the man and the woman] should be separated during the whole night[440].

Another treatment. If all these medicaments do not help her and the pain is not even diminished, then we should apply various bandages made of grains to her. Take *pollen*, which is barley flour[441], bitter vetch, cumin, boiled and pounded figs and terbentine. Bandage her, and it will succeed with the help of God[442]. A helpful bath for this [ailment]. Take laurel, pennyroyal, marrubium, artemisia, scopa regia[443], centaury and mint. Boil all these in water and bathe the place continuously. This treatment has to be done immediately be-

---

[434] The London text of the treatise breaks off at this point, due to the loss of several leaves. The remaining passages are based exclusively on the Parma Ms.

[435] DPM B: "Omnes autem collectiones in corpore mulierum cum maturate, aperiende sunt".

[436] The Hebrew text omits the following sentence: "Si uero feruor affuerit, spongia sublata linteolo in oleo dulci intinctis sinum ipse comple".

[437] DPM B: "tetrafarmacon"; P: *tetra farmaqa*. See Radicchi, *La Gynaecia di Muscione*, pp. 481-482.

[438] The translator misunderstood the Latin, which refers to the use of a speculum: "neque organo patefacto oculis uideri possit".

[439] DPM B: "pessariorum calasticorum"; P: *qalastinqas*. See: *ibid.*, p. 309.

[440] The last sentence was added by the Hebrew translator or a later scribe.

[441] DPM B: "polline ordei"; P: "*polegni*, which is barley flour".

[442] The last sentence is the Hebrew translator's addition.

[443] DPM B: "scopa regia"; P: *esqoparegia*. See: Radicchi, *La Gynaecia di Muscione*, pp. 467-468.

cause if the collection rests for a long time, it is harmful to the womb and it might damage it[444].

A suppository. Take butter, hyssop juice, chicken fat, nitron and fried raisins. Pound all these, prepare a suppository and apply it on the above-mentioned collections, which occur suddenly and develop very quickly, so that the humours [P. 30] flow out through another part [of the body], and sometimes even break the skin. Every time it breaks inside the womb, it is purified through the womb[445]. If it occurs outside [the womb], the proper treatment is to apply an emollient bandage and then to remove it from its roots with a scalpel.

Another [prescription] for pregnancy[446], which is wonderful. Take bile of a bull, wind wool around it and place it in her uterine orifice, a short time [after] her menstruation. She will remove it at night and sleep with her husband, and she will become pregnant with God's help.

For pregnancy. [Take] two dirhems balsam, two dirhems *frazrani*[447], one dirhem gander fat, a quarter dirhem myrrh, one dirhem deer [P. 35] brain and opoponac, pound all these in rose oil and place it there [in the womb] for three successive hours; then she should remove it and lie with her husband. But she will conceive only if it is used constantly.

Another [prescription] for pregnancy. Take bile of a she-goat and cumin, and mix it with rose oil [P. 49v] [and] green oil[448] and apply it properly.

Another [prescription] for pregnancy. Pound [...]

On lesions of the womb[449]. Sometimes it [the womb] is scorched and diseased [in a manner similar to the effect] of vinegar.

{Following are the signs. Pain of} the head and the afflicted area. The humour flows with pain {and smells, at times abundantly} and

---

[444] The following prescription was omitted in the Hebrew text: "Vtimur etiam pessariis que maturent et rumpatur, scilicet adipis anserini et ficus diligenter trite, ana + .i. terebentine + i. rute 3 .iii. yris illiricis + .ii. nitri 3 .ii.". [+ means drachme].

[445] DPM B: "ita ut humor ipse per partes mulierum foras excludatur".

[446] The following prescriptions for facilitating pregnancy were added by the Hebrew translator or one of the scribes.

[447] I could not identify the term.

[448] P: *finzuit*, which is probably a deformation of *omphacinum*, L. and *onfacino*, It. See: Radicchi, *La Gynaecia di Muscione*, p. 418-419.

[449] DPM B: "De uulneribus in matricis".

at times in a small quantities. If the disease is in the lower places[450], the pain is very strong; [P. 5] {if the lesion occurs} in the cervix[451], it causes a fever and a strong inflammation, the pulse becomes strong and the humour scanty; {if there is filth} in the lesion, then it diminishes[452] and the humour becomes leaden-coloured and as if {it was abundant with *rasuris*.

If it becomes} cancerous, the evil smell that occurs there is unbearable, the blood flows continuously, and she will suffer from {black corrupted blood}, headache and pain in the neck, the eyes and the interior parts of the eyes.

The treatment. Purifying the dirty {lesion by applying} a tisane made of a lot of honey and tetrapharmacum, both dissolved in {frankincense} oil [P.10] {Or} boil {in honeyed water} fenugreek, wheat bran and lentil. Wash the lesion well with it. If there {filth remains}, place upon it marrubium, barley flour and iris. Also place bandages on the external part [made of] barley {flour} and green oil. If a cancer has developed there, you should apply all the proper medicaments for cancer. If the cancer is inside, it is a grave and dangerous ailment, since we cannot apply the proper medicaments there. In this case, you should apply light medicaments, such as various lukewarm bathes[453], with a lot of honey and a small quantity of oil, as well as fenugreek [P.15] mixed with water and dates, all these pounded well[454], and add a small quantity of good wine or vinegar. If the cancer becomes larger, we have to boil pomegranate peels, rose leaves, olive branches, quince, alum, acacia and lycium and try to place it inside. If the ailment is cleansed, we will give her tasty food and good wine.

---

450 DPM B: "Si autem in feruore fuerit". The Hebrew translator may possibly have read *in inferiori*.

451 The translator omits: "uel collo matricis".

452 DPM B: "dolor quidem minuitur"

453 DPM B: "Quare leuibus intus uti debemus medicaminibus".

454 The Hebrew text omits: "Admixto modico panis, et calida imponito. Sucus herbe plantaginis, et uue lupine et intube...".

THE HEBREW TRANSLATION OF *LIBER DE SINTHOMATIBUS MULIERUM*, 3 [1]

Jews' College, Ms. Montefiore, 440, fols. 60r-62r.

[f. 60r] [...] [..]של אפיסת הלב הנקרא שינק[ופיש] [...] [ול]פעמים יקרא לה בסבת החולי כפיפות גו[ף] [...] יאבד הדבור ממנה. והחוטם ושפתיה יתעקמו [...] גבה למעלה. **וספר גאלינוס** על אשה אחת [...] בדמה ונמנע ממנה הדפק כלו ממנה והיתה [...] ולא נשאר לה מבחוץ אות חיים. ואולם הטבע השאיר קצת חום סבי[ב] הלב ורוב הרופאים דנוה למות ובא גאלינוס עצמו ולקח צמר רך וזך [ושם] קרוב לנשימת פיה וראה הצמר נע והכיר בתנועתו כי עוד יש בה רוח חיים. וזה החולי יקרא אל האשה בסבת שפעת הזרע וכאשר ישחת הזרע יתהפך בטבע ארס. וזה יקרה להם בהפסקתם ממשכבי זכר ויותר אל האלמנות שהרגילו משכב. ויקרה אל הבתולות בהגיעם לבגר ולא תתענגו במשכב זכר בשאלת הטבע מהם כי אז ישפיע הזרע בהן הוא הנקרא אֱשְׁפֶּרְמַא. ירצה הטבע לגרשו ולא יוכל ומשפעת הזרע יולד עשן ויעלה אל החלקים הנקראים קוֹרְנֵילְיאֶש ואז יקרה מצוק אל כנפי הקאה[2] ואל הלב. ושאר כלי הקול עד שיגיע מצוק אל הלשון ואל הדבור. ותחילת זה החולי רגיל להולד מאפיסת הפרחים. ואם ישפיע הזרע יוסיף החולי ויכבד וי[ות]ר בהתאחדו בחלקים העליונים הם כלי הדבור.

העזר אל החולי הזה יתכן לחכך רגליה בחוזקה בשמן לַבְּרִין וידיה בנחת ויניחו לאפיה דברים אשר ריחם קשה כמו קשתור גַלְבֵּי[..] גֵימַא שרופה צמר שרוף עור חרוך ודומיהם. ולמשוח הערוה במשיחות אשר ריחם קשה כמו אִירֵילְיאוֹן נַרְדִילֵיאוֹן כי אלה ימשכו ויעוררו נדות. ולבתולות ישימו כוסות המציצה עלי ערותן ובפנים וסביב מבחוץ ימשחו בשמן אשר ריחו טוב. ובערב יתנו לה מן דִיאַה סִימִינוס עם מיץ אפי. או עם אישרוף העשוי מקַלַמֵינט. ויעשו לה משקה העשוי כן תקח גֻוֹשְׁקִיאַמִי. קשתור. פלפל לבן. [f. 60v] [...] וימזוג הכל ביין מתוק ות[אכל] [...] כנגד

---

[1] The openly section of the translation was lost due to loss of several leaves of the manuscript. The title may have been that mentioned by the anonymous translator is *Sefer ha-seter* (Book on the Hidden [places]).

[2] Read: הריאה

זה החולי לקחת כמון וליבשו ולקג[..] במשקה. ואמר לקחת קבת שועל או צב[ין] [...] אבק ולעשות ממנה מוך. ואמר אוֹרִיבַש לבשל מן [5] זרע הפשתן ומיץ כרובות ותשליך לפנים. או שורש גִימַבְדֵרִי טוב נכון מאד לבשל ולכתוש ולשום על הבטן והטבור.

מירידת האם אחר לדתה. לפעמים תנוח[3] האם ממקומה ויורדת ולפעמים יוצאת חוץ מן הערוה. וזה יקרה ברפיון גידיה ברב שפעת הליחות וקרירות אשר [10] ישפיעו בפנים. והיה זה בסבת האויר הקר הנכנס מלמטה בעמדה לאויר גלויה או שבת על אבנים. או יקרה במרחץ מים קרים ואז תחלש האם [ותנוע] ממקומה. או בהתחזקה ללדת תצא ממקומה ותרד. והיה העזר אל החולי הזה כן. יתכן לחלח אותה החולי ולחמם ואחר כ[ן] תניעה. ואם תרד האם ולא תצא תשים לאפיה להריח בשמים אשר [15] [רי]חם טוב כמו בשמי מושק אשפיק אשתורקש ודומיהם. [והק]טירוה למטא בדברים אשר ריחם רע כמו בגד שרוף והאחרים שהזכרנו. ותטבול טבורה בצמר טבול ביין ושמן.

העזר אל האם היוצאת. תקח אמוניאק ותמזוג אותו במיץ אישנץ ותמשח הבטן בנוצה אחת. ואחר כן תקח קשא פשתולא [20] ורודא ארטיטיקא בשוה ותבשל הכל ביין עד כלות שני החלקים והחלק השלישי ותן לה לשתות. ותניח על הבטן ועל הטבור חטים צלויים. אך תחלת לפני כל דבר ינתן להחזיר האם לפנים למקומה ואחר כן תכנס במרחץ שנתבשלו בו רושש בלישטיאִש. קלפת רמון ומינטה כתושה. סומק קליפת גלנץ. קליפת אֹגָרִיג או אגוז שיפריש. עדשים. ואחר כן לעשות לה מרחץ יבש ויועילו אליה מאד. [f. 61r] שאלה דונג או פחם ינתן לה סוקרי עם פולים מבושלים. ובהתקרב זמן לידתה תרחץ תמיד ותמשח גופה בשמן זית ויהיו מאכליה קלים וממהרים לבשל. ואם יעלה נפח ברגליה תמשח בשמן ורד וחומץ ואחרי שאר מאכליה תאכל עופות חבושים ורמונים אם הבטן יתפשנו ויעלה בו נפח בסבת רוח יתכן לעזור [5] אליה.

העזר אל הנפח תקח זרע אפיי מדאטרי מינטא איריאוס ד׳ אוקי׳ בשוה משתיק גירופלי קרדמומו. שרש רודא הגדולה משקל ג׳ פשו׳ מכל אחד. סוקרי ו׳ אוקי׳ ויעשה מהן אבק דק מאד וירקח עם דבש ויתנו לה אוקי׳ עם יין והרפואה הזאת תסיר הרוחות יומים שלא יועיל.

בבא עתה ללדת בהיות העובר נע מאד [10] ומתחזק לצאת אז יתכן להפתח שני הערוה בעבור שימצא העובר מקום רחב ואשר יתגרש העובר ממטתו כפי כח הטבע. ויש מהן אשר בעצבון תלדנה ומקשה מאד ללכת ופעמים גופם כפוף ולא עצרו כח. וזה יקרה בסבות רבות. לפעמים יולד חום גדול מאד ואין טבעי סביבות הטבעת מאשר תקשה לידתה באין שיעור. ופעמים יקרה בהיות מוצא האם [15] קצר מאד. ופעמים בהיות האשה שמינה יותר מדאי. ופעמים יקרה בסבת העובר שמת בבטן ולא יוכל לעזור אל היציאה בתנועתו. וזה יקרה תמיד אל הנערות בלדתן

[3] Read: תנוע

בחורף אשר בטבעם רחמם קצר ויותר מפני הקור. ולפעמים תתקרר האשה ולא תעצור כח לעזור לעצמה להמלט.

העזר להמלט יהיה כן יעשו לה מרחץ מים שנתבשלו [20] בהם מלבה פין גריק זרע פשתן שעורים. ותמשח פניה וצדדיה וירכותיה וערותה בשמן זית. ושתתגרד היטב וישקנה אוקי׳ וסוכרי ויתנו לה אבק מינטא אוקי׳ אחת עם יין ויביאו לה עיטוש באבק לבונה מושם בנחירים ותנהגיה לאט במקום מדרון. והעומדות סביבותיה לא יביטו אותה בפנים פן תתביש ויחלש כוחה ויאות לחזקה בדברים.

בהתהפך העובר לצאת שלא כדרכו אם יוציא הזרוע [f. 61v] או השוק תחלה יתכן להיות המילדת זריזה לעמוד אליה ופיה[4] קטנה וחלק. וטבילה בבישול פין גריק וזרע פשתן תחזיר אותו האבר שהוציא לפנים ותתקן אותו בסדר ישר ונכון.

לגרש העובר המת יתכן לתת לה מיץ רודא וארסמישא או אישינץ ופלפל [5] נתון ביין יועיל לה גם סטריגא כתושה קשורה על הבטן ובענין זה יצא העובר חי או מת.

לגרש אותו חי או מת תקח מרשצל לבן תעשה ממנו ג׳ צלעות דקות למדת האצבע הארוך ותעמוד על ברכיה כאלו רוצה להשתין ותכניסם בתוך הרחם על פי האם ויהיו שם מן הבקר עד הערב. **עזר אחר** תקח [10] ברבינק כתושה או המיץ ביין ותתן לה לשתות. או תקח מים מלוחים או מי ורדים וחלב חמה ותתן לה לשתות.

עזר אחר תכתוב אלה השמות שאטור ארפיטיציר אופיא רוטהץ על גבינה או על מאכל אחר וינתן לה. או תערב חמאה ודבש ויין ותתן לה לשתות. ואם בזה לא תצא תשקה שנית רודא וארטמיסא ותשקנה חלב [15] אשה אחרת בשמן ותמלט. ותקח אישנץ ורינתול עם סוכרי ועם מעט שמן ויונח סביב הערוה מן הצדדין גם יחגרוה בעור נחש אותו שהפשיט בקיץ. גם יקשרו לה שורש וירוגה הוא דלוע על הירכות ויסירו אותו מהר אחר שתמלט פן תצא אחרי העובר וכל הענינים נבחנו ונודע אמתתם.

בהשאר השליא בפנים הנקראת סקודינא יתכן למהר [20] צאתה וימהרו להביא לה עטוש ותסגור הפה והנחירים גם יעשו לה לישיב אמרניון קר ויערבו בו אבק זרע מלבא אוקי׳ ויתנו לה לשתות ואחר כן תקיא מהר או יתנו לה אבק זרע מלבא במים חמים ותקיא גם יועיל מאד אם נעשית קטרת מלמטה מעיני דגים מלוחים. או עם צפורן סוס או עם צאת חתול או כלב. כי בכל אלה יביאו השליא ויגרשנה. או ינתן לה לשתות זרע פשתן מבושל [f.62r] ביין ואם לא תצא הדם אחרי השליא יתכן לעשות לה מה שזכרנו לעורר דם הנדות.

אם תכאב האם אחר שהמליטה תקח אשתורק ולבונה בשוה אוקי׳ וגרעיני ענבים שחורים ב׳ אוקי׳ ותתן על גחלים ותקבל ההקטרה מלמטה.

---

[4] Read: וידה

להכיר אם תלד זכר תקח מי מעין ותוציא האשה טפה אחת דם מן הצד הימני ותשים במים ואם יורד למטה היא הרה זכר ואם צפה למעלה יולדת בת. ואמר אבוקרט כי האשה שהיה היה זכר צבעה נאה והדד הימני יותר מן השמאלי ואם היא הרה בת יהיה ההפך.

המקשה ללדת בסבת צרות פי הרחם. נאמר כי ג׳ ירחים קודם נידתה יתכן להרגיל עצמה במאכלים קלים וממהרים לבשל האברים כמו תרנגולים קטנים פדריץ פיושנץ דגי סנפיר במרק טוב ותמיד לבא במרחץ מים מתוקים. וישיבו שם עשבים מלחלחים כמו מלוא שטרי שאר. ותרחץ במרחץ מים ובמרחץ יבש ובצאתה מן המרחץ יאות למשוח אותה מן הטבור ולמטה במשיחות חמות בשמן קאמומינה שמן הניט שמן זרע פשתן שומן אווז או תרנגולת בלא מנה.

איך ראויה להתנהג ביום לדתה יתכן להזמין עצמה כמנהג הנהוג בחכמת המילדות ותתן לה עטוש ותסגור פיה וחוטמה כדי ללבת כל הפה לפנים גם ינתן לה מן בצק כעיסת קדישול פניגריג או בבשול זרע פשתן גם יתנו לה מעט צרי או דיאושראון ביין שנתבשל בו ארטמיסיא. דא יעשו לה הקטרה מן גלנגני ומן אשא פטידא עם רודא או עם מירא ויקטירוהו לו פיה בדבר שריחו טוב אך למטה יכולים לה להקטירה בכל דבר טוב אשר ריחו טוב כי אם בו ומואסת הריח הרע ולענין זה ישכים הסמים שריחם טוב כמו מושק ענבר לינאלובי ודומי׳ ומהעשבים כמו שומר מינטא אורינגא ודומיהם.

נסיונות אשר [f. 62v] נעלמו טעמם. אמרו שתקח המילדת בידה אבן מגניט ותשתה אבק אבורי ויועיל מאד. גם קורל אדום תולין לה בצוארה ויתנו לה לשתות אותו הלובן הנמצא בצואר אסתור הוא העוף הדורס גם יקחו קן צפור דרור וירחצו אותו מבית ומבחוץ ויתנו לה המים לשתות ויועיל לה מאד. גם בבטן צפור דרור הנולד ראשון נמצאת אבן וירחצו אותה ותשתה המים והיא מופלאה והיא טובה לדברים רבים. תם ונשלם שבח לאל עולם.

English translation

[f. 60r] [...] a weakness of the heart called *sinc[opin]*.[5] At times, because of this ailment, a contraction of the body occurs [and she is] unable to speak. Her nose and her lips become distorted {she grits her teeth, and her chest is unnaturally elevated} upwards.

---

5 The Hebrew text omits: "et ita pulsus euanescit".

Galen told about a woman {who suffered from this disease} [...] in her blood[6], she did not have any pulse nor any exterior signs of life. But nature left {a small amount of heat near} the heart. Most physicians consigned her to death. Galen himself came, he took a piece of soft and pure wool, and put it near to her mouth's breath[7]. Thanks to its movement, he recognized that she was alive.

This sickness occurs to women because of an abundance of sperm. When this sperm becomes corrupted, its nature is transformed into a poison. It happens to them when they stop having sexual relations, especially widows, who were used to coitus. It happens to virgins when they reach maturity if they do not enjoy sexual relations with a male, as nature demands[8]. Therefore, they have an abundance of semen, called *esperma*, that nature desires to expel but cannot. From that abundance of sperm smoke[9] is created, which ascends to the organs called collaterals[10] and causes suffocation to the wings of the lung, to the heart and to the other instruments of the voice[11], until the suffocation reaches the tongue and affects the speech. Usually, the origin of this ailment is the want of flowers[12]; if the sperm is abundant, the ailment becomes more serious, and even more so if it afflicts the superior organs, which are the speech instruments[13].

The treatment for this ailment. Rub her legs and hands forcefully with laurel oil, apply things that have a strong smell, such as castor, galbanum, burnt gum[14], burnt wool, burnt linen cloth, scorched leather and the like to her nose. Anoint her pubes with strong smelling ointments, such as those based on iris[15] and nard[16], since they draw and provoke menstruation. For virgins[17], put cup-

---

6 Addition of the Hebrew text.

7 LSM 3: "naribus et ori eius apposuit".

8 LSM 3: "Virginibus etiam solet euenire cum ad annos nubiles peruenerunt et uiris uti non possunt".

9 LSM 3: "frigida fumositas".

10 LSM 3: "... ad quasdam partes que a vulgo corniles apellantur"; L: *cornilias*.

11 LSM 3: "... que quia uicine sunt pulmoni et cordi et ceteri instrumentis uocis".

12 Influenced by Latin terminology, some of the Hebrew medical texts employed the word "flowers" for "mensrtuation".

13 LSM 3: "et maxime quando partes occupat altiores".

14 LSM 3: "pix".

15 LSM 3: "yreleon"; L: *ireleon*.

16 LSM 3: "nardileon"; L: *nardileon*. The Hebrew version omitted the other preparations mentioned in the Latin: "camomileon, musceleon".

17 The Latin text does not specify that this treatment is to be applied to virgins.

ping glasses on their pubes, and anoint them inside with good-smelling oil, and all around outside. In the evening, give them a preparation on the basis of cumin[18] with celery juice, or with syrup made of wild basil[19]. Or prepare a beverage for her made as follows: Take one dirhem each of henbane[20], castor, white pepper, [f. 60v] {kust, mint and celery} and mix them with sweet wine, and give her {one dirhem.

Justian the physician recommends} against this sickness: Take cumin, dry it, and {put one dirhem or two spoons} in a drink. He [also] said to take the stomach[21] of a fox or a deer, powder it and make it into a suppository. Oribasius[22] said to boil {germander and fenugreek roots, or} linen seeds and cabbage juice, and to put them inside her. Or it is very good to boil and pound root of germander[23] and to put it on the belly and the navel.

On the womb's descent. At times, after giving birth, the womb moves out of its place, it descends and goes out the pubes[24]. This is due to the feebleness of its nerves, the abundance of humours, and a coldness inside.

The cause is the cold air that enters from below when she is exposed to the air, or when she sits on a stone, or it may happen, if she takes a cold bath, that the womb weakens and moves out of place. Or if she has had hard labor pains, and the womb moves out of its place and descends. The treatment of this sickness is the following: You have to wet the affected place, to warm it, and then to make her [the woman] move[25]. If the womb descends but does not move out, give her perfumes which have a pleasant odour to smell, such as[26] musk, nard, storax and the like. Also fumigate her from below with bad smelling things, such as burnt cloth and others such as we have mentioned before. And anoint her navel with wool immersed in wine and oil.

---

[18] LSM 3: "diaciminum"; L: *diah siminus*.

[19] The Hebrew text omits: "uel nepita".

[20] LSM 3: "iusquiami"; L: *jisquiami*. See Radicchi, *La Gynaecia di Muscione*, pp. 380-381.

[21] LSM 3: "penis"

[22] L: *Oribas*.

[23] LSM 3: "radix leuistici"

[24] LSM 3: "nimis inferius descendere"

[25] In the Latin text, this sentence appears at the beginning of the paragraph.

[26] The Hebrew text omits "balsamus"

The treatment of a womb that protrudes. Take ammoniac and mix it with absinthe juice and rub the belly with a feather. Then take equal amounts each of Indian laburnum, [20] rue and southern-wood[27], boil them in wine until two parts are evaporated and give her the third part to drink. And put roasted wheat on her belly. But before all, restore the womb to its place; she must get into a bath in which there have been boiled roses, flowers of pomegranate, peel of pomegranate, pounded mint, sumac, bark of gall oak, bark of ballota oak or of cypress and lentils. Then give her a dry bath[28], which could be very useful for her. [f. 61r] [...][29] which are wax or coal, given her with sugar with boiled beans.

When the hour of birth approaches, wash her regularly and anoint her body with olive oil. Her food should be light and easy to digest. If her feet are swollen, anoint them with rose oil and vinegar, and she should eat fowl, cydonia and pomegranate. If an inflammation occurs in her belly because of winds, you should help [5] her.

The treatment of the inflammation. Take four ounces[30] each of celery seed, myrtle, mint, iris, mastic, a weight of three grains each[31] of clove, cardamom, root of rue[32], six ounces of sugar, pound them all into a fine powder, and mix with honey [which is] to be given to her with wine. This medicament makes the winds disappear; [it should be taken for] two days, if others are not efficient[33].

When the hour of birth arrives, and the foetus is agitated [10] and makes an effort to get out, then the orifice of the vulva should open in order to give him ample place to leave his bed, as is natural. But there are some women who give birth painfully, they can hardly

---

[27] LSM 3: "arthimesiam"; L: *ruda artetiqa*; written as if the two words compose one name.

[28] LSM 3: "stupha".

[29] The Hebrew translation of this section is interrupted at the end of the folio, and several leaves are missing. As a result, about 30 sections have been lost; these pertain to the following diseases and their cures: the means to return the womb to its place; on the movement of the womb from its place, neither upwards nor its exit through the orifice; on inflations which occur in the womb; on changes in the uterine temperaments; uterine ulcers; on itches in the vulva; on sterility of both women and men; how to conceive a male.

[30] LSM 3: "dirhems".

[31] The Hebrew text omits: "cinnamomi, nucis muscati, castorei, zedoarii, yris illirica ana pondus .ii. den.".

[32] LSM 3: "radicis rubee maioris".

[33] The last part of the sentence is not clear. MLS 3: "Hec medicina aufert uentositatem et aborsum".

walk, and at times their bodies are very feeble and they have no strength. This happens for many reasons. Sometimes there occurs an excessive and unnatural heat around the anus and it makes giving birth very difficult. At times the womb's opening is very short[34], and in other cases the woman is too fat. At times it happens because the foetus died in the belly and he cannot help himself by his movement. It generally occurs to young women in wintertime, since they have a short womb, which becomes even shorter because of the cold[35]. Sometimes the woman catches a cold and does not have enough strength to help herself.

The treatment [20] **for birth giving should be as follows**. Make a bath for her in which there have been boiled mallow, fenugreek, linen seed and barley; anoint her face[36], her sides, her feet and her pubes with olive oil. She should scratch herself well; and give her one ounce of sugar and one ounce of mint powder to drink with wine. Then make her sneeze with frankincense powder placed in her nose, and make her walk in a steep place[37]. The women who surround her should not look at her face, since she might be ashamed and it might weaken her; [thus] it would be proper to give her things to strengthen her.[38]

When the foetus turns to move out unnaturally. If the arm [f. 41v] or the leg comes out first, the midwife should attend her quickly, and with her small smooth hand, anointed with boiled fenugreek and linen seed, return that member[39] to its place, and arrange him in a straight and proper position.

To expel the dead foetus, give her juice of rue and absinthe with pepper, [5] in wine[40]. It would also be helpful to tie a herb of savory on her belly, since it expels the foetus alive or dead.

To expel it alive or dead. Take a white onion and make three thin pieces of it, as long as the long finger; the woman has to kneel on her knees, as if to urinate; and put these onion pieces inside the womb, close to the orifice. Do not remove them from morning until even-

---

[34] LSM 3: "nimis angustus est".

[35] LSM 3: "Cum enim strictum habeat uuluam, adhoc amplius hiemale frigore constringitur".

[36] Addition made in the Hebrew text.

[37] LSM 3: "Ducatur lento passu per decliuia".

[38] The remark that "it would weaken her" and the recommendation "to give her things to strengthen her" are additions made in the Hebrew text.

[39] The Latin text refers to the foetus.

[40] LSM 3: "arthemesia et terantur simul et bibat succum".

ing.[41] **Another treatment**. Take [5] pounded verbena or its juice, mixed with wine, and give this to her to drink. Or else, take salty water or rose water[42] and hot milk, and give it to her to drink.

Another treament. Write these names on cheese or on another food: *sator, arpeticia, ospera, rotas*[43], and give it to her. Or mix butter, honey and wine, and give this to her to drink. If it does not come out, give her another drink, of rue and absinthe[44], and give her the milk of [15] another woman, mixed with oil, to drink, and she will give birth.

Take frankincense[45] and pound it with sugar and a small amount of oil, and rub her pubes on the sides. Also bind her loins with a skin shed from a snake in the summer. Also tie roots of *virugah*[46], which is gourd, on her kidneys and remove it quickly after she gives birth, since the other internal parts might come out after the foetus. All these treatments have been tested and are known to be true.[47]

When the placenta, which is called *secundina*[48], **remains inside**. We should take it out [20] quickly; [to do] so, we have to make her sneeze at once, with her mouth and nose closed. We should seat her in cold *amarnion*[49], and mix powder of mallow seed in it; give it to her to drink and she will quickly vomit. Also, give her potions in order to provoke her vomiting[50]. It would be very useful to fumigate her from below with the eyes of salty fish, or with a horse's hoof, or with the dung of a cat or a dog, since these [substances] bring [out] and expel the placenta. Or give her linen seed boiled [f. 62r] in wine to drink. If the blood does not flow after the placenta has been discharged, treat her as we mentioned to provoke the menstrual blood.

If she has pains in the womb after birth, take one ounce each of storax and frankincense, two ounces of black grape pips, and put them on burning coals and fumigate her from below. [5]

To know whether she will beget a male. Take spring water and put in it one drop of blood, taken from her right side. If the drop

---

41 The last section is an addition made in the Hebrew text.
42 Addition made in the Hebrew text.
43 LSM 3: " sator + arepo + tenet + opera + rotas".
44 The last sentence is an addition made in the Hebrew text.
45 LSM 3: "butirum".
46 LSM 3: "cucurbite".
47 Addition made in the Hebrew text.
48 L: *sequdina*.
49 LSM 3: "Fiat lexiua de frigido cinere...".
50 Addition made in the Hebrew text.

sinks, it is a male; if the drop floats, she will beget a daughter. Hippocrates said that if the woman begets a male, her colour is fine and her right breast is larger than the left one. If she begets a daughter, it would be the opposite[51].

On [a woman] who has a difficult birth, because her womb is narrow.[52] Three months before giving birth, she has to eat light food, which is easily digested and enlarges the members, such as soup[53] made of young chickens, partridge, pheasant and fish in a good soup[54]. She has to bathe regularly in sweet water. Also place moistening herbs there, such as mallow and centaury. And she should bathe in water and in a dry bath. After bathing, anoint her from the navel downwards with hot ointments such as camomile oil, anise oil, linen seed oil, gander fat or hen fat.

How to treat her on the day she gives birth. She has to be treated according to the knowledge of the midwife. Make her sneeze while she closes her mouth and nose, so that all the force produced is directed downwards. Also give her a kind of dough, [20] which is produced after cooking fenugreek or linen seeds. Give her some medicament or *diatessaron*[55] with wine in which artemisia has been boiled. Then fumigate her with asa fetida, rue or myrrh. She has to be fumigated in her mouth with something that has a good odor, but from below with everything that has a good odor, because the womb is attracted by the good smells and abhors bad ones[56]. For that reason, use good-smelling drugs, such as musk, amber, aloe and the like, and herbs such as fennel, mint, oregano and the like.

Experiments which [f. 62v] were conducted for unknown reasons[57]. They say that if a woman holds a magnet stone in her right hand while giving birth, and drinks powder of ivory, it could be very useful. They also hang a red coral on her neck, and give her the white [matter] that is found in the neck[58] of a bird of prey, called

---

[51] Two short sections were omitted in the Hebrew text.

[52] This section is abbreviated in the Hebrew version.

[53] LSM 3: "iuscella".

[54] LSM 3: "cum bono condimento".

[55] L: *diosareon.*

[56] Undoubtedly, this is a scribe error. LSM 3: "Sed ad matricis orificium tucius possit fieri, quia ipsa matrix sequitur odorifera et fugit fetida".

[57] LSM 3: "Item sunt quedam phisica remedia quorum uirtus est nobis occulta".

[58] Probably a scribe error, i.e., *be-zavar* (in the neck) instead of *be-zoat* (in the dung); the Latin states "dung".

anceps[59], to drink. They also take a nest of a sparrow, and wash it [5] inside and out, and give her the water to drink, which is very useful for her.

Also, in the belly of a first born-sparrow, there is a stone; they wash it and she drinks the water. It is marvellous and good for many things. Ended and completed. Thanks be to God of the Universe.[60]

---

[59] LSM 3: "in stercore ancipitris"; L: *astor*.

[60] Addition made by the Hebrew translator. LSM 3: "Et hec de sinthomatibus mulierum sufficiant".

MEDICAMENT FOR PREGNANCY CALLED THE HEAD SHIELD

Oxford, Bodleian Library, Ms. Or. 2142, fols. 251v-257v.

תרופות להריון נקרא מגן הראש. [f. 251v] **להריון**. רפואה להריון נעשתה על ידי הנשיא רבנא ששת ז״ל ועלתה בידו. פעמים שלש נעתקה מפי החכם ר׳ יהודה חריזי ז״ל ונקרא מגן הראש. קח אשפיק משטיק זעפראן קשיא ליגאני קאנילה חזקה מאד קושט מתוק קנאבוס זרע קרמומי אגוז מושקטא מאשיש זנגביל גלנגר פלפל שחור וארוך לבונה זכה ליגנוס אלואיש גאליאה מושקאדא קלפת אתרוג יבש וכן מחבושים יבשים טריאנגלי מקולף וקליפת פשטוקש. ואם לא ימצא. יותן תחתיו לינגא פאשירינא אניסון מא׳ חצי או׳ סא׳ משקל פשיט גירופלי טוב ב׳ או׳ סא׳ כד׳ פשיטים ויונף ויובלל בשמן מושלין אחרי אשר יעורב בשמן ההוא משקל פשיט מר דדור וחצי פשיט עמברא. אחר כל זה יולש הכל כדי ספקו משקה שושנים הוא אישרוף רושאד מובחר ומבושל עד תכונתו ועשוי עם סוקרי לא עם דבש ויושם בכלי זכוכית זך למשמרת ועליו צמיד פתיל ויהיה סתום היטב ויעמוד ב חדשים או חדש ואחר כן יאכלו ממנו קודם אכילה בכל יום כמות לוז גדולה בבקר ואחר אכילה ולערב יעשו ויצליחו בגה׳. ויש לו תועלות רבות לחזק תאות המשגל ולהוליד עקרות ולתקן כל מדוי הרחמים וכל מדוי האצטומ׳ וכל מדוי הראש ונקר׳ מגן הראש.

להריון לקוח ארשימישאה פוליגריאל מא׳ אגודה זרע /רל׳ ניזיליאה/ לכמות אניז יבושל ב׳ רביעים יין לבן עד ישוב לשתי ידות. ומזה תשתה ט׳ בקרים בכל בקר חצי כוס. גם בעת שתותו זה המשקה תקח מרקוריא ארשימישאה ודבש וכמון ומעט קצח ביין הכל לכמות ביצה ומזה תעשה ט׳ כדורים הנקר׳ בירוקש. ואם ה[...] [f. 252r] בערב מהעשב מהשבוע הבאה תעשה הקזה מהקרסול מאי זה רגל שתרצה. ואחר שבילתה יום או יומים תעשה מרחץ יבושל בו בשק אחד רומנייל וורדים וניפיטא וסובין מלא שיבאדייד ובצאתה מהמרחץ בקר וערב תשתה כמות שקד קיבת ארנבת עם יין אדום חצי כוס כה תעשה ג׳ ימים רצופים ותכף תשמש.

אחר עבור ב׳ ימים מהמרחץ תעשה מושב מיין בושל וורדים גלאטאש סומקא קלפת רמונים מא׳ ב׳ או׳ הדס ב׳ אוגדות. אלום דפלימא אוקיא

וחצי כל זה יבושל עד החצי או קרוב ובזה תשב ז׳ או ח׳ לילות רצופות כמו חצי שעה או יותר אך יהיה היין חם ותכף תשמש.

לאשה שאינה יכולה להתעבר מחמת כשוף. [...] אא׳ אני ערב בדבר זה שאם ישתה האיש עשב מרובי הוא עשב פרסה גדולה הנקראת אונגולא קאבאלינא י׳ ימים. והאשה תשתה עשב טורינא י׳ ימים וישמש עמה תתעבר מיד. כשתבעל האשה ביום רביעי מטהרתה תהר מזכר. ובחמישי נקבה ובששי זכר ובשביעי נקבה. ובח׳ זכר ובט׳ נקבה ובי׳ זכר וביא׳ אנדרוגינוס ואם יהיה על החילוף זה על המעט ובפליאה והאל ית׳ יביא את אשר יחפוץ.

להריון. תקח גרעיני מנדריגולא וישרם ט׳ ימים ביין לבן ויחליפנו בכל יום ואחר עבור הט׳ ימים יקח מושק נבחר ויערב הכל עם טריפא מגנא חשובה ותעשה כדור קטן ותשימנו תוך מקורה ט׳ ימים ולא תסירנו ואף אם תשמש ואם לא יפול מאליו תהר בלי ספק. והנה הוא מנוסה בנשים רבות ובתוכן באשה אחת בת חמשים [f. 252v] שנה שלא קבלה הריון מימיה ונתעברה בזה העניין.

להגיר וסת בחזקה דבר טוב ומקובל ומנוסה. קח שקדים מרים וקלוף ושים ושים *[sic]* באותו מקום פתילה. **עוד** אחרת קח מררת כבש בדבש מא׳ בשוה בשל יחד עד שיתקשה ויעשה פתילה ושים תוך רחמה ותכסנה בבגדים עד שיזיע ותרד הדם. אחרת קח שרש אורטינאש ברבאנאש וכתוש אותם וינתן לשתות עם יין לבן וזה בדוק כפי מה שהגיר גויה אחת.

להגיר וסת. מירה אליבורי ניגרי אופיפונאמי מא׳ חצי או׳ פילי׳ טאברי קוש יעשה בדמות משיחה.

עוד ריצי׳. גלבני גלבני מירא טרושישיש קאבלי דיקוטי מא׳ פיל טאבריני קוד שופישיט אד אינקורפורנדום. עוד אחרת גלבני ארמוניאסי אשה פיטידא יעשה פתילה. עוד ארישטולוגיאה עגולה שאויני נשטורשי מא׳ חלקים שוים עוצמו עם מררת שור. עוד אלקיטראן מונח.

משקה מגיר. אבק ראדישיש דיפטאמי אלבי עם מי שאוינא וארטימישיאיאי ואברוטני. עוד ריצי׳ אופופונאסי ארמוניאסי מא׳ חצי או׳ גלבני ב׳ דר׳ זרע ניגיללי א׳ דר׳ קשטוריאי א׳ דר׳ וחצי טריבינטי׳ קוד שופישיט איט פיאט מאשא לפתילות.

לנקות האם ריצי׳ טריפירי מגני שים אופיאו אוקיא. אגרצי אלבי דר׳ תאנים שמנות חצי או׳ קמח ניגיללי אשקרי׳ אבק אנישי אבק שומר מא׳ חצי דר׳ גיראפיגרא גאליאני ב׳ אשקרי׳ אבק ארטימישאיאה יבשה חצי דר׳ יעשה מאשא עם מיץ ארטימישיאה ועשה פתילה.

[f. 253r] **עוגות** לעשון ופתילות מחזקות האם. חצי אליפטי מושקאטי ט׳ או׳ אשטוראשיש קאלאמיטי לפדאני אשפיצי נרדי מא׳ כ׳ דר׳ מושי פיני אשקרי׳ גאריאופי א׳ דר׳ נוסי מושקאטי ב׳ אשקרי׳ יעשה מאשא במי ורד יעשה עוגות לעשון. ופתילות לחזק האם מרקחת לזה זה תארו. ריצ׳ פולויש דיאה סימיני פולויש דיאנישיאון אנא דר׳ שימי׳

פולויש דיאה גלנגי' איט דיאה אשפירמאטון אני' דר' אוני' פולויש דיאמאנאריטון פילי' דיאה אמברי אני' דר' שימי' רקוח סיטיראנגולירום רקוח [10] קורטישיש סיטרי רקוח שיטריאוניש ואירינגורום זינזיביריש ויריריש מא' או' סינאמומי וזינזיברי לבן גראנא פאררידישי מא' דר' מושק חשוב אשקרי. סוקרי כמספיק יעשה מרקחת לחתיכות.

הנהגה אחרת להריון מבשל מגיר. ריצי' בישטוטי ראדישיש [15] גריאופילטי מגוריש אני' קרטום או' שמשומי מילישי פוליגו ריאלי איסאופי אוריגאני קאלאמינטי אני' מאני' שימי רושטי פורשיני פיריש קולי מביני אני' קרטום אני' פלרום אנטוש אשטיקאדוס אנא' או' אוני' אינדויאי מאניפולום שימיש ראדישיש אי רינגורום מאניפי' [20] אוני' זוקרי אלבי קרטוש טריש פיאט שירופוש אדליבר' או' איט שימיש ינתן לשתות עם מי בשול מינטא נוסי מושקאטי ריפטי בלשאמיטי.

עשון לזה אחרי שהרתה. אוליפטי מושקאטא או' אשטוראשיש קאלאמינטי לפדני אשפיצי נרדי אני' דר' דוא' נוסי. מושקאטי אשקריפ' דואיש יעשו טרישיקש.

[f. 253v] **מרקחת** לזה אחרי שהרתה. ריצי' פלויש דיאה סימיני איט דיאנישון פולויש דיאה גאלנגי איט דיאה אשפרמאטו' פולויש טריפירא מאגאנא אני' דר' או' פאניש זוקארי קוד שופושיש פיאט איליקטואריאום אד [5] מודום מאנום קריסטי.

להשקיט כאבי היולדת ריצי' ארטימישאי פוליאורום לאברי אשפילאום שירפינטוניש יבושל הכל במים ויעשה תחבושת.

שלא תפיל. קח דונג ולוש בחלב סוסיא וכרוך בעור צבי וקשור על בטנה ולא תפיל. ובעת לידתה הססר מעליה [10] ואם תרצה לנסות אם אמת הדבר קשור בבטן תרנגולת ולא תלד כל זמן שיהיה עליו. **לשליא** תעשן רחמה בצואת חתול הרבה מאד.

להביא הוסת ג' פעמים בג' ימים תתעשן על גבי לבנה בגחלים מצואת פרה יבשה. עוד להביא הנדות והוא מנוסה. [15] קח מגוראנה ארטימישאה רוביאה מאגור מא' מלא כף יבושל בחצי קרטון יין לבן ותשתה מזה האשה כוס קטן ט' בקרים. אחר כן תאכל כמות לוז או ערמון מזה קח דבש רבי' ליט' תבשלהו עד שיתעבה וערב בו מקניליידא וכרכום מא' ב' דר' או יותר ומאבק קלפות שקדים ב' דר' ומפליא לעשות. [20] לשופעת אבק קרן צבי שרוף שתוי עם מי פלנטאגי ובורטולייגא חם. עוד לעצור דם נידות. לוס דרוקא ד' או' אלומיני גימאני או' מים ליט' יבושל הכל עד ימוחו האלומש ומזה ירחץ תוך הרחם וזה מנוסה.

לעצור דם נידות מנוסה ובדוק כי ניסיתיו קח ליקנום אלואיש ג' דר' עשה שלשה חלקים [f. 254r] ותתן לשתות בכל בקר דר' אחת מעוצמת עם מי פלנטאגי. קח שרשי המרגארידאש ויאכל ממנו ג' ימים ויעצור.

להפיל טאבונאריאה משקל ח' זוזים מפיל העובר חי או מת. וחצי הזוז מגיר הוסת. ועשרה זוזים [5] ממית. **להפיל** קח האבן השואבת דר' עשה אבק ותשתה אותה עם מי ארשימישאה או עם מי רוגא ומפליא.

לשמור העובר. אם תתלה הקקברי על האשה ההרה ישמור העובר. גם אם יוחק באבן טבעת צורת עקרב ותשאנה האשה לא תפיל.

למקשה לילד בחון מפי ישמעלית זה העשון. קח נוצת פרדיש וזפת שחורה שלא נשתמשה בה מעולם וישים על גחלים ותקבל העשן ותלד מיד וזה מנוסה. **עוד** נסיון אחר מופלג קח ארסיניק שושלימאט וזבל החמור ואלקיטראן מא׳ בשוה יעושן מזה דרך שפורפרת. גם אם תקח בידה השמאלית האבן המושכת הברזל תכף תלד. עוד תשתה מיץ מינטא. עוד אם תשתה מיץ זקני הכרתי ודעהו ודי.

לחלי הרחם אם תשב האשה בבשול הכרתי יועיל מצרות הרחם והקושי בו. להצר הרחם. אמר בוזינא האיבפורכי מצר הרחם צרות חזק עד שימנע הסמים העוזרים להפיל העובר.

למנוע הריון. קח העלים והפרחים והתפוחים משלזיר ועשה מהם מים ומהמים ההם תשתה האשה ולא תלד לעולם ומימיו יעצרו דם.

לכאבי האם ולחליה מסוגל והוא ומנוסה. ריצי׳. רודא אגודה פרח קאמומילי׳ חצי דר׳ אניש או׳ באקארוס לאברי עשהם כמספר יוכתשו ויבושלו בשמן ועשה חוקן עד חצי כוס.

[f. 254v] **לטהר האם** מהזוהמה הלבנה הנגרת. קח טריפא מגנא או׳ שמן מושקשילני או׳ או׳ כוליאנטור איט פיאט שופשאינטורי עם מוך וישים בתוך רחמה. **להשיב** האם למקומה. תחבשת מסוגל קח איבפורבי או׳ או׳ שירי או׳ דואי׳ אולאי קומיניש קוד שופישיש משיאנטור.

למקשה לילד. השקנה עשב בירבינא שחוקה היטב נתונה ביין. לאשה שמת עוברה במעיה השקה אותה חלב כלבתא וכבש ביין חם. גם החלב ההוא טוב להתעבר אם האשה תרחץ רחמה ג׳ ימים וג׳ לילות ולא תשמש אותם הג׳ ימים וג׳ לילות ואחר יזדוגו. עוד לקושי הלידה ראשונה צוה למילדת לקשור האם אל ירכותיה אחר לידת הולד למען לא תעלה מעלה וזהו עקרון גדול. ואחר קח סיקלאמין הנק׳ פאן כורסין וקשור בירכותיה ותצא השליא. גם האבן השואבת קשורה בירך. עוד אריסטולוגיאה מבושלת ומונחת כגון קטאפלשמא על הטבור. עוד חלב כלבתא שתוי יגרש השליא.

אחרי זה אם לא יועיל יוקח זבל כלב לבן ינתן לה לשתות עם ארשימישאה ומי פרח שמבוק ומי אישניץ. עוד אריסטולוגיאה מאובקת תשתה עם המימות הנזכרות משקל ה׳ דר׳. אפופונאק סינאמומי מא׳ אשקריי׳ ושחק ויערב עם מיץ פונילויי ומיץ אפי ומיץ אישניץ ומי רוביאה. עוד אחרת קרדמומי סינמומי רודא ארטימישאיאי מא׳ חצי דר׳ ינתן עם מי בישול רוביאה ומי שוינא. עוד [f. 255r] עלי לאבייר כתוש ומונח על הטבור.

עוד לעורר אליה הקיא. עא׳ עשון מלמטה בהפשטת נחש וצואת יונים וזבל כלב וחתול. עא׳ מיץ קאלאמינט כשיונח חם על הטבור או על פי האם עם בגד פשתן. עוד אבק סינאמומי עם יין מזוג וישתה ויועיל.

עא׳ קח פלאנטאגי ושים על חזה האשה ותלד מיד ואחר הלידה קחנה מעליה מהרה. עוד אם תקשור אישטוראק ליקידי בירך לא תרגיש כאב.

עשון למקשה לילד. קח נוצת פרדיש וזפת שחורה חדשה וסובין מא׳ חלק שוה ושים על הגחלים ותקבל העשן ותלד מהרה נוסה. עוד תשתה מיץ פשתן לח. עא׳ מיץ מינטא כתושה ושתויי עם יין לבן. עא׳ ביטונוקא שתוייה עם מים חמים. עא׳ טוניס וקארואי ואיקינינטי שתויים. עד׳ אבן הנשר הנמצא בקנה כמאמר אלטברי שהוא כמו אגוז וישמע בתוכה כקול ענבל תשימנה הנשר בקינה להקל לידת ביציה. ואם יושם תחת המקשה ימהר לידתה. גם האלום הכרכומי קשור בירך. גם העשון בגללי בקר יפיל השליא ויוציא העובר המת. גם עצם התמרים ועצם האפרסקים וקלפת קשיא פושטילא כתושים ושתויים.

תחבושת חזק לגרש העובר המת. ריצי׳ מיץ רוטי חצי ליט׳ מירא מאובקת ג׳ דר׳ בשר קולוקונטירא די הספק עד שיתעצם יעורב הכל ויעשה תחבושת לח על הבטן. בעוד חם. אחר מעולה מאד קח מירא קשטור אשטוראק קאלאמיטי מא׳ חצי דר׳ סינאמומי שאויני מא׳ חצי פשיט יעשה אבק ויולש עם דבש ויעשו גרגרים יקח מהם האשה כשתרגיש חבליה.

[f. 255v] אם תכתוב זאת הצורה על עור בהמה ותשב עליה האשה המקשה תלד מיד והזהר שלא יפול בה טעות בזה

שנים	שלשה	ארבעה
ארבעה	שנים	שלשה

להחזיר חלב לאשה. קח אבן אלמוגים והדק לעפר יתן לה לשתות עם חלב ויחזיר לה חלבה. קח זבל עכבר גינגיברי לבן קאנילא גירופלי ערב הכל יחד ויהיה הזבל בכמות האחרים וינתן לה לשתות עם מרק בשר להשפיע החלב. גם לזה קח זרע אינדויאה אנישי מראטרי מוליאום שיליש קאראוי מא׳ חצי או׳ קרישטמאליי פיפרי מא׳ ג׳ דר׳ עשה אבק ותתנהו לשתות עם יין או מרק.

להרבות החלב. ריצי׳. אנישי מראטרי קארואי א א א׳ קרישטאלי אוקי׳ וחצי סינמומי נבחר או׳ וחצי לאקטושי חצי או׳ זנגביל לבן אוקיא סוקרי חצי רביע יעשה אבק דק ויקח ממנו דר׳ עם מרק או עם ביצה ומושת וישן. **להשיב** החלב אחר שברח. ריצי׳. זנבות אשטינקו חצי או׳ בראנא פאראדישי ה׳ דר׳ אגוז מושקאד׳ פלפל ארוך מא׳ ב׳ דר׳ גירופלי קרישטאליי מא׳ דר׳ זעפראן ב׳ דר׳ זנגביל לבן אוקי׳ יעשה אבק ויתן לשתות עם מרק או ביצה מנוסה.

להבריחו ולהתיכו להבריח ולהתיך החלב. קח עדשים מבושלים רביע ליט׳ מינטא אגודה אחת יבושל יחד ואחר הבשול יזה עליהם חומץ מעט ויחבוש על השדים ויברח החלב. אחרת קח מלא הכף [f. 256r] מינטא יבשלהו בקדרה ואחר בשולה תתן האשה הדד על פי הקדרה לקבל העשן ויותך החלב. **להרבות** חלב. אבק קרישטאליי אבק גלדא מא׳ או׳ ערב שני

האבקים וישתה אותו האשה ג׳ ימים אחר הלידה. ואם יבושל האישיניש בדבש ותניחהו למטה.

בהוצאת השליא וניקוי האם אחרי הלידה. רפואה מנוסה קח זרע פיא הנלקט בחדש מאיי אותו אוכלים הבהמות ושירוהו בקערה גדולה עם מים רבים על האש וירתח הרבה רתיחה אחר רתיחה ואחר ישים המים בעודם רותחים בקערה גדולה וישים הקערה תחת כסא נקוב ותשב האשה על הכסא ותקבל העשן כפי היכלת ותוציא השליא ותזהר האשה שלא יגעו המים ברחם ויריחו אליה בעוד שתקבל העשן דבר נמאס.

אחרת. יושם לה שורש האינטריוידיל הוא הנקר׳ בשם אחר פלאמולא כשכל השדרה כנגד האם ותכף תצא אחרת ינתן לה לשתות מעלי האגרימוניא כתושים במיים ויין. להוציא העובר חי או מת. השקה האשה ביין עם אבק קליפת לשיא פושטולא עם אבק גרעיני תמרים. להחזיר האם למקומה. קח לבונה לבנה ונדיטורס ובגאש דלאבר ודוק הכל ושים בשעוה והנח על הבטן ואם היא יוצאת כלה תחזירנה למקומה בדוק ומנוסה.

למנוע מהפיל. קח בולי ארמיטשי דם תנין משטיגי לובן ביצה הדק היטב וערב הכל עם לובן ביצה ועשה תחבושת והנח מאחריה על השדרה. לאשה זבה והיא מבולבלת במעיה בדוק ומנוסה [f. 256v] קח שומים קלופים ומנוקים מלוא הכף תוך שמן בשול חזק ואחר שים עליהם שלשה ביצים ויטוגנו הביצים שמה ותאכל שמה ג׳ בקרים רצופים ותרפא.

לחולי השד שנסטרטן ולא היה מנוגע. זאת ההנהגה עשה רופא גדול וחכם לאשה בעד סרטן בא אליה בשד ועשה זאת הרישיפטא קודם שנשתחן. ריצי׳ טוטיא פירפאראטי או׳ שי׳ פלימם אושטי שירושאי אני׳ דר׳ דו׳ טוריש או׳ שימיש שירי קוט שופיזויט. ולאחר ההשחנה עשה זאת הרישיפטא. ריצי׳ טוטיאי פירפאראטי או׳ או׳ שירושא או׳ דו׳ ליטארגיה אברי איט ארגינטי אנא או׳ שימ׳ קנפורא דר׳ דואש שמן שולי או׳ שי׳ פיאט די קוקשיאו קום אקא רושא שיאה איט אקשיפי דיקטא די קוקשיאוני ליב׳ או׳ אוליאי ויאולאשיאי ליב׳ או׳ פלומבי אושטי או׳ או׳ משיאנטור איט פיאט אונגינט. אד מודום אונגיטו׳ אלבום. גם המימות האלה עשה לרחוץ הנגע. ריצי׳ אקי פלנטאגיני׳ אקי רושאשיאה אקא קורקוביתו. אני׳ ליב׳ שימי׳ אד דאטור סומאק ברבאריש שמן סיטיניאורו׳ שמן שילי גומי דרגנטי אני׳ דר׳ דו׳ פוננטור אין פאננוליני איט אישפומטור.

לסדיקת השדים ריצי׳ פישיט נאבליש או׳ או׳ טי׳ שיני דר׳ אונאי׳ אוליא מרטילורים או׳ שי׳ משי אנטור איט פיאט אד מודום אונגינטו׳ עוד לזה. ריצי׳ ליטארנירי פולוירישאטי פולואורום מירטי אני׳ דר׳ דואי׳ אוליאי רושאשי אוליאי מירטילורום [f. 257r] אני׳ דר׳ טריש ששירי אלבי קוט שופישיט משיאנטור אאיט פיאט אונגיטי׳.

לקושי השד קח עלי אפרסקין ועלי רוטא לחה יודקו יחד וירטה בהם. עוד קח פופליאן ולמשוח בו הדדים ואחר לקח עלי שמבוק ולטגנם

במחבת כלי שמן ולשומם על הדדים בעודו חם וזה יתיך כל החלב דרך הפטמות תוך ב׳ ימים. **אחרת** קח מוח לחם לבן ובשל עם יין לבן ואחר קח מיץ גושפתו וערב הכל יחד ועשה תחבשת על השד והפטמת יהיה חוץ ויתיך כל החלב כמו שיהיה באלמפיק.

לנאצור בשר האשה בשד האשה. רחץ תמיד הנגע ביין חי שנתבשל בו מיררא ואחר ינוגב ואחר כן קח סרקקוללא אלואין יאובקו ויעורבו עם דבש ויכרוך בו הפתילה ויכניסה בנאצור. וזהו מסודות הנאצור לרפאתו בגה׳. לפי הדד הנפוח והמאוכל זהראבי. להסיר הנפח. מי אפר גפנים שרוי יום ולילה ומסונן ומעורב עם מעט חומץ ובגדים שרויים וסחוטים מונחים שם ולפי הדד המאוכל או עלי עפצים לחים עם שמן ורדים או מי מברילאה או כולי ארמיניצי ושמן פולין ואלואין ורדים וחול ומוח לחם ואגוז.

ומפי המנסה בחון אפר ביצה יודק לו קלחי הכרוב אחרי היניקה בהיות פי השד פתוח ורטוב יזרוק עליו מן האפר ההוא וירפא תוך ג׳ או ד׳ ימים.

בקווץ הוא אישפאשמי מפי מומחה. ריצי׳ אוליאו קאמומיללי אוליאו אנישי אאא׳ אוליאו לבריני אוליאו קשטוריאי אנ׳ או׳ שימיי׳ משטיציש שלויאה קאמומיללי אנישי אא׳ דזאשי׳ שירי דר׳ דו׳ משיאנטו איט פיאט אונגיני[f. 257] ומשח כל השדרה מקדקד עד הקצה התחתון ממנו וזה מחזק העצבים כלם. וזכור לך כי האישפאשמי שהוא עם ליחות או בעד דם מאי זה ליחה שיהיה סבתו הוא יותר בטוח מאותו שהוא כלו ליחה כי רפואת הראשון בהרקת הליחה דרך הקזה או בדרך אחרת. ורפואת האשפאיימי החלקיי שאינו בכל הגוף רק באבר אחד רפואתו לכרות אותו עצב שהוא הסבה או את אותו אבר שהוא בו שאם לא יכרות אותו יתפשט האשפאשמי בכל הגוף. וזכור לך כי מהאישפאשמי ג׳ מינים. האחד שלא יכפפו ולא יתנועעו האברים לפנים ויתנועעו לאחור. השני שיהיה בהפך. השלישי שלא יתנועעו לא לפנים ולא לאחור רק שיעמדו במתיחה שוה.

English translation

[f. 251v] **Medicament for Pregnancy Called the Head Shield**. **For pregnancy**. A medicament for pregnancy has been prepared successfully by the Head of the community, our Rabbi Sheshet of blessed memory. It was copied three times from the wise Rabbi Yehudah Ḥarizi of blessed memory, and it is called the Head Shield.

Take nard, mastic, saffron, cassia, a very hard canella wood, sweet costus, hemp, cardamom seed, the fruit of nutmeg, male ginger, galangal, black and long pepper, pure frankincense, aloe wood, tamarisk, nutmeg, peel of dry citron, dry cydonias, peeled *trianguli*[1] and peel of pistachio. If you cannot find any [of these], replace them with half an ounce each or the weight of a small coin[2] of bird tongue[3] wood and anise and two ounces or the weight of four small coins of good stock. Mix them all and immerse in mucilan[4] oil, which has been mixed with the weight of one small coin of sweet marjoram[5] and the weight of half a small coin of ambar. Then knead them all in a sufficient quantity of rose liquid, which is best as a rose syrup[6], well- cooked and made with sugar, but not with honey. Put this in a clear glass vessel, well-sealed with a cord, so that it is perfectly closed. It should stay like that two months or [at least] one; then they will eat the amount of a big nut, before and after breakfast, and in the evening as well, and it will succeed with the help of God. It provides many benefits, such as strengthening sexual desire, curing sterility, repairing all the ailments of the womb, of the stomach and the head, and it is called the Head Shield.

For pregnancy. Take one pack each of absinthe and water pepper, the seed of Arabian costus and the same amount of anise, cook them in two-quarts of white wine until half remains. She should drink from it every morning for nine mornings. While drinking this beverage, she should also take mercury, absinthe, honey and cumin, and a little quantity of Arabian costus in wine, all of them in the amount of an egg, and prepare nine balls called "warts"[7]. And if [...][8] [f. 252r] at evening of the herb, during the next week, let blood from her ankle from whatever foot you prefer. After one day or two, make a bath in which there were boiled, in one sack, rosemary, roses, naphta, whole bran and white alum[9]. When she gets out of the bath, in the morning and in the evening, she has to drink an amount as little as a nut of rabbit stomach with half a glass of red wine. She should do

---

[1] I could not identify this plant.

[2] Aramaic: *pshita*

[3] Spanish: *passerina* or *lengua passarina*. See *Menor daño de la medicina de Alonso de Chirino*, p. 284.

[4] The author probably refers to the vegetal substance, called *mucilage* in French, used in the Middle Ages for different preparations. See *Platéarius, Le livre des simples médecines*, p. 357.

[5] Arabic: مرددوش. See *Tuḥfat al-aḥbâb*, no. 253.

[6] Spanish: *axrab rosado*. See *Menor daño de la medicina de Alonso de Chirino*, pp. 313-314.

[7] Spanish: *verruga* and *berruga*. See *ibid.*, p. 312.

[8] A lacuna of a few words in the manuscript.

[9] Arabic: شب ابيض. See *El libro del 'Amal man ṭabba li-man ḥabba*, p. 9.

this for three days successively, and then immediately have sexual relations.

Another [one]. Two days after having a bath, she should sit in wine in which there have been boiled two ounces each of roses, chestnut, tanner's summac and pomegranate peel, and two packs of myrtle, [as well as] a half ounce each of alum and diapalma[10]. Cook all these until there remains half or so of it, and she should sit in this during seven or eight successive nights, for half an hour or more, but the wine has to be hot, and afterwards she should immediately have sexual relations.

For a woman who cannot conceive because of sorcery, God forbid, amen, amen. I guarantee that if the man drinks of the horehound herb, which is the big horseshoe herb called *ongula caballina*[11], for ten days, and if the woman drinks of the bull herb[12] for ten days, and they have sexual relations, she will immediately conceive.

When the woman has sexual intercourse four days after her purification, she will conceive a male; on the fifth day a female; on the sixth, a male, on the seventh a female, on the eighth a male, on the ninth a female; on the tenth, a male; and on the eleventh, an hermaphrodite. The reverse cases are rare and extraordinary. In fact God, be He blessed, brings about whatever He wishes.

For pregnancy. Take grains of mandrake[13], immerse them in white wine for nine days, change the wine every day, and after the nine days, take selected musk, mix them all with grey truffle, and make a little ball. Put it in her source[14] for nine days and do not take it out even if she has sexual intercourse. If the ball does not fall, she will undoubtedly conceive. It has been experimented on many women, including one aged fifty [f. 252v] years, who was never pregnant, and she conceived with this treatment.

For menstruation. To [make it] flow strongly, [a recipe that] is good, accepted and tried. Take bitter almonds, peel and put them in that place as a suppository.

---

[10] Hebrew text: *dipalima*, Spanish: *diapalma*, a preparation made on a base of palm juice. See *Menor daño de la medicina de Alonso de Chirino*, p. 269.

[11] The author used three terms for the same plant. The second is a Hebrew translation of the Spanish: *ungula cavallina*, or *uña de cavallo*; See Cobarruvias, *Tesoro de la lengua castellana o española*, p.987.

[12] Romance: *torina*, or *taurina*

[13] Romance: *mandragola.*

[14] The author employs the Hebrew term *maqor*, originating in the Bible (Levit. 20:18) and frequently used in the Talmudic literature.

Another one: Take the same quantity of lamb gall and honey, cook them together [5] until it [the mixture] becomes thick, make a suppository and put it in her womb. Cover her with cloths till she sweats, and the blood flows. Another one: take roots of roman-nettle[15] and vervain[16], pound them and give her this to drink with white wine, and it is tried, since it provoked menstruation in one Gentile woman.

To [cause the] flow of menstruation. [Take] half an ounce each of myrrh, black hellebore, opoponax, [10] and bull gall[17], pound them sufficiently and make an electuary.

Another. Take [...][18] each of galbanum, myrrh, melted horse pill[19] and bull gall, and pound sufficiently till they become integrated[20]. Another [remedy. Take] galbanum, amoniac and asafoetida, and make a suppository. Another [remedy. Take] round aristoloch, savin and watercress, an equal quantity of each, [15] strengthened with bull gall. Another [one] is applied pitch.

A beverage to provoke the flow. The powder of white mint roots, savin water, absinthe and abrotanum. Another [remedy]. Take half an ounce each of opoponax and amoniac, two dirhems of galbanum, one dirhem of black cumin seed, one dirhem of castor, and half a dirhem terbentine. Pound sufficiently and make [20] a dough[21] for suppositories.

To clean the womb. Take trefoil with one ounce of opium, one dirhem of white agaric, half an ounce of fat figs, one scruple of black cumin powder, half a dirhem each of anise powder and fennel powder, two scruples of the powder of a clove-tree, half a dirhem of dry absinthe; make a dough with absinthe juice and [then] make a suppository.

[f. 253r] **Cakes** to fumigate and suppositories which strengthen the womb. Half eliptic muscade, nine ounces storax, twenty dirhems each of pennyroyal, cress, nard, one scruple fine duck weed, one dirhem clove tree, two scruples muscade nut; knead them in rose

---

15 Romance: *ortigas.*

16 Romance: *vervena.* See Cobarruvias, *Tesoro de la lengua castellana o española*, p. 1001.

17 Latin: *fel tauri.*

18 A lacuna of few words.

19 Latin: *trocicus caballi.* See Radicchi, *La Gynaecia di Muscione*, p. 485.

20 Latin: *fel taurini cud sufficit ad incorporandum.*

21 Latin: *cud sufficit et fiat masa...*

water and make cakes for fumigation [5] and suppositories to strengthen the womb.

A preparation for the same [purpose]. Its description: Take one dirhem each of the powder of diacyminum[22], the powder of dianiseon[23], one dirhem each of the powder of diagalanga[24] and diaspermaton[25], powder of diamargueriton[26] and dia ambra; one dirhem in equal parts each of "angels concoction", [10] "bark concoction", "citron concoction"; one ounce each of ginger electuary [?] and verdigris; one dirhem each of cinnamon, white ginger and paradise grains[27]; one scruple musk[28]; and enough sugar to make pieces of medicaments.

Another **treatment** to conceive, [and to] cause the [menses] to flow. Take one-quarter ounce [each of] the roots of [15] bistort, a big clove tree; one quarter ounce each of sweet marjoram, balm, pennyroyal, hyssop, marjoram, mint; a handful of seed of pork rose [?][29], geranium[30]; one ounce of flowers of lavender[31]; a handful of endive, a handful of radish seed electuary, [20] add three-quarters of white sugar, and make one and a half pounds of syrup. Give her this to drink with water in which there have been boiled mint, muscade nut, dittany and balsam.

---

[22] A preparation based on cumin. See *Platéarius, Le livre des simples médecines*, p. 355.

[23] A preparation based on anise.

[24] A preparation based on galanga (*Alpinia galanga*. L.)

[25] A preparation based on plant seeds. See Radicchi, *La Gynaecia di Muscione*, pp. 343-344.

[26] A preparation based on pearl powder. See *Platéarius, Le livre des simples médecines*, p. 355.

[27] *Aframomum granum-paradisi*, L. See *Platéarius, Le livre des simples médecines*, p. 335.

[28] Latin: *rece. pulvis dia cymuni pulvis dianiseon ana dr. semi. pulvis galangi. et dia aspermaton an. dr. un. pulvis diamanariton pulvis dia ambari an. dr. semi. [concoction] sitirangelorum [concoction] cortisis sitri [concoction] citreonis heiringorum zinzibris verdigris [one ounce of each] cinamumi [white] zinzibri grana paradisi...* The bracketed words appear in Hebrew.

[29] The text says: *semi rosati porcini.* I could not identify the plant.

[30] Hebrew text: *pedis colombini*. In the Middle Ages this term referred to various kinds of *geranium*. See *Platéarius, Le livre des simples médecines*, p. 341.

[31] The Hebrew text states: *esticados arabici*; it is *lavandula stoechas*, L., called *sticados arabici* in the Middle Ages. The addition of the "e" before the "s" at the beginning of the word is typical of Romance languages. See *Platéarius, Le livre des simples médecines*, p. 334.

A fumigation treatment after conception. [Take] two dirhems each of eliptic muscade, mint, ladanum, nard; two scruples of muscade nut; and make pills.

[f. 253v] **A confection** for a woman after she has conceived. Take one dirhem each of the powder of diacyminum and dianiseon, the powder of diagalanga and diaspermaton, the powder of great trefoil and aromatic roses, sugar bread, pound them sufficiently and make an electuary in the [5] form of Christ's hand[32].

To tranquillize delivery pains. Take fine flour of absinthe, hellebore, asphodel and snake-plant. Boil them all in water and make a bandage.

To prevent abortion. Take wax, knead it in mare milk, bind it with deer leather, tie it on her belly and she will not abort. And when she delivers, take it off. [10] If you wish to experiment [and to see] if it really works, tie it to the belly of a hen and it will not deliver as long as it is tied on.

For the placenta. Fumigate her womb with cat dung for a long time.

To make the menses flow. She should be fumigated three times a day for three days with cow dung on burning coals. Another [remedy] which has been tried to make menses flow. [15] Take a handful each of sweet marjoram, absinthe, madder, to be boiled in a half-quarter litre of white wine; the woman should drink a small glass of it for nine mornings. Then she should eat a nut- or chestnut-amount of the following [preparation]: Take a quarter litre of honey, cook it until it is thickened, mix it with two dirhems or more cinnamon and saffron, two dirhems of powder from almond peels, and it acts wonderfully.

[20] For [a woman who suffers from] a surplus [of menstruation]: [Take] powder of burnt deer horn, drunk with waybread water and hot purslane. Another [remedy] to stop the menstruation blood. [Take] four ounces of lily and dragon-tree, one ounce of aloe resin, one litre of water, cook them all [together] until the aloe disappears, wash her womb with it; it has been tried.

To stop menstrual blood, I myself have tried and tested it. Take three dirhems of aloe wood, divide it in three parts [f. 254r] and give her one dirhem of this to drink in the morning, strengthened with waybread water. Take marguerite roots, give [them to] her to eat for three days, and it stops [the flow].

---

[32] Latin: *cud sufficit fiat electuarium ad modum manum christi.*

To abort. The weight of eight *zuz*[33] of soapwort will abort the foetus, alive or dead. Half a *zuz* [of it] make menses flow. Ten *zuz* [of it] causes [5] death.

To abort. Take one dirhem of lodestone, pound it and give it to her to drink with absinthe liquid or with lettuce juice; it does wonders.

To keep the foetus. If you hang the tuber of colocynth[34] on the pregnant woman, it will keep the foetus [from aborting]. Also the image of a scorpion engraved on a round piece of stone, if carried by the woman, [then] she will not abort.

A fumigation for a difficult delivery, tested and transmitted by an Ismaelite woman. [10] Take a partridge feather and an equal quantity each of black pitch that has never been used, and bran; put [them] on burning coals, and after she receives the smoke [below] she will deliver immediately; it is tried. Another excellent experiment: Take an equal quantity each of arsenic sulfur, donkey dung and pitch, and fumigate her with that through a tube. Also, if she takes the stone that attracts the iron in her hand, she will deliver immediately. Another [remedy], is to drink mint juice. Another [remedy]: if she would drink leek juice. You should know [all this] and it will be sufficient.

For the ailment of the womb. If the woman sits in water in which leek was boiled, it will be helpful for all womb troubles and its hardness.

To narrow the womb. Ibn Sina said that spurge greatly narrows the womb, so that it prevents the function of abortive drugs.

[20] **To prevent** pregnancy. Take the leaves, the flowers and the fruits of *salzir*[35], make a potion of them; and if the woman drinks from this she will never conceive and the potion [also] stops the blood.

For pains of the womb and its ailments, efficient and experimented. Take a pack of rue, half a dirhem of camomile flower, one ounce of anise and the same quantity of hellebore grains. Pound and boil them in oil, and prepare a clyster of not more than half a glass.

---

[33] Ancient Hebrew weight and coin, about three grams.

[34] Arabic: ككابري. See Mosheh ben Maimon, *(Medical) Aphorisms of Moses in Twenty Five Treatises*, p. 262.

[35] I could not identify this plant.

[f. 254v] **To purify the womb** from the flowing white filth. Take one ounce of great trefoil, one ounce of muslage oil, warm them, make a suppository and put it in her womb.

To return the womb to its place. An efficient bandage: Take one ounce [5] of spurge, two ounces each of wax and cumin oil, pound [them] sufficiently and rub.

For a difficult delivery. Give her well-pounded vervain herb in wine to drink. For a woman whose foetus died in her intestines, give her the milk of a bitch and a sheep in warm wine to drink. That milk is also good for conceiving, [10] if the woman washes her womb with it for three days and three nights. She should not have sexual intercourse during these three days and nights, but she should afterwards.

More on the difficulty of a first delivery: Order the midwife to tie the womb to her hips after the baby is born, in order to prevent it from ascending upwards, and this is an important principle. Then take cyclamen[36], which is called the pork bread[37], tie it onto her hips and the placenta will [15] come out. For the same [problem], use a magnet tied onto her hips. Another [treatment]: [Take] boiled aristoloch and place it as a bandage[38] on the navel. Another [remedy] is to drink bitch milk and it expels the placenta. If this [treatment] is not efficient, take the dung of a white dog and give it to her to drink with absinthe, sap of danewort flower and the juice of frankincense. Another [remedy]: [20] give her to drink aristoloch powder with a weight of five dirhems of the above-mentioned liquid. Another [remedy]: [Give her] to drink leek juice; it has been tried. Another [remedy] for a difficult delivery: [Take] one scruple each of myrrh, opoponax and cinnamon, pound them and mix with *potlavii*[39] juice, opium juice, frankincense juice and madder liquid. Another [remedy]: Take half a dirhem each of garden cress, cinnamon, rue and absinthe, give these to her with water in which madder was boiled, and savin juice. Another [remedy]: Take [255r] laurel leaves, pound [these] and put [them] on her navel. It is also useful to provoke vomiting. Another [remedy is] a fumigation from below: use snake skin, pigeons' excrement and dung of a dog and a cat. Another [remedy]: Put warm mint juice with a linen cloth on her navel or in

---

[36] Hebrew text: *siqlamen.* It is the *Cyclamen Europaeum*, L.
[37] Hebrew text: *pan porcin.*
[38] Hebrew text: *qataplasma.*
[39] I could not identify this term.

her womb's orifice. Another [remedy]: Give her to drink cinnamon powder [5] mixed with perfumed wine, and it will be useful. Another [remedy]: Take waybread and put it on the woman's chest, and she will give birth immediately. After the birth, remove it quickly. Another [remedy]: If you tie liquid storax[40] onto her hips she will not feel pain.

A fumigation for a difficult birth. Take a partridge[41] feather, new black pitch and bran, and put them on burning coals; when she receives the smoke [below], she will [10] give birth quickly; it has been tested. Another [remedy is] to drink fresh linen juice. Another [remedy is] to drink juice of crushed mint with white wine. Another [remedy is] to drink black bryony[42] with hot water. Another [remedy is] to drink savin, caraway and hyacinth[43].

Another [remedy], according to al-Tabari, is an eagle stone which has been found in its nest, appears like a nut and sounds like clapper. The eagle puts it in the nest in order to facilitate its egg-laying. If it is placed under a woman who is having a difficult delivery, it accelerates [15] the birth[44]. Also, [use] a yellow aloe tied to the hip. Also, fumigation with cattle excrement drops the placenta and removes the dead foetus. Also, [give her to] drink pounded kernels of dates and peaches, and the bark of pudding-pipe tree[45].

A strong **bandage** to expel the dead foetus. Take half a litre of rue[46], three dirhems [20] of myrrh powder, enough colocynth[47] to make it thick, mix all these, prepare a wet bandage and put it on her

---

40 Hebrew text: *istoraq liquidi.*

41 Hebrew text: *pardis.*

42 Hebrew text: *bituniqa.* It is probably the Romance term *butania.* See *Menor daño de la medicina de Alonso de Chirino*, p. 259.

43 Hebrew text: *savanis* and *qarqvi'i* and *iqininti.*

44 This practice was very popular in the Middle Ages. It is found in the tenth-century work "Book of Virtues", written by al-Haitham, and elaborated in "The Book of Medical Experiences", attributed to Abraham ibn Ezra (See *Sefer Hanisyonot, The Book of Experiences Attributed to Abraham Ibn Ezra*, pp. 316; 240-241). Also, it has been integrated into the Moroccan Arabic Glossary of Medical Materials - *Tuḫfat al-aḫbâb* : "*Iktamakt.* On l'appelle *hajar an-nasr* [the eagle stone] et *hajar at-talq* [the delivery stone]. Si on l'agit, on entend un bruit de clochette. Voici une de ses propriétés: si on l'attache a une femme en travail d'enfant, l'accouchement s'effectue proprement, avec la permission de Dieu très haut" (no. 49).

45 Hebrew text: *qasia fistula.*

46 Hebrew text: *ruti.*

47 Hebrew text: *qoloqontida.*

belly when it is still warm. Another [remedy], which is an excellent [one]: take half a dirhem each of myrrh castor, storax and water-mint, the weight of half a small coin each of cinnamon and savin, make a powder, knead with honey and prepare grains, and give them to the woman when she feels birth-pangs.

[f. 255v] If you write this formula on cattle leather and the woman who is having a difficult delivery sits on it, she will immediately give birth, but be careful that a mistake does not creep in:

two	three	four
four	two	three

[5] To recover mother milk. Take coral, pound it to a powder, and give her this to drink with milk, and it will restore her milk.

To provoke woman's milk. Take mouse dung, ginger, white canella and clove; the quantity of the dung should be equal to that of the other materials. Mix them all together, and give her this to drink with meat soup and she will have an abundance of milk. For the same [purpose]: Take half an ounce each of [10] endive seed, anise, myrtle oil, fenugreek and caraway, three dirhems each of crystal[48] and pepper[49], make a powder and give [her this] to drink with wine or soup.

To increase the [quantity of] milk. Take one ounce each of anise, myrtle and caraway, an ounce and a half of crystal, an ounce and a half of fine cinnamon, half an ounce of lettuce, an ounce of white ginger and half a quart of sugar, finely pound them and give her one dirhem with soup or with an egg. It is a tried and ancient [prescription].

To recover the milk after it has disappeared. Take half an ounce of root of scincus[50], five dirhems of paradise grain, two dirhems each of nutmeg and long pepper, two dirhems each of clove and cristal, two dirhems [20] of saffron, and one ounce of white ginger. Pound them all and give this to her to drink with soup or an egg.

To stop [the milk] and to make it watery. Take a quarter litre of boiled lentils and a pack of mint, boil them together, then sprinkle [on it] a small amount of vinegar, bandage her breasts with it, and the milk will disappear. Another [remedy]: Take a handful [f. 256r]

---

[48] Hebrew text: *qristalii.*

[49] Hebrew text: *piperi.*

[50] Hebrew text: *estinco*, derived from *stincs*, it is the *scincus officinalis*, L. See *Platéarius, Le livre des simples médecines*, pp. 349, 347.

of mint, boil it in a pot, then the woman should put her breast over the pot to receive the vapour and the milk will become watery.

To increase the milk. [Take] one ounce each of crystal powder and acorn powder, mix them together; the woman should drink it three days after the birth. [Also], knead frankincense with honey and put it below [the woman].

On removing the placenta and cleaning the womb after birth, a tried medicament: Take peony[51] seed, which is collected in May to feed the cattle, immerse it in a big bowl full of water, boil it for a long time, in successive boilings. Then take the water still boiling in the bowl, and put it under a holed chair. The woman has to sit on the chair and receive the vapour as much as she can, but she must be careful to prevent the water from touching the womb. Also, while she is receiving the vapour, give her something stinking to smell.

Another [remedy]: Apply roots of *enterividel*, which also has another name: *palmola*[52]. Put the smoke against the womb, and the placenta will immediately come out.

Another [remedy]. Let her drink pounded agrimony leaves [mixed] in water and wine.

To expel the foetus alive or dead. Give the woman wine with powder of pudding-pipe tree[53] peel and the powder of date stones [to drink]. To return the womb to its place. Take white frankincense, *naditores*[54] and laurel grains, pound them all, mix with wax, and put this mixture on her belly. If the whole [womb] is outside, return it to its place. Tested and experimented.

To prevent abortion. Take cola, absinthe, resin of dragon-tree, and mastic, pound them well and mix with an egg white. Make a bandage with the mixture and put it on her back, on the spinal column.

For a woman suffering from discharge and confused intestines, tested and experimented. [f. 256v] Take a handful of peeled and cleaned garlic, boil it well in oil and add three eggs. When the eggs are fried, she should eat them during three successive mornings, and she will be cured.

---

51 Hebrew text: *pia.*

52 Spanish: *palomilla*, it is the *fumaria officinalis*, L. See Cobarruvias, *Tesoro de la lengua castellana o Española*, p. 847.

53 The manuscript says *lasia fustula*, a corruption of *cassia fistula*.

54 I could not identify the term.

For a cancerous breast, which was not previously afflicted. This is a treatment provided by [5] a great and wise physician, for a woman who found cancer had developed in her breast. He prepared this recipe before the breast was inflamed. [Take] one ounce of zinc oxide[55] preparation[56], three dirhems each of lead and burnt white lead, two dirhems each of pounded stone and stone flour, one ounce of incense, and half an [ounce] of wax, and pound [all] sufficiently[57]. After the inflammation, [10] make the following recipe[58]: [Take] one ounce zinc oxide preparation, two ounces of lead, one ounce each of gold and silver litharge, two dirhems of camphor seed, one ounce of fenugreek oil, and thicken them all together with rose water. Take one pound of the said concoction, one pound of violet oil and one ounce of burnt [15] lead, knead them and prepare an ointment in the manner of the white ointment[59].

Also make the following liquids to wash the afflicted place. Take one pound each of waybread water, rose water and gourd water, add two dirhems each of tanner's sumach, centaury oil, fenugreek oil and astragal gum. Put them in a linen cloth [20] and apply [to the breasts][60].

For cracked breasts. Take one ounce of *pisit navalis*[61], one ounce each of incense and astragal resin, one dirhem cumin, one ounce of myrtle oil, mix and prepare them in the form of an ointment[62]. Another [remedy] for that [ailment]. Take two dirhems each of litharge powder and myrtle powder, three dirhems each of rose oil and myrtle

---

[55] Arabic: توتيا. See *Tuḥfat al-aḥbâb*, no. 403.

[56] On this preparation, called also *Alexandrian tuthi*, See *Platéarius, Le livre des simples médecines*, p. 359.

[57] Latin: *rec. tutia preparati o. si. plomum usti cerusai an. dr. du. tri. lapidis cudis lapidinis muliandis an. dr. du. turis un. semis ciri cud sufficit.*

[58] Latin: *recepta.*

[59] Latin: *rece. tutia preparati un. on. cerosa o. du. lethargia aurei et argenti ana o. sem. qanphora dr. duas [oil] scili o.si. fiat de quqcio cum aqua rosatea et accipi dicta de quqceoni lib. u. olei violatei lib. u. plombi usti u. o. maciantur et fiat unguent. ad modum unguentum album.*

[60] Latin: *rece. aqui plantagini aqui rosasia aqua qurqubitu un. lib. semi. ad datur sumac barberis centaurum [oil] scili [oil] guma darganti an. dr. du. funantur in pannulini et isfumatur.*

[61] I could not identify the term.

[62] Latin: *rece. pisit navalis un. o. turis mastici sarqaqola un. o. se. cin. dr. una. olea martilorum o. se. maciantur et fiat ad modum unguentu.*

oil, [f. 257r] a sufficient quantity of white wax, knead them and make an ointment[63].

For hardness of the breast. Take peach leaves and green rue leaves, pound them together and put on as a plaster. More: Take populeon ointment[64] and anoint the breasts with it, [5] then take elder leaves, fry them in a pan without oil and, while they are hot, put them on the breasts. This will melt all the milk through the nipples in two days. Another [remedy]: Take the inner part of white bread, boil it with white wine and then take *gusbato*[65] juice, mix them all together and place a bandage on the breast and the nipple, and it will melt [10] the milk as musk.

For a fistula[66] in the flesh of the woman's breast. Frequently wash the afflicted place with wine boiled with myrrh. Then dry it, take sarcocolla and aloe, pound them and mix with honey, roll this into a suppository and put in the fistula. This is one of the secret treatments of the fistula, with God's help.

[15] For swollen and consumed nipples, [according] to al-Zahrawi. To cure the swelling, immerse ashes of a vine in water during one day and one night. Filter this and mix with a small quantity of vinegar, and place it on the consumed nipple with immersed and squeezed cloths. Or [use] the green leaves of gall nuts with rose oil or quince[67] juice, or Armenian vinegar, beans, laurel, earth, the inner part of a bread and a nut.

[The following recipe] was given by the [physician who] tried it, and so it is tested: [Take] egg ashes mixed with [20] a head of cabbage, sprinkle the ashes on the nipple immediately after sucking, while the nipple is still open and wet; it will be cured in three or four days.

On contraction, it is *espasma*[68], [a prescription] given by a specialist. Take one ounce each of camomile oil, anise oil, one ounce [each of] seeds of mastic, sage[69], camomile, anise, two dirhems di-

---

[63] Latin: *rece. lithargiri pulvurisati pulvorum mirti an. dr. dua. olei rosasi olei mirtilorum an. dr. tres ciri albi cod sufficit maciantur et fiat unguent.*

[64] Hebrew text: *popileon.*

[65] I could not identify the term.

[66] Arabic: باصور.

[67] Spanish: *menbrillo*; it is *cydonia vulgaris*, L., see: *Menor daño de la medicina de Alonso de Chirino*, p. 288.

[68] Hebrew text: *espasmi.*

[69] Spanish Arabic: شلبية. It is the *Salvia officinalis*, L. See *Tuḥfat al-aḥbâb*, no. 30.

ascordium[70] wax, pound them and make an ointment[71]. [f. 257v] Anoint the whole spinal cord, from the head to the tip, and it will strengthen all the muscles. Remember that the *espasma* which occurs with humours or with blood, caused by any of the humours, is safer than that which is humourous, because the treatment of the first case involves the evacuation of the humour by letting [blood] [5] or by any other means.[72] The treatment of partial *espasma* is to cut the muscle which causes the ailment or even the limb itself, whereas if we do not cut it, the *espasma* will spread all over the body.

Remember that there are three kinds of *espasma*: In the first one, the members do not bind, neither do they move forward, they move only backwards. In the second, it is the opposite. In the third, they do not move forward or backward, they are simply straight.

---

[70] The Hebrew text used an abbreviation: *dias.*, so the identification is doubtful.

[71] Latin: *rece. oleo camomili oleo anisi a.u.o. oleo labrini oleo castorei un. dr. seme. masticis salvia camomili anisi u. o. dias. ciri dr. du. maciantur et fiat unguen.*

[72] The meaning of this passage is quiet obscure.

THE TREATISE ON PROCREATION CALLED THE SECRET OF CONCEPTION, AND IT IS DIVIDED INTO THREE PARTS

Bodleian Library, Oxford, Ms. Or. 2142, ff. 248v-250(ii)v.

המאמר בתולדה נקרא סוד העבור ונחלק לשלשה חלקים. להיות אהבתך אחי הקדומה בנפשי חקוקה ורשומה למה שכבר ראיתיך מיום אשר ידעתיך שלם בכל [f. 249r] מדע וחכמה ולכל דבר שבקדושה זרועך נטויה וידך רמה מצוק היות טבעך טבע קיים מתדמה לטבע המקור אשר ממנו חוצבת גזע היחס ושרש האמונה זאת ועוד אחרת לאהבה המחוייבת עלי מצד הקירבה העצמיית היא היא עם הכבודה אשת חיל נוה צדקך אחותי וגברתי עוררתני אהבתכם העצומה לחבר לך מאמר קצר ונבחר מאד מועיל בתולדה ומיישיר למנוע סבות העקרות בכל מה שאפשר עם העזר האלוהי שילוה עליך להביאך ברכה ושלום אחריך תראה זרע יאריך ימים בנפשך החשוכה מגזע היחס חצובה ונפש הדל באלפי נע ונד בארץ מולדתי פה אברינגא ארץ מנוס ועתה אתחיל בהעתקת המאמר ומהשם אשאל העזר יהיה עם פי ולשוני וישמררני מכל שגיאה ואומר כי המאמר הזה נחלק לשלשה חלקים. **הא**. בהנהגה הכוללת המועילה בתולדה. **הב**. ברפואות הפרטיות המונעות סבות העקרות בכל אופני האפשר. **הג**. בסגולות המיוחסות על זה הדרוש על פי גדולי הרופאים הקדמונים.

הראשון בהנהגה ונאמר כי באמת היותר הכרחי בזה הדרוש הוא ההנהגה במאכלים ובמשקים כי עם המאכלים הנאותים יאותו המזגים לקבול התולדה. לכן אחי וגבירי איעצך ראשונה תרגיל עצמך עם חברתך הטהורה לאכול מיני מתיקה בכל מה שאפשר כמו תמרים צמוקים תאנים שמנות מעורבות עם לוזים ושקדים קלויים. גם פיטייונש פאשטינאכאש מסוגלים בזה הדרוש ויין משתך גם כן יהיה נוטה למתיקות עב מעט בלתי לבן ולחם חוקך יהיה שוה החמוץ כי כל חמוץ יותר מן הראוי מנגד מאד בזה הדרוש גם תרגיל עצמך עם [f. 249v] חברתך הטהורה במיני השמחות ונסו יגון ואנחות כי בזולת זה לא יושג ענין התולדת בשום צד. והנה כל מיני החלמוני מועילים מאד בזה הדרוש ותרחיק מאד כל מיני הגבינות היבשות והמלוחות וכל מיני מליח כי זה מתנגד מאד אם לא שיהיה הגבינה חדשה שמנה ומתוקה. והבצל

המבושל הוא טוב מאד בזה הדרוש גם הזרעונים הלבנים הם היותר נכון שבמיני קטנות. ובשר הכבש השמן הוא היותר נכון שבבשרים והיותר מועיל בתולדה ומהבשמים היותר נבחרים גינגיבר לבן קנילא נבחרת פלפל ארוך נוסי מושקאדא גלנגי קרדמומי פרח קנילא גירופלי עם מעט סיטואל והנה באחרית זה המאמר אסדר לך תאר פומינט מעולה מאד חברו השלם מאיי ארנבט דוילא נובא לאדוננו המלך רובירט נאויעא והנה יכנס בשער סדר ההנהגה גם כן אופן התשמיש וזה שאתה אחי צריך שתזהר מאד מהשנות לשמש מטתך בלילה אחת כי השנית תפסיד הראשונה בלי ספק גם קודם המשגל בעת [שכ]בה לימינך תעוררה במיני השמחות גם במיני המשוש כי זה הענין הוא מהסוד הרפואיי ולזה רמזו רז״ל באמרם אסור לבוא על אשתו כשהיא ישנה כי בעת השינה לא יושג ענין התולדה בשום פנים. גם היא תהיה נשמרת מאד אחר התשמיש לבל תטה עצמה ימין ושמאל כמו שעה אחת או יותר כי אחוש שתהיה כבולעה כך פולטה אם לא בזה האופן ובמה שזכרתי לך בהנהגה הכוללת מספיק בזה העזר הדרוש ואתחיל בשער השני ברפואות הפרטיות העוזרות בעיני התולדה ומונעות סבות העקרות בעזרת האל היכול כל ואומר.

השני אומר כי לפי האמת [f. 250(i)r] יראה בעיני כי טבע צלעתך קר ולח וטבעך אחי קר ויבש והנה האיכות הלח עם היבש הוא נאות בעניני ההולדה מאד כי בהתמזגם ישתוו אכן שתי האיכויות הקרים הנמצאים בכל אחד מכם היא היא הסבה המונעת לזה הדרוש. לכן אחי אסדר לך במאמר זה הרפואיי התרופות המנוסות בזה הדרוש רובם תרגיל לכבודה צלעתך וקצתם תרגילו יחד. והנה אסדר לך ראשונה המצטרך אליה ואומר כי היא תצטרך על כל פנים לנקות גופה לעת פרימא וירא או אבטון ולעשות לה זה המשקה אשר זה תארו. ריצי׳. ראדישיש בוגלישי איט פוליאורום איגוש ארטימישי ביטוניסי פוליג ריאל מא׳ ב׳ אגודות שתו גושכירט פנוייל אפי גראמיני פאניקאבט מא׳ חצי אגודה פוליפודי קארסיני פרח רומאנייל ובוראייש וזרעי פאשטינגאש טימי אופטיסי אניטי קרואי מא׳ חצי אגודה נוסי סיפרישי מינטא מא׳ חצי או׳ ליקאריציאה צמוקים מתוקים מא׳ ב׳ או׳ יושרה כל זה ביין לבן חשוב לילה אחת די הספק מן היין כדי שיוכל לכסות העניינים ובבקר תוסיף בו מים מתוקים די ספקו ויבושל הרבה מאד ויסונן ובסנון ההוא יושם דבש לבן מקוצף ה׳ רביעים ואחר יבושל עם הדבש גינגיברי לבן סינאמומי גירופלי אשפיק נרדי סיטואל גלנגי פלפל ארוך מכא׳ חצי דר׳ יונחו כל אלה הבשמים תוך בגד דק צרור תלוי תוך הדבש עד יבושל כל צרכו ויעשה אישרוף לליט׳ וחצי ינתן לה בבקרים ד׳ כפות קטנות מהאישרוף וח׳ כפות ממי בישול הזרעונים השחורים ואחר השלמה לשתות האישרוף תתן אליה אלו הפילולא [f. 250(i)v] בעת שכב בתחילת הלילה וזה תארם.

פילולאש ריצי׳ פילולאש קוגיאש לראזי פילולאש אגריקון מא׳ דר׳ ינוסכו עם מעט יין מבושל ויעשה לה פילולאש ינתן לה מהם יז׳ או יט׳ לעת שכב ותשן עליהם כל הלילה. ואחר הניקוי הכללי יעשה לה מוכים לנקות הרחם מהליחות הלבניות וזה תארם נוסח אחר מבלוטות מנוסה יעשה פועל הבלוטות המחזקו׳ הרחם ומכינות להריון. וזה תארם. גטלא מושקאדא אקוטי לבונה זכה מא׳ חצי או׳ קושטי משטיצי שנדאלי מושקא שיליני סיפה אשפיק נרדי ורדים אדומות מא׳ ב׳ דר׳ יאובק כל זה ויולש עם יין חשוב צימוקיי ר״ל יין לבן שבושלו בו צמוקים הרבה ויעשה מזה בלוטות עם בגד פשתן לבן חלק כלוח. שיהיה ישן בלול עם האבקים המולשים ביין הצמוקי או מצמר גפן בלול באופן הנזכר וקודם הנחת הבליטא תרחץ ביין הצמוקיי בין סתריה.

נוסח אחר. ריצי׳. עלי ארטימישאה עלי מר קוריאל קצות קאלה מינט מא׳ ב׳ דר׳ טריפא מגנא הנעשית מדבש בב׳ או׳ יולש הכל עם הטריפא מגנא אחר הכתישה הרבה ויעשו בלוטות צרורות עם בגד משי דק באורך חצי אצבע קטנה יונחו אחת אחת בתחלת הלילה עד הבקר וזה תתמיד שבוע אחת רצופה קודם הטהרה מטומאתה. ושתי הנוסחאות הנזכרות אמתיות הן. אמנם כתבתי שתיהן למען תרגיל פעם זאת ופעם זאת ואחר אלו הבלוטות הנזכר׳ יעשה לה זה המרחץ אשר תארו׳ ריצי׳ שוינא ריחני אשפיק ענפי פינייאש עם הפינייאש אגוז סיפריש וענפיו פרי גולא ענפי הדס מא׳ חלק שוה שיספיק [f. 250(ii)r] ויעשה מרחץ ג׳ ימים רצופים או ד׳ ואחר המרחץ והטבילה יעשו לה אלו הבלוטות המחזקות הרחם ומכינות להריון מונעות סבת העקרות כפי האפשר וזה תארם. ריצי׳. אשטורק ליקידי קשטוריאי גלביול אופופונאסי קושטי אשפיק נרדי דיליאו קרפיו בלשמו זרע מושליני מא׳ חצי או׳ יאובק כל זה ויולש ביין ריחני חשוב מאד ועשה מזה בלוטות באורך אצבע קטנה עם פתיל תלוי בכל אחת מהנה ימשכו מחוץ עם הפתיל לעת הצרך ומאלו הבלוטות יונח אחת בתחלת הלילה ותעמוד שם כמו ב׳ שעות קודם התשמיש ואחר תוסר כל אותו הלילה עד לילה שנית גם מאחת מהנה אפשר להשתמש שנים ושלשה פעמים בשלשה לילות לא יותר.

גם יורגל לכבודתה צלעתך המרקחת אשר כבר סדרתי אליך אחי ולמען ימצא הכל מסודר במאמר אזכיר לך פה נוסח המרקחת אשר זה תוארו בשר תמרים חשובים פינייוש פאשטינאגאש לוזים ושקדים קלויים מעט מא׳ חצי ליט׳ גינגיבר לבן ב׳ או׳ טושי מושקא גלנגי פלפל קרדמומי בשטותוי סינאמומי מא׳ חצי או׳ גירופלי מאסיש גראנא פאראדישאי קונובארוס מא׳ ב׳ דר׳ פרח רומני מינטא יבשה שמשומי מא׳ חצי או׳ סיטרונשי קונדיטי רבי׳ ליט׳ דבש לבן מקוצף ב׳ ליטר. ועשה מרקחת וזה המרקחת תרגילו יחד לעת שכב גם תרגילו יחד זה הפומינט שבחו החכם השלם ברפואה מאיי ארנאבט דוילא נובא וזה תארו. ריצי׳. מינטה יבשה ג׳ דר׳ זרע שומר זנגביל גירופלי קנילא נבחרת

קרדמומי מא׳ ב׳ דר׳ לאבישטיצי אשפיק נרדי זידואה פלפל לבן קוביבארוס מא׳ חצי דר׳ גלנגי אניטי קארואי נוסי מושקאטא וורדים רוביאה מינור. מא׳ דר׳ [f. 250(ii)v] דבש לבן די שיהיה ערב לפי כמות היין ועשה פומינט יורגל לעת שכב עם המרקחת הרמוז ועשה אחרי כן לכבודה זה התחבושת יונח על השדרה והטבור לחזק האם וזה תארו. ריצי׳. ארמנישי איפופונאשי מא׳ חצי רביע אנישי מארובי אשארי זידואה בושטותוי מא׳ ב׳ דר׳ אמברא קקבה מא׳ חצי או׳ לדנום שעוה מא׳ או׳ טרבינטי ב׳ דר׳ עשה תחבשת על השדרה והטבור. והנה לך במה שזכרתי בתרופות העוזרות אל ההריון לפי ההקש הרפואי.

השלישי עתה אזכור לך מה שהסכימו גדולי הרופאים ומונעות סבות העקרות ואומר הסכימו רופאים רבים כי קיבת הארנבת שתויית ביין או מונחת תוך הרחם מולשת עם מעט חמאת בקר מי תקבל ההריון וכן הסכימו הרופאים שהטריאק הגדול אם תקח ממנו האשה חצי דר׳ עם משקל דר׳ נסורת שן הפיל בלוגמא או יין לבן והיא לא ילדה מעולם יהיה זה סבה שתהר בזה גם יש מגדולי הרופאים שאמרו שאם יקח מררת הצבי וביצי השועל ופלפל ארוך וזרע גרגיר ומררת השור מא׳ דר׳ תערב הכל עם ב׳ דר׳ דבש ויונח בלוטא תוך בית סתריה וישכב עמה בעלה מיד ותהר. עוד אמרו פרח האכרינאש שתוי או מורח יעורר תאות המשגל לנשים ויכינם להריון ברצון הבורא יתב׳ אשר לו בלבד עלילות ומאתו לבדו נשפעות כל הטובות יתי׳ ויתי׳ אמן. ובזה נשלם המאמר הקצר הנקרא מאמר בתולדה בנלכ.

English translation

Since your abiding love, my brother, is engraved and inscribed in my soul, and [because] from the first day I became acquainted with you, I saw that you have a perfect knowledge of all [f. 249r] the sciences and wisdom, and that you treat every holy matter with a strong arm and a hand higher[1] than a cliff. Your nature is similar to the nature from which you were carved, a noble race and the root of faith. Moreover, I am motivated by the binding love which was engendered by my closeness to that honourable woman of valour[2], your temple[3], my sister and mistress.

Your mighty love has inspired me to compose a short and excellent treatise on procreation for you, one that is very efficient in eliminating the causes of sterility, as much as is possible, with the

[1] Paraphrase on Deuteronomy. 4:34.
[2] Proverb. 12:4; 31:10.
[3] Job 8:6.

help of God. May He accompany you and bring benediction and peace upon you[4], so that you may be able to see in your temperate soul, [10] carved from a noble race, a long line of offspring[5].

My humble soul is wandering in my homeland, here in Orange, a land of refuge[6]. And now I will begin writing the treatise, while beseeching God to help my mouth and my tongue, and to preserve me from any error. I would advise you that this treatise is divided into three parts: the first on the general regime useful for procreation; the second on particular medicaments which overcome the causes of sterility in any [number of] possible ways; the third on the virtues [15] attributed to different [ingredients] by the greatest ancient physicians in order to achieve [procreation].

The first, on regime. I would say that indeed the most important [means] for achieving this [aim] is a regime of food and drink, since with proper food the temperaments will enable procreation. Therefore, my brother and master, [20] I advise you, in the first place, to accustom yourself and your pure mate to eat sweet things, such as dates, raisins, and fat figs mixed with almonds and roasted almonds[7], as much as possible. Also useful to this end are pine-kernels[8] and cow-cakes[9]. The wine you drink should be red, tending to sweetness, and somewhat thick. Your daily bread should be of moderate sourness, because anything too sour contradicts this end.

You should make it a habit for yourself [f. 249v] and your pure mate [to partake] in various kinds of joy, then sorrow and sighing shall flee away[10], since without that [joy], procreation can never be achieved.

In fact, all kinds of yolks are very useful to this end. Keep away from all types of dry and salty cheeses and anything salty, because they strongly counteract [conception]. You may eat cheese, [5] but it has to be fresh, fat and sweet. Boiled onion is very good for our purpose and the same is true of white seeds, since they are the best of all

---

[4] The origin of this expression is Samuel II, 8:10.

[5] Isaiah 53:10.

[6] Hebrew text: *manos*, which indeed means refuge. The word may also be an abbreviation of *Manosque*, the region in which the city of Orange was located.

[7] The author uses two different Hebrew terms to designate almonds: *luz* and *shaqued*, which are the fruits of *Prunus amygdalus*, L.

[8] Hebrew text: *pityones*, a distortion of the Spanish: *piñones*.

[9] Spanish: *pastinacas*. See Cobarruvias, *Tesoro de la lengua castellana o Española*, p. 856.

[10] Isaiah 35:10.

the delicacies. Fat lamb meat is the most perfect of all meats, and it is the most useful for procreation.

The most select perfumes are white ginger[11], fine Chinese cinnamon[12], [10] long pepper, muscade nuts[13], galanga, cardamom, Chinese cinnamon flower, cloves with a small quantity of centaury[14]. At the end of this treatise I will write you a description of an excellent fomentation[15] composed by the perfect Master, Arnold of Villanova, for our lord, the King Robert.

This section on regime must also include the manner of coitus. In this respect, you should be very careful, my brother, [15] not to have sexual intercourse twice on the same night, since the second undoubtedly spoils the first. Also, before having intercourse, while she is lying on your right, you should excite her with different kinds of joys and caresses, for it is this medical secret, to which our sages of blessed memory referred, when they said: "It is prohibited to come upon your wife while she is sleeping"; since when she sleeps procreation absolutely cannot be achieved.

[20] She has to be very careful not to move to the right or to the left for one hour or more after coitus, since I fear that if she does not behave in this manner, she will expel [the sperm] as soon as she receives it. All that I have mentioned up to this point on general regime is sufficient. I will [now] begin the second part, on special medicaments that aid in procreation and prevent the causes of sterility, with the help of God, the Omnipotent.

The second [on medicaments]. I would truly say [f. 250(i)r] that it seems to me that the nature of your honorable rib[16] is cold and wet, while your nature, my brother, is cold and dry. In fact, the two qualities, wet with dry, are very apt in the matter of procreation, for when they merge together they equilibrate one another. The two cold qualities found in each of you are indeed the causes that prevent conception. [5] Therefore, my brother, I will prescribe for you, in this medical treatise [some] medicaments that have been tried for

---

[11] Spanish: *gingibre.* See *Menor daño de la medicina de Alonso de Chirino*, p. 279.

[12] Spanish: *canela.* See *ibid.*, p. 260.

[13] Spanish: *nuez muscada.*

[14] Hebrew text: *cetual*, probably a distortion of *centauri.*

[15] The Hebrew text employs the Latin form: *fumentum.*

[16] The author evidently refers to the creation of woman from Adam's rib. See Genesis 2:21.

this purpose. Most of them should be given to the honourable [woman], your rib, while some are for the two of you.

First, I will indicate her treatment. At the start, she has to clean her body in the springtime[17] or in autumn[18]; prepare the following drink for her: Take two packets each of roots of bugloss[19] [10] and waterpepper, iris, absinthe, carnation and pennyroyal; one packet each of marjoram, quince, *nesta*[20], *nereo*[21], waybread, mint, oregano; half a packet each of antimony[22], *goskhirat*[23], fennel[24], opium, dog's-tooth grass[25] and common eryngo[26]. [Then add] half a packet each of polypody, ers[27], flowers of rosemary and borage[28], seeds of pastinaca, thyme, dodder of thyme, [15] anise; half an ounce each of cypress nuts and mint, two ounces each of liquorice root and sweet raisins. Immerse all these in fine white wine in sufficient quantity to cover all the ingredients during one night. Add sweet water in the morning and boil them for a long time. Then filter [the concoction] and, in the meantime, add five quarters[29] of foamy [20] white honey. Then boil the honey mixture with half a dirhem each of white ginger, cinnamon, lavender, centaury, galangal and long pepper. Put all these herbs in a fine cloth, then immerse them in the honey [mixture] until it is well boiled. Reduce it to one and a half litres of syrup; she should drink four small spoons of it in the morning, along with eight spoons of water in which black seeds have been boiled.

---

17 Spanish: *primavera.*

18 Hebrew text: *avton*, probably influenced by old French.

19 Hebrew text: *buglisi*, French: *buglosse*, it is the *anchusa officinalis*, L. See *Platéarius, Le livre des simples médecines*, p. 320.

20 I could not identify this term.

21 I could not identify this term.

22 Read: *stibi* = *stibium*, L.

23 I could not identify this term.

24 French: *fenouil*, *Foeniculum volgare*, L. See *Platéarius, Le livre des simples médecines*, p. 327.

25 Latin and French: *Gramen*, *Cyndon dactylon*, L. See *ibid.*, p. 323.

26 French: *Panicaut.* See *ibid.*, p. 341.

27 The origin of the term is Arabic: كرسنة, from which the Spanish term: *alcarceña*, *Ervum erivilia*, L. is derived. See Dozy, *Supplément aux dictionnaires arabes*, II, p. 464.

28 French: *bourache*, *Borrago officinalis*, L. See *Platéarius, Le livre des simples médecines*, p. 320.

29 Hebrew text: *revi'im*, *ravi'* (sing.). An ancient Hebrew liquid measure originating from the Bible (Exodus 29:40). In post-Biblical times it signified a quarter of a *log;* one log contained six eggs.

Once she has finished the syrup, give her the following pills [f. 250(i)v] when she goes to bed, at the onset of night. Following is their description: Take one dirhem each of *arkaghanis*[30] pills, attributed to al-Razi, and agaric[31] pills, mix them with a small quantity of boiled wine and prepare pills [from this mixture]. Give her seventeen or eighteen [pills] when she goes to bed; she must also sleep on them [the remainder] throughout the night. After a general cleansing, [5] prepare suppositories for her to clean the womb of white humours; this is their description[32].

Another version is to prepare tried suppositories for strengthening the womb and to accommodate pregnancy. This is their composition: Take half an ounce each of agnus castus[33], muscade, aconite and pure frankincense; and two dirhems each of costus, mastic, sandal, musk, catchfly, onion, nard and red roses. Pound them all together [10] and knead them with fine resinous wine, meaning white wine in which a considerable quantity of resins were boiled; make them into grains, to be put in a white and smooth linen cloth. The cloth has to be an old one, permeated with these powders kneaded with resinous wine, or [prepare it] with cotton blended [with the same ingredients] as mentioned. Before you apply the suppositories, she should wash her secret places with the resinous wine.

Another variant: Take half a packet each of absinthe leaves, [15] myrrh, coral and watermint; half a quart of fat figs; two dirhems each of cumin and ash tree; and two ounces of tamarisks made with honey. Knead all [the ingredients] with the tamarisks, after pounding, and prepare suppositories wrapped in fine silk cloths, at a length of half a little finger. Put them in successively, one by one, from the beginning of the evening until morning. [20] She must continue this treatment the whole week before she is purified of her impurity. These two versions are indeed true, I wrote them both so that you may apply first one, and then the second.

After the mentioned suppositories, make a bath for her as follows: Take an equal part each of sweet smelling savin, nard,

---

[30] Arabic: اركغانيس. See *El libro del 'Amal man ṭabba li-man ḥabba*, p. 12.

[31] Hebrew text: *agariqon*. It is *Agaricus officinalis*, L. See *Tuḥfat al-aḥbâb*, no. 435.

[32] The description of the first preparation appears later on in the text.

[33] French: *gattlier, Vitex agnus-castus*, L. During the Middle Ages, this plant served as a symbol of cleanliness and purity. See *Platéarius, Le livre des simples médecines*, p. 329.

branches of cow-cakes[34] and its fruits, cypress nut and its branches, cola nut and its branches, and myrtle branches, [f. 250(ii)r] and prepare a bath for her for three or four successive days.

After the bath and the dipping, prepare the following suppositories for her, which strengthen the womb, prepare it for pregnancy, and prevent the causes of sterility, as much as is possible. This is their description: Take half an ounce each of the liquid resins of a sweet gum-tree, castor, iris, opoponax, costus, nard, resin of bdellium tree, dandelion, [5] balsam and *mutelline*[35] seed, pound them all and knead them with very fine perfumed wine. From these, make suppositories [the size] of half a little finger, with a cord tied to each, so that it may be possible to pull them out if necessary. Put one of these suppositories in at the beginning of the night, where it should remain until about two hours before coitus. Then pull it out for the rest of the night until the following evening. [10] You may use [the same suppository] twice or three times over three nights, but not more.

You should apply to your honorable rib the ointment which I have already prepared for you, my brother, but I will also describe it here in order for this treatise to be tidy. Here is a description of the ointment: [Take] half a litre each of fine figs, pine seeds, cow-cakes, fried almonds; [15] two ounces of white ginger; half an ounce each of frankincense, musk, galangal, pepper, cardamon, *bastutavi*[36] and cinnamon; two dirhems each of clove, nutmeg[37], paradise grain and gherkin[38]; half an ounce each of pomegranate flower, dry mint and sesame; a quarter of a litre each of citron and perfumed wine[39]; and three litres of foamy white honey. Prepare an ointment [20] to be used by both of you when you lie [together]. Also use, in common, the following ointment, which was praised by the perfect erudite in medicine, Master Arnold of Villanova. This is its description: Take three dirhems of dry mint; two dirhems each of fennel[40] seed,

---

[34] French: *panais, Pastinaca sativa*, L. See *ibid.*, p. 340.

[35] French: *mutelline.* It is the *Ligusticum mutelina*, L. See *Platéarius, Le livre des simples médecines*, p. 337.

[36] I could not identify this term.

[37] Hebrew text: *masis*= *macis*, the fruit of *Myristica fragrans*. See *Platéarius, Le livre des simples médecines*, p. 335.

[38] Spanish: *cobonbro*, it is the *Cucumis sativus*, L. See *Menor daño de la medicina de Alonso de Chirino*, p. 264.

[39] Hebrew text: *conditi*, Latin: *conditum.*

[40] The author employs the Arabic term: شمار. (*Foeniculum vulgaris*, L.).

zangwill, clove, fine cassia and cardamon; half a dirhem each of tachylite stone[41], nard, zedoary[42], white pepper and gherkin; one dirhem each of galangal, anise, caraway, nutmeg, roses and cleavers; [f. 250(ii)v] and enough white honey to make it agreeable when mixed with the wine. Make an ointment and apply it with the previously mentioned one when you lie [together].

Then prepare for the honourable [your wife] the following bandage, to be applied to the spinal column and the navel in order to strengthen the womb. This is its description: Take half a quarter each of cupreous oxide[43] and opoponax; two dirhems each of [5] anise, horehound, asarabacca[44], zedoary and *bastutavi*; half an ounce each of amber and caraway; one ounce each of ladanum and wax; two dirhems of terebinth, and make a bandage for the spinal column. Up to this point I have mentioned the medicaments which assist pregnancy, according to medical logic[45].

The third [part on preventing sterility]. Now I will mention [medicaments] preventing [10] the causes of sterility, on which the prominent physicians have agreed. I say many physicians have agreed that if the woman drinks a rabbit stomach with wine or if it is kneaded with butter and laid in the womb, she will immediately conceive. The physicians also agreed that if a woman takes half a dirhem of the great theriac[46] mixed with ivory powder, and drinks it with white wine, she will conceive even if she has never been pregnant.

[15] Some of the prominent physicians state that if you take one dirhem each of deer bile, fox testicles, long pepper, rocket[47] seed and ox bile; and mix them with two dirhems of honey; and put a suppository in her secret place; and her husband then immediately lies with

---

[41] Hebrew text: *lapistizi*, it is the *lapis taccie*. See *Lapidario de Alfonso X*, introducción, edición y vocabulario de S. A. M. Montalvo, Madrid, 1981, p. 118.

[42] French: *zédoaire*, it is *Curcum zedoaria*, L. See *Platéarius, Le livre des simples médecines*, p. 351.

[43] Latin: *Armenicus*, also called Armenian stone. See *ibid.*, p. 341.

[44] Latin: *Asarum*, it is *Asarum europaeum*, L. See *Tuḥfat al-aḥbâb*, no. 30.

[45] The medieval Hebrew expression: *hequesh refu'i*, means "logical" or "scientific" medicine.

[46] The origin of the term is Greek: *thêr*, wild animal, and *akeomai*, I cure. By tradition it is attributed to the Greek poet and priest Nicander of Colophon (2nd century B. C.). It was the most famous medical preparation throughout Antiquity and the Middle Ages, and was considered a "universal medicament", thought to cure almost every illness and was considered especially efficient against poisons.

[47] Arabic: جرجير, it is the *Eruca sativa*, L. See *Tuḥfat al-aḥbâb*, no. 95.

her; she will become pregnant. They also say that the flower of the acrion, when drunk [by her] or rubbed in [her secret place], provokes a woman's sexual desire and prepares her for pregnancy [20], with the Creator's will, may He be blessed, since He does mighty deeds, and from Him only all goodness emanates. May He be blessed, May He be blessed, Amen. And this completes the short treatise, called the Treatise on Procreation. Blessed be He who gives strength to the weary.

SOURCES AND BIBLIOGRAPHY

I. UNPUBLISHED SOURCES

'Ezer elohi ma'mar be-'ipush ha-avir ve-ha-dever (A Treatise on the Corruption of the Air and the Plague), Paris, Bibliothèque Nationale, ms. héb. 1191, f. 142r-146r.

Genecea cleopatre ad deodatam, Paris, Bibliothèque Nationale, Ms. lat. 7056, ff. 87r-89r.

Guerem ha-ma'alot, Paris, Bibliothèque Nationale, ms. héb. 1143, f. 86r

Ha-ma'mar ba-toladah niqra sod ha-'ibbur (The Treatise on Generation, Called the Secret of Conception), Oxford, Bodleian Library, Ms. or. 2142, ff. 248v-250(ii)v.

Kitab majannat al-ṭâ'ûn wa-l-wabâ' (Book on Epidemy and Plague), Dublin, ms. 3676,6, ff. 185r-216r.

Liqutei Rabbenu Moshéh be-'inyanei vesset ve-herayon (Our Rabbai Moshe's Compilation on Menstruation and Pregnancy), Parma, Ms. 1339/2 {3169}, ff. 185r-186v.

Me'asef le-kol ha-maḥanot (The Collected Book of All the Fields), Paris, Bibliothèque Nationale, ms. héb. 1116, f. 12r.

Miqoshi ha-ledah (On the Difficulties of Birth), London, British Library, Ms. or. 10766, ff. 9r-9v; Bibliothèque Nationale, Ms. héb. 1122, ff. 66r-67r.

Oxford, Bodleian Library, Or. 2142.

Paris, Bibliothèque Nationale, ms. héb. 1190, ff. 44r-46r.

Sefer agor ,Paris, Bibliothéque Nationale, ms. héb. 1116, f. 12v-22r; ms. héb. 1191, ff. 103r-124r

Sefer Dinah le-khol 'inyan ha-reḥem ve-ḥolayehah (Dinah's Book on All that Concerns the Womb and its Sicknesses), London, British Museum, or. 10539/4.

Sefer ha-kibusim ve-ha-ṭaharot ha-gufaniyot (Book on Purgations and Purifications of the Body), Paris, Bibliothèque Nationale, ms. héb. 1120, f.1r-24v; ms. héb. 1128, ff. 128r-165v.

Sefer ha-dofeq (The Book on the Pulse), Paris, Bibliothèque Nationale, ms. héb. 1190, f.111r.

Sefer ha-em el Galenus (Galen's Book on the Womb), Jews' College, Ms. Montefiore, 440, fol. 53v-59v

Sefer Ḥaguan, (Introductory book on the art of medicine), Paris, Bibliothèque Nationale, ms. héb. 1190, f. 46v-110v.

Sefer ha-mis'adim (Book on Foods), Paris, Bibliothèque Nationale, ms. héb. 1128, ff.1r-33r.

Sefer ha-qadaḥat (Book on Fever), Paris, Bibliothèque Nationale, ms. héb. 1126.
Sefer ha-qadaḥot ha-divriot (Book on Plagues), Parma, ms. 1365/7.
Sefer haqdamat ha-yedi'ah (Book on Introductory Knowledge), Paris, Bibliothèque Nationale, ms. héb. 1191, ff.124r-134r; ms. héb. 1106, ff. 141r-202r.
Sefer ha-riquaḥ ha-qaṭan (An Abridged Book on Pharmacology), Paris, Bibliothèque Nationale, ms. héb. 1128, ff. 60r-94v.
Sefer ha-sheten (Book on Urine), Paris, Bibliothèque Nationale, ms. héb. 1125.
Sefer hashlamat ha-teva' ve-ha-mezeg (Book on the Perfection of Nature and Temperament), Paris, Bibliothèque Nationale, ms. héb. 1171, ff. 5r-29r.
Sefer ha-toledeth (Book on Generation) Vatican, heb. 360; heb. 366, 4; London, Jews College, Montefiore, 440, ff. 25v-53r.
Sefer iohanitio (Iohanes' Book) Paris, Bibliothèque Nationale, ms. héb. 1116, ff. 1r-12r.
Sefer le-Abûqrât be-herayon, (Hippocrates' Book on Pregnancy), Parma, ms. 3040 (Rossi, 150/4), ff. 26r-30v.
Sefer yeṣirat ha-'ubar ve-hanhagat ha-harot ve-hanoladim (Book on the Creation of the Foetus and the Treatment of Pregnant Women and Babies), Munich, Ms. 295, ff. 30v-32v; Ms. 220, ff. 64v-65r.
The Hebrew Translation of *Liber sinthomatibus mulierum*, = *Sefer ha-seter* (Book on the Hidden [places]) ?, London, Jews' College, Montefiore Ms. 440. ff. 60r.-62r.
Terufut le-herayon (Medicaments for Pregnancy), Oxford, Bodleian Library, Ms. Or. 2142, fols. 251v-257v.
The surgical treatise of al-Zahrâwî (Abulcasis): *Kitâb al-tasrîf li-man 'ajiza 'an al-tasnîf)*, Paris, Bibliothèque Nationale, ms. héb. 1163.
Zikhron ha-ḥolayim ha-hovim bi-khlei ha-herayon (A Record of the Diseases Occuring in the Genital Members), London, Jews College, Montefiore, 440, ff. 15v-25r.

II. PUBLISHED SOURCES

Abraham ibn 'Ezra, *Sefer yesod mora*, Jerusalem, 1970.
Aristotle, *De la génération des animaux*, texte établi et traduit par P. Louis, Paris, 1961.
A. Arjona Castro, *El libro de la generación del feto, el tratamiento de las mujeres embarazadas y de los recién nacidos de 'Arib Ibn Sa'id* (Tratado de obstetricia y pediatría hispano árabe del siglo X), Córdoba, 1983.
Beḥyah ibn Paquda, *Sefer ḥovot ha-levavot*, Zifroni edition, Jerusalem, 1969.
El libro del 'Amal man ṭabba li-man ḥabba de Muhammad b. 'Abdalllah b. al-Jatîb, ed. C. Vázquez de Benito, Salamanca, 1972.
Hippocrates Pseudepigraphic Writings, ed. and trans. with an Introduction by W. D. Smith, Leiden, 1990, p. 71.
Hippocrates: On Superfoetation, edited and translated with introduction, notes and glossary by J. N. Mattock, Cambridge, 1968.

Ibn Rushd, *Kitâb al-kullîyyât fi l-tibb*, edición y notas por M. Fórneas Besteiro y C. Alvarez de Morales, Madrid, 1987, 2 vols.

Lapidario de Alfonso X, introducción, edición y vocabulario de S. A. M. Montalvo, Madrid, 1981.

Le livre de la génération du fœtus et le traitement des femmes enceintes et des nouveau-nés, publié, traduit et annoté par H. Jahier et A. Noureddine, Algier, 1956.

Maimonides' Medical Writings, published by S. Muntner, Jerusalem, 1987 , 4 vols. (Hebrew).

Maimonides, *Mishneh Torah hu ha-yad ha-ḥazaqah*, Hilkhot 'avodah zarah.

I. Mazzini and G. Flamini, *De Conceptu: Estratti di un'antica traduzione latina del Peri Gynaikeion pseudoippocratico libro I*, Introduzone di I. Mazzini, testo critico di G. Flammini, revisto da I. Mazzini, Bologna, 1983.

J. Ma. Millás Vallicrosa, *Abraham bar Ḥiia, Llibre Revelador, Meguillat Hamegallé*, Segons l'edició del text revisat i prologat per J. Guttmann, versió de l'hebreu per J. Millás I Vallicrosa, Barcelona, 1925.

Me'ir Zabara, *Sefer ha-sha'shu'im*, Berlin, 1925 (Hebrew).

Menor daño de la medicina de Alonso de Chirino, edición crítica y glosario, por M. Teresa Herrera, Salamanca, 1973.

M. Meyerhof, *L'explication des noms de drogues - un glossaire de matière médicale composé par Maïmonide*, Cairo, 1940.

Mosheh ibn 'Ezra, *Kitâb al-muḥ â darah wa-l-mudhâkarah*, edición y traducción por M. Abumalham, Madrid, 1986, vol. II.

S. Muntner, *The Medical Writings of Rabbi Shabtai Donnolo*, Jerusalem, 1949 (Hebrew).

——, *Introduction to the Book of Asaph the Physician - the Oldest Existing Text of a Medical Book Written in Hebrew*, Jerusalem, 1957 (Hebrew)

——, "Asaph the Physician - 'Sefer ha-refuoth'", *Koroth*, 4 (1966), pp. 11-40; 4 (1967), pp. 170-207, 389-443; 4 (1968), pp. 531-572) (Hebrew).

Platéarius, *Le livre des simples médecines*, translated and adaptated by G. Malandin *et al.* Paris, 1986.

Responsa of Rabbi Shelomoh ben Adret from Barcelona, Benei-Braq, 1968 (Hebrew).

V. Rose, *Sorani Gynaeciorum vetus translatio latina*, Leipzig, 1882.

R. Radicchi, *La Gynaecia di Muscione: manuale per le ostetriche e le mamme del VI sec. d. C.*, Traduzione italiana e note con testo latino tratto dai codici e ampio glossario, Pisa, 1970.

Sefer Hanisyonot, The Book of Experiences Attributed to Abraham ibn Ezra, Edited, translated and commented by J. O. Leibowitz and S. Marcus, Jerusalem, 1984.

Soranos d'Éphèse: maladies des femmes, texte établi, traduit et commenté par P. Burguière, D. Gourevitch et Y. Malinas, Paris 1988 (I), 1990 (II).

W. Steinberg and S. Muntner, "Maimonides' Views on Gynecology and Obstetrics - English Translation of Chapter Sixteen of his Treatise 'Pirke Moshe' (Medical Aphorisms)", *American Journal of Obstetrics and Gynecology*, 91 (1965), pp. 443-448.

Tuḥfat al-aḥbâb, glossaire de la matière médicale marocaine, texte publié pour la première fois avec traduction, notes et index par H. P. J. Renaud et G. S Colin, Paris, 1934.

III. BIBLIOGRAPHY

A. Alteman and S. Stern, *Isaac Israeli. A Neoplatonic Philosopher of the Early Tenth Century. His Works, Translated with Comments and an Outline of his Philosophy*, Oxford, 1958.

R. Arié, *Historia de España (III), España musulmana (siglos VIII-XV)*, Barcelona, 1982.

E. Ashtor, *The Jews of Moslem Spain*, translated from the Hebrew by A. Klein and J. Machlowitz Klein, Philadelphia, 1973.

I. F. Baer, *A History of the Jews in Christian Spain*, translated by L. Schoffman, Philadelphia, 1961, vol. II.

A. Bar Sela and H. E. Hoff, "Isaac Israeli's Fifty Admonitions to the Physicians", *Journal of the History of Medicine and Allied Sciences*, 17 (1962), pp. 245-257.

R. Barkaï: "Astrologie juive au moyen âge: aspects théoriques et pratiques", *Le moyen âge*, 93 (1987), pp. 323-348.

——, "A Medieval Hebrew Treatise on Obstetrics", *Medical History*, 33 (1988), pp. 111-112.

——, *Les infortunes de Dinah, ou la gynécologie juive au moyen âge*, Paris 1991.

——, "The Hebrew and Judeo-Arabic Versions of al-Majûsî", in C. Burnett and D. Jacquart (eds.), *Constantine the African and 'Alî ibn al-'Abbâs al-Majûsî*, Brill, Leiden, New York and Köln, 1994, pp. 57-70.

——, "Between East and West: A Jewish Doctor from Spain", *Mediterranean Historical Review*, 10 (1995), pp. 42-64.

Augusto Beccaria: "Potio utilis valde ad universas causas mulierum" *(I codici di medicina del periodo presalernitano (secoli IX, X e XI)*, Rome, 1956).

Benton, "Trotula, Woman's Problems, and the Professionalization of Medicine in the Middle Ages", *Bulletin of the History of Medicine*, 59 (1985), pp. 30-53.

D. Bercovy, "Quelques reflexions sur la gynécologie et l'obstétrique dans l'Aphorismes de Maïmonide'", *Revue d'histore de la médecine hébraïque*, 19 (1966), pp. 123-129.

——, "Un nome illustre parmi les médecins juifs de Provence: Ibn Tibbon", *Revue d'histoire de la médecine hébraïque*, 20 (1967), pp. 169-176.

C. Burnett and D. Jacquart (eds.), *Constantine the African and 'Alî ibn al-'Abbâs al-Majûsî*, Brill, Leiden, New York and Köln, 1994.

J. Chr. Brügel, *Averroes, contra Galenum*, Göttingen, 1967.

J. Cadden, *Meanings of Sex Difference in the Middle Ages Medicine, Science and Culture*, Cambridge, 1993.

S. de Cobarruvias, *Tesoro de la lengua castellana o Española*, Madrid, 1611, fasc. edition, Madrid, 1977.

L. Demaitre, *Doctor Bernard of Gordon: Professor and Practitioner*, Toronto, 1980.

F. Díaz Esteban (ed.), *Abraham ibn Ezra and his Age,* Proceedings of the International Symposium, Madrid, Tudela, Toledo, February 1-8, 1989, Madrid, 1990.

R. Dozy, *Supplément aux dictionnaires arabes*, Leiden, 1881, 2 vols.

R. Drory, *The Emergence of Jewish-Arabic Literary Contacts in the Beginning of the Tenth Century*, Tel Aviv, 1988 (Hebrew).

——, "'Words beautifully put', Hebrew versus Arabic in tenth-century Jewish Literature", in J. Blau and S. C. Reif (eds.), *Genizah Research after Ninety Years: The Case of Judeo-Arabic*, Cambridge, 1992, pp. 53-66.

C. E. Dubler y E. Terés, *La versión árabe de la "Materia Médica" de Dioscórides*. Estudio de la transcripción de los nombres griegos al árabe y comparación de las versiones griega, árabe y castellana, Tetuán y Barcelona, 1952-1957.

R. Y. Ebied, *Bibliography of Medieval Arabic and Jewish Medicine and Allied Sciences*, London, 1971.

B. Flood, "The Medieval Herbal Tradition of Macer Floridus", *Pharmacy in History*, 18 (1976), pp. 62-66.

E. Fontana, "Il capitolo sulle urine del 'Fasciculo de medicina", *Pagine di storia della medicina*, 13 (1969), pp. 37-42.

L. García Ballester, *Galeno, en la sociedad y en la ciencia de su tiempo*, Madrid, 1972

——, *Los moriscos y la medicina. Un capítulo de la medicina y la ciencia marginadas en la España del siglo XVI*, Barcelona, 1984.

L. García Ballester and C. Vázquez de Benito, "Los médicos judíos castellanos del siglo XIV y el galenismo árabe: El kitab al-tibb al-qastali al-maluki (Libro de medicina castellana regia) (c. 1312)", *Asclepio: Archivo iberoamericano de historia de la medicina y antropología médica*, 1 (1990) pp. 119-147.

F. H. Garrison, "Bibliographie der Arbeiten Moritz Stenschneider zur Geschichte der Medizin und Naturwissenschaften", *Archiv für Geschichte der Medizin*, 25 (1932), pp. 249-278.

J. S. Gil, *La escuela de traductores de Toledo y sus colaboradores judíos*, Toledo, 1985.

R. Graves and R. Patai, *Les mythes hébreux*, Paris, 1987.

M. H. Green, *The Transmission of Ancient Theories of Female Physiology and Disease Through the Early Middle Ages*, Ph. D. dissertation, Princeton University, 1985.

——, "The De Genecia attributed to Constantine the African", *Speculum*, 62 (1987), pp. 299-323.

——, "Women's Medical Practice and Health Care in the Middle Ages", *Signs*, vol. 12 (1989), pp. 434-473.

——, "The Development of the *Trotula*", *Revue d'Histoire des Textes*, 26 (1996), pp. 119-203.

H. Grensemann, *Hippokratische Gynäkologie: Die gynäkologischen Texte des Autors C nach den pseudohippokratischen Schriften De mulieribus I, II und De sterilibus*, Weisbaden, 1982.

A. S. Halkin, "Translations and Translators", *Encyclopaedia Judaica*, vol. 15, 1971, cols. 1318-1329.

A. E. Hanson and M. H. Green, "Soranus of Ephesus: Methodicorum princeps", in: W. Hasse and H. Temporini (eds.), *Rise and Decline of the Roman World*, Part II, Principate, vol. 37.2, Berlin and New York, 1994, pp. 968-1073.

A. E. Hanson, "Hippocrates: "Diseases of Women I", *Signs*, I (1975), pp. 567-584.

T. Hunt, *Popular Medicine in Thirteenth-Century England*, Cambridge, 1990,

A. Issa, *Dictionnaire des noms des plants en latin, français, anglais et arabe*, Cairo, 1926.

D. Jacquart, *Le milieu médical en France du XIIe au XVe siècle: En annexe 2e supplément au "Dictionnaire" d' Ernest Wickersheimer*, Geneva, 1981.

D. Jacquart et F. Micheau, *La médecine arabe et l'occident médiéval*, Paris, 1990.

D. Jacquart and C. Thomasset, *Sexualité et savoir médical au moyen âge*, Paris, 1985.

R. Jalby, *Sorcellerie, médecine populaire et pratique médico-magique en Languedoc*, Lyons, 1974.

S. Jarcho, "Guide for Physicians (Musar Harofim) by Isaac Judaeus (880?-932?), Translated from the Hebrew with Introduction", *Bulletin of the History of Medicine*, 15 (1944), pp. 180-188.

M. Jordan, "The Fortune of Constantine's *Pantegni*", in Burnett and Jacquart (eds.), *Constantine the African and 'Alî ibn al-'Abbâs al-Majûsî*, pp. 286-302.

P. Kibre, "Hippocrates Latinus: Repertorium of Hippocratic Writings in the Latin Middle Ages", *Traditio*, 31 (1975), pp. 99-126; 32 (1976), pp. 257-292; 33 (1977), pp. 253-295; 34 (1978); pp. 193-226; 36 (1980), pp. 347-372.

P. Sj. van Koningsveld, "Andalusian-Arabic Manuscripts from Christian Spain: A Comparative Intercultural Approach", *Israel Oriental Studies*, 12 (1992), pp. 75-110.

P. O. Kristeller, "The School of Salerno: Its Development and Its Contribution to the History of Learning", in his *Studies in Renaissance Thought and Letters*, 2nd ed., Rome, 1969, pp. 495-551.

——, "Bartholomaeus, Musandinus and Maurus of Salerno and other Early Commentators of the *Articella* with a Tentative List of texts and Manuscripts", *Italia medioevale et umanistica*, 19 (1976), pp. 57-87.

——, *Studi sulla scuola medica salernitana*, Naples, 1986.

D. J. Latham, "Isaac Israeli's Kitâb al-ḥummayât and the Latin and Castilian Texts", *Journal of Semitic Studies*, 14 (1969), pp. 80-95.

S. Laurent, *Naître au Moyen Age, de la conception à la naissance: la grossesse et l'accouchement*, Paris, 1989.

P. J. Llamas, *Ishaq Israeli: Tratado de las fiebras*, edición de la versión castellana y estudio, Madrid, 1945.

G. E. R. Lloyd, "The Hippocratic Question", *Classical Quarterly*, 25 (1975), pp. 175-192.

——, *Science, Folklore and Ideology. Studies in the Life Sciences in Ancient Greece*, Cambridge, 1983.

A. C. López, "Vida y obra del famoso polígrafo cordobés del s. X 'Arîb ibn Sa'îd", in *Ciencias de la naturaleza en Al-Andalus, textos y estudios*, ed. E. García Sánchez, Granada, 1990, pp. 317-347.

I. Löw, *Die Flora der Juden*, Vienna, 1934.

A. Lutz, "Der verschollene frühsalernitanische Antidotarius magnus in einer Basler Handschrift aus dem 12. Jahrhundert und das Antidotarium Nicolai", *Die Vorträge der Hauptversammlung der Internationalen Gesellschaft für Geschichte der Pharmazie*, XVI, Stuttgart, 1960.

Gregor Maurach, "Johannicius: Isagoge ad Techne Galieni", *Sudhoffs Archiv*, 67 (1978), pp. 148-174.

J. Ma. Millás Vallicrosa, "La obra enciclopédica de R. Abraham bar Ḥiyya", in his *Estudios sobre historia de la ciencia española*, Barcelona, 1949, vol. I, pp. 219-262 (a new facsimile edition, Madrid, 1987).

M. S. Micalé, "Hysteria and its Historiography: A Review of Past and Present Writings (1), *History of Science*, 37 (1989), pp. 223-261.

S. Muntner, "Ya'qob ha-Qatan, the Anonymous Translator of the 13th Century", *Tarbitz*, 18 (1947), pp. 192-193. (Hebrew).

——, "Donnolo et la contribution des juifs aux premières oeuvres de la médecine salernitaine", *Revue d'histoire de la médecine hébraïque*, 32 (1956), pp. 155-161.

——, "Galen's Books Listed by Maimonides in His Aphorisms", in *Homenaje a Millàs-Vallicrosa*, Jerusalem, 1956, vol. II, pp. 119-130. [Hebrew].

G. Nebbia, *Donnolo, medico e sapiente ebreo di Oria in provincia di Brindisi,* Verona, 1963.

F. Newton, "Constantine the African and Monte Cassino: New Elements and the Text of the *Isagoge*", in Burnett and Jacquart (eds.), *Constantine the African and 'Alî ibn al-'Abbâs al-Majûsî*, pp. 16-42.

P. G. Ottosson, *Scholastic Medicine and Philosophy, A Study of Commentaries on Galen's "Tegni" (ca. 1300-1450)*, Naples, 1984

J. Peine, *Die Harnschrift des Isaac Judaeus*, Berlin, 1919.

S. Pines, "Razi, critique de Galien", in *International Kongress der Geschichte der Naturwissenschaften*, 7 (1953), pp. 480-487;

P. Porter, "Herophilus of Chalcedon; An Assessment of his Place in the History of Anatomy", *Bulletin of the History of Medicine*, 50 (1976), pp. 45-60.

J. Preuss, *Biblische talmudische Medizin, Beiträge zur Geschichte der Heilkunde und der Kulture überhaupt*, 1st. ed. 1911, latest ed. New York, 1971; translated into English by F. Rosner, New York and London, 1978.

E. Renan, *Ecrivans juifs français du XIVeme siècle*, Paris, 1893.

B. Richler, "Manuscripts of Avicenna's Kanon in Hebrew Translation: A Revised and Up-to-date List", *Koroth*, 8 (1982), pp. 145-168 (Hebrew).

J. M. Riddle, "Dioscorides", in *Catalogus translationum et commentariorum: Medieval and Renaissance Translations and Commentaries*, edited by P. O. Kristeller et al., Washington, D. C., IV (1980), pp. 6-8.

T. Rosen-Moqued, "La poésie juive espagnole", in R. Barkaï (ed.), *Chrétiens, musulmans et juifs dans l'Espagne médiévale, De la convergence à l'expulsion*, Paris, 1994, pp. 103-133.

N. Roth, "Jewish Collaborators in Alfonso's Scientific Work", in R. I. Burns, S. J., *Emperor of Culture. Alfonso X the Learned of Castile and His Thirteenth-Century Renaissance*, Philadelphia, 1990, pp. 59-71.

J.-P. Rothschild, "Motivations et méthodes des traductions en hébreu du milieu du XIIe à la fin du XVe siècle", *Traduction et traducteurs au Moyen Age*, Actes du colloque international du CNRS, Paris 1986. Textes réunis par G. Contamine, Paris, 1989, pp. 279-302.

J. Schacht and M. Meyerhof, "Maimonides Against Galen on Philosophy and Cosmogony", *Bulletin of the Faculty of Arts*, Cairo, vol. V (1937), pp. 53-88.

H. Schipperges, *La medicina árabe en el Medioevo Latino*, Toledo, 1989.

A. Schippers, *Arabic Tradition and Hebrew Innovation: Arabic Themes in Hebrew Andalusian Poetry*, Amsterdam, 1988.

F. Sezgin, *Geschichte des arabischen Schrifttums*, Band III, Leiden, 1970.

J. Shatzmiller, "On Becoming a Jewish Doctor in the High Middle Ages", *Sefarad*, 43 (1983), pp. 239-250.

——, "Médecins et expertise médicale dans la ville médiévale: Manosque 1280-1348" in *Vie privée et ordre public à la fin du moyen âge: Etudes sur Manosque, la Provence, et le Piémont (1250-1450)*, ed. M. Hérbert, Aix-en-Provence, 1987, pp. 105-117.

——, *Médecine et justice en Provence médiévale: Documents de Manosque, 1216-1348*, Aix-en Provence, 1989;

——, "Etudiants juifs à la faculté de médecine de Montpellier, dernier quart du XIV siècle", *Jewish History*, 6 (1992), pp. 243-254.

——, *Jews, Medicine, and Medieval Society*, Berkeley, Los Angeles and London, 1994.

H. Sigerist, "Early Medieval Medical Texts in Manuscripts of Vendôme", *Bulletin of the History of Medicine*, 14 (1943), pp. 68-113

W. D. Smith, *The Hippocratic Tradition*, Ithaca and London, 1979.

H. von Staden, *Herophilus. The Art of Medicine in Early Alexandria*, Cambridge, 1989.

M. Steinschneider, "Medicinische Handschriften im Besitz des Herrn Halberstam", *Magazin für die Wissenschaft des Judenthums*, 1883, pp. 108-112.

——, "Medizinische Handschriften", *Magazin für die Wissenschaft des Judentums*, 10, 1883.

——, *Die hebraeischen Übersetzungen des Mittelalters und die Juden als Dolmetscher*, Berlin, 1893, reprinted at Gratz, 1956.

——, "Jüdische Aertze", *Zeitschrift für hebraeische Bibliographie*, 17 (1914), pp. 63-96; 121-167; 18 (1915), pp. 25-57.

——, *Abraham Judaeus, Savasorda und Ibn Esra zur Geschichte der mathematischen Wissenschaften im 12. Jahrhundert* , in: *Gesammelte Schriften*, I, Berlin,1925, pp. 327-387.

M. Steinschneider and H. Friedenwald, "Manuscript Copies of the Medical Works of Isaac Israeli", in *The Jews and Medicine*, Essays, vol. I, Baltimore, 1944.

O. Temkin, "Celsus' 'On Medicine' and the Ancient Medical Sects", *Bulletin of the Institute of the History of Medicine*, 3 (1935), pp. 249-264.

——, *Soranus' Gynecology*, Baltimore, 1956 (reprint, 1991).

——, *Galenism: The Rise and Decline of a Medical Philosophy*, Ithaca and London, 1973;

M. Ullmann, *Islamic Medicine*, Edinburgh, 1978.

C. Vázquez de Benito and Ma. T. Herrera, *Los arabismos de los textos médicos latinos y castellanos de la edad media y de la modernidad*, Madrid, 1989.

——, "Dos capítulos ginecológicos: árabe y castellano", *Asclepio: Archivo iberoamericano de historia de la medicina y antropología médica*, 33 (1981), pp. 183-241.

J. Vernét, *La cultura hispanoárabe en Oriente y Occidente*, Barcelona, 1978.

M. Wack, "'Alî ibn al-'Abbâs al-Magûsî and Constantine on Love, and the Evolution of the *Practica Pantegni*", in Burnett and Jacquart (eds.), *Constantine the African and 'Alî ibn al-'Abbâs al-Majûsî*, pp. 178-184.

R. Walzer, *Galen on Jews and Christians*, Oxford, 1949.

INDEX

Subjects, Names and Places

Materia Medica

BRILL'S SERIES IN JEWISH STUDIES

1. COHEN, R. *Jews in Another Environment.* Surinam in the Second Half of the Eighteenth Century. 1991. ISBN 90 04 09373 7
2. PRAWER, S.S. *Israel at Vanity Fair.* Jews and Judaism in the Writings of W.M. Thackeray. 1992. ISBN 90 04 09403 2
3. PRICE, J.J. *Jerusalem under Siege.* The Collapse of the Jewish State 66-70 C.E. 1992. ISBN 90 04 09471 7
4. ZINGUER, I. *L'hébreu au temps de la Renaissance.* 1992. ISBN 90 04 09557 8
5. GUTWEIN, D. *The Divided Elite.* Economics, Politics and Anglo-Jewry, 1882-1917. 1992. ISBN 90 04 09447 4
6. ERAQI KLORMAN, B.-Z. *The Jews of Yemen in the Nineteenth Century.* A Portrait of a Messianic Community. 1993. ISBN 90 04 09684 1
7. BEN-DOV, N. *Agnon's Art of Indirection.* Uncovering Latent Content in the Fiction of S.Y. Agnon. 1993. ISBN 90 04 09863 1
8. GERA, D. *Judaea and Mediterranean Politics,* 219-161 B.C.E. 1998. ISBN 90 04 09441 5
9. COUDERT, A.P. *The Impact of the Kabbalah in the 17th Century.* ISBN 90 04 09844 5. *In preparation*
10. GROSS, A. *Iberian Jewry from Twilight to Dawn.* The World of Rabbi Abraham Saba. 1995. ISBN 90 04 10053 9
12. AHRONI, R. *The Jews of the British Crown Colony of Aden.* History, Culture, and Ethnic Relations. 1994. ISBN 90 04 10110 1
13. DEUTSCH, N. *The Gnostic Imagination.* Gnosticism, Mandaeism and Merkabah Mysticism. 1995. ISBN 90 04 10264 7
14. ARBEL, B. *Trading Nations.* Jews and Venetians in the Early Modern Eastern Mediterranean. 1995. ISBN 90 04 10057 1
15. LEVENSON, D. *Julian and Jerusalem.* The Sources and Tradition. 1996. ISBN 90 04 105441
16. MENACHE, S. (ed.). *Communication in the Jewish Diaspora.* The Pre-Modern World. 1996. ISBN 90 04 10189 6
17. PARFITT, T. *The Road to Redemption.* The Jews of the Yemen 1900-1950. 1996. ISBN 90 04 10544 1
18. ASSIS, Y.T. *Jewish Economy in the Medieval Crown of Aragon, 1213-1327.* Money and Power. 1997. ISBN 90 04 10615 4
19. STILLMAN, Y.K. & STILLMAN, N.A. (eds.). *From Iberia to Diaspora.* Studies in Sephardic History and Culture. 1998. ISBN 90 04 10720 7
20. BARKAI, R. *A History of Jewish Gynaecological Texts in the Middle Ages.* 1998. ISBN 90 04 10995 1

GENERAL THEOLOGICAL SEMINARY
NEW YORK

DATE DUE

1/19/19			

HIGHSMITH #45230
Printed in USA

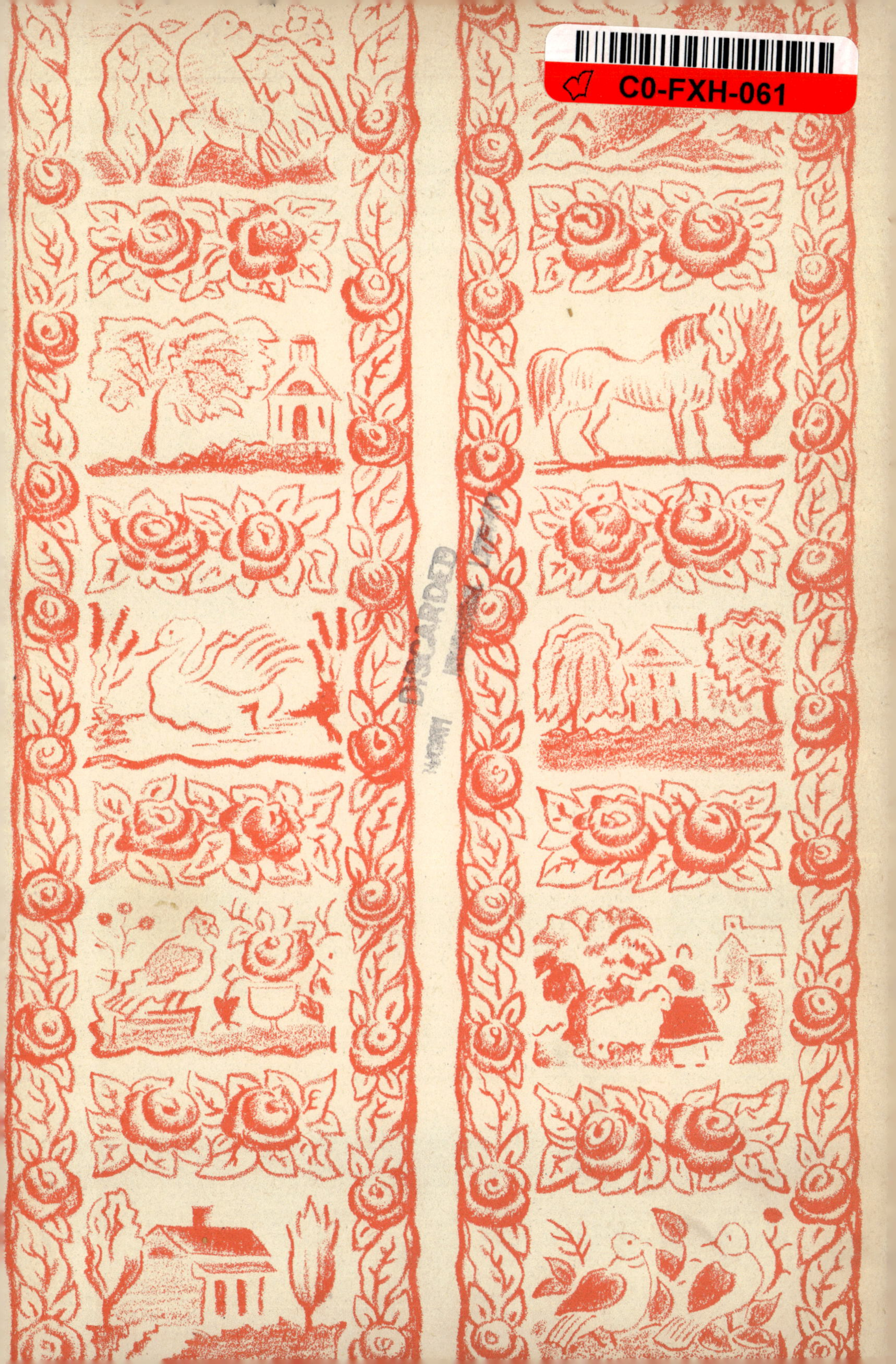

C0-FXH-061
DISCARDED

PIONEER ART IN AMERICA

BY CAROLYN SHERWIN BAILEY

Girls have always prized autograph albums. And once in early America a girl designed and sewed together colorful pages of an album, in which none other than Henry Wadsworth Longfellow, as well as all her school friends, were to wish her luck. She is only one of many girls and boys with whom you will become acquainted here.

You will enjoy Rebecca who loved to make crisp doughnuts for Johnny Lincoln and who, with him, had an amazing adventure with an Indian scouting party. You will like Eliza whose handsome admirer painted her portrait on the parlor wall. And as you watch two friends dye fabrics into beautiful colors—into pink made from boiled-down scrapings from old bricks, into blue from indigo, into moss green—you will be truly fascinated as these soft shades are woven into gaily patterned rugs.

Other girls, as well as boys, await you in the enchanting stories of this captivating book.

Charles Brown
Guilderland, NY

Purchased August 1986
at Buckham Library
in Faribault, Minn.

Pioneer Art in America

Also by Carolyn Sherwin Bailey

and illustrated by Grace Paull

CHILDREN OF THE HANDCRAFTS

TOPS AND WHISTLES
TRUE STORIES OF AMERICAN TOYS AND CHILDREN

HOMESPUN PLAYDAYS

COUNTRY-STOP

PIONEER ART IN AMERICA

CAROLYN SHERWIN BAILEY

WITH LITHOGRAPHS BY GRACE PAULL

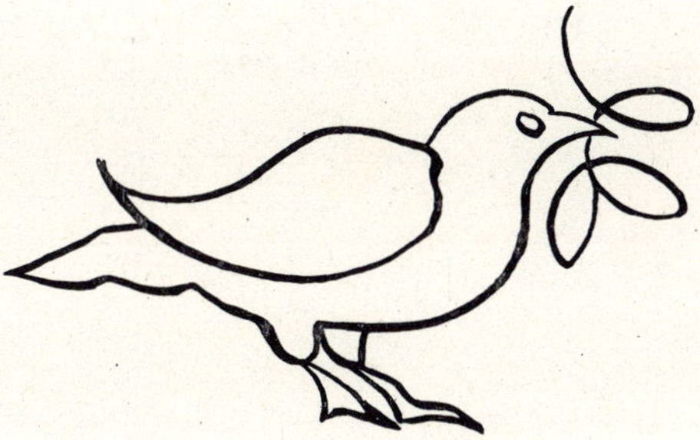

THE JUNIOR LITERARY GUILD
AND
THE VIKING PRESS NEW YORK

1944

THIS EDITION IS PRODUCED IN FULL COMPLIANCE WITH
ALL WAR PRODUCTION BOARD CONSERVATION ORDERS

COPYRIGHT 1944 BY CAROLYN SHERWIN BAILEY
FIRST PUBLISHED BY THE VIKING PRESS IN OCTOBER 1944
PUBLISHED ON THE SAME DAY IN THE DOMINION OF CANADA BY
THE MACMILLAN COMPANY OF CANADA LIMITED

J 745
B 151

PRINTED IN THE UNITED STATES OF AMERICA

For Peter, Guy, and Dennis

45775

Contents

Full-Page Illustrations

Illustrator's Note

Grateful acknowledgment is made to The Museum of the City of New York, The Museum of the American Indian, The American History Museum, The Metropolitan Museum of Art, and the Picture Collection of The New York Public Library for the very real and generous assistance given in my search for reference material which would make these illustrations historically accurate.

G. P.

Pioneer Art in America

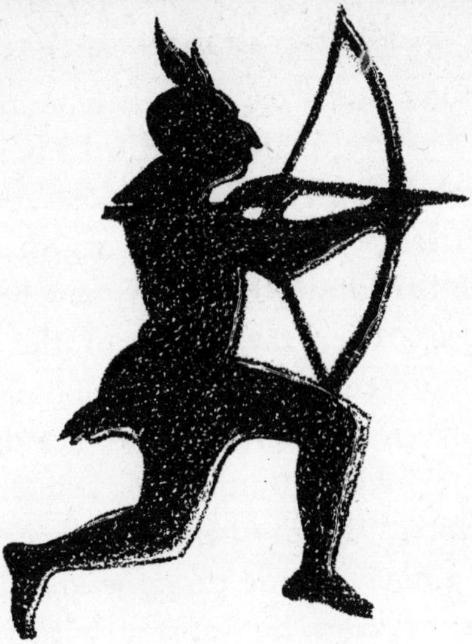

THE WEATHERVANE

Rebecca started as the knocker clanged. She waited a moment, then opened only the upper half of the door, peering out furtively. Then her face broke into smiles.

"Johnny Lincoln!" She let him into the house. "I foresaw that you would forget us here in Coventry. How comes it that you have left your fine new house at Exeter to call on your playmate?"

The boy grinned. "Your baking scented the air all the way from the forge. Father can't resist the smithy even if he has sold it. He rode over to work a bit today, the new smith being on his way to Philadelphia with a load of ironware. I rode behind him." He sniffed eagerly. "This brisk autumn air gives one an appetite."

Rebecca Flowers, a housewifely figure in her indigo-dyed homespun and long calico apron, dipped into a kettle of sizzling fat, took out a crisp cruller on the long iron fork and laid it on a pewter plate. She filled a porringer with apple sauce and a goblet with milk.

"Stoke yourself, Johnny," she urged. "How is Master Mordecai's health? I heard that your new house is showy with your father's art, even the hinges of the barn doors being forged in the butterfly design, and the house doors hinged in Holy Lord pattern to frighten away the devil."

"That is so." Johnny dunked his cruller in the milk and took luscious bites. "I truly believe, Rebecca, that my father built so large a house, made of stone and having gable windows, in order to show his artistry with iron. Some of the hinges are wrought in a pattern of a double dragon or a fleur-de-lis. The hearth dogs are shaped like soldiers in red coats. Even the bread shovel that hangs beside the fireplace has a cunningly shaped tulip by which to hold it. The lanterns are pierced in designs. The foot scraper beside the front door is a dragon, wings facing outward. The trivet upon which the teapot rests is made of slender iron in leaf form."

"I mind me of something Master Mordecai once said to me when I was watching him working here at his Coventry forge," Rebecca said. "He was hammering out a set of sleigh bells in ball shape the better to carry their chiming. 'Rebecca,' he said, 'whatever is useful may also be wrought in beauty. It is my belief that decoration is natural to the temperament of iron.' I can't say exactly what Master Mordecai meant but I love to look at his works."

" 'He has an eye for art and hands to make dreams come true.' I am quoting Squire Boone," Johnny explained. "The elders at the meeting house were minded to rebuke my father for his enjoyment of fancy, but Squire Boone would have none of it. 'Let Mordecai Lincoln forge as he likes,' said the Squire. 'If he hammers the weaver's knocker in the pattern of a flax flower and stem, or forges a garden gate that has a spry squirrel and his nut tree for its design, may we not be blamed for envy, we who have not the artist's vision?' "

"True," Rebecca agreed. "Spoken with the wisdom of your fourteen years. Here is another cruller."

Was Rebecca making sport of him, Johnny wondered? She was a housewifely girl of old Pennsylvania, and almost as skillful at swimming, fishing and woodcraft as he. It was a wild but lovely countryside there where the Susquehanna River cut through a range of hills and made a fertile valley, where apples and grapes, corn, wheat, and pastureland blessed the earth. There was stone for building comfortable homes, timber for raising the great Dutch barns, iron for the forges that lighted the villages for miles. It was the year 1730. The land lay basking in the harvest sun. A scent of boiling preserves and cider, apple butter and spiced fruits lay heavily everywhere. Turnips and winter squash, bonfires and swathes of grain added their pungent odors. Rebecca Flowers, ten years old this autumn, alone, for her parents had gone to Philadelphia by wagon with produce, took off her apron and put on her sunbonnet and cloak.

"I think Master Mordecai might like a new cheese and a loaf of apple cake, if he is at work in the smithy. Also, I wouldn't be averse to taking a walk, Johnny. I have made ready for the folks. I have spun, chopped the sausage meat, and baked. Come, Johnny. Let us go, but wait! Every day since I have been alone I have cut a small notch in the door cheek and on the Sabbath a double one, to keep tally of the days." She took a knife from the table.

"Hold on; let me!" Johnny took his hunting knife out of his belt. "My father made and gave me this knife. There isn't another blade so keen in all Bucks County. It would cut a hair."

Rebecca shivered as she watched the sharp point slip into hard wood as if it were butter. "I heard that the Iroquois are marching again for Conestoga scalps," she said. "The kindly Conestogas, so anxious to raise their corn and pumpkins, help the wagoners and live in peace with us!"

"The Iroquois aim to be conquerors," Johnny said. "All the trails from the north, even as far as our land, are guarded by one of the Iroquois sachems. A good runner of their tribes can make a hundred miles a day, my father says. The Iroquois have a kind of examination they give the Indians hereabouts, the good Conestogas particularly. It has to do with the rules of their Long House and if it is not passed, they scalp and steal. It is because of their nature and their feeling of greatness."

"Well, let us speed on," Rebecca urged. "How pleasant the day is!"

She raised her head and breathed the crisp air. Johnny, too, struck out in his moccasins. They were two young settlers, she in her working garb, he in his tanned leather breeches, calfskin boots and coonskin cap. All about them lay the glory of the season, gardens and roadsides bright with the last flowers, orchards, harvest fields and the purple of vineyards. The hills were folded in a colored damask of the autumn leaves, and there was no sound. The small stone houses they passed, whose eaves drooped like sleepy eyebrows, basked in peace. It was a prosperous land. Coventry was not far from Reading, and Reading led to Philadelphia where incoming

vessels from Europe and the Indies brought spices and household goods, stuffs and finery for which the loads of Pennsylvania ore and timber were exchanged. The Indian trails to the east had been broadened by pack animals, then widened into roads by the wagon trains.

Master Mordecai Lincoln, the honored smith of Coventry, had recently built an even better road to Philadelphia. He was a man of means and honor. His new house at near-by Exeter was a delight to Johnny's mother and the little girls, his sisters, but Master Mordecai was still a smith at heart. He drew and wrought designs in iron; tulip-shaped sconces, waffle irons that turned out fancifully stamped cakes, gracefully curved sleigh runners, hearth forks having vines and flowers and twisted curls for their handles. That was why the Coventry smithy still lured him, why he was there now.

Nuts dropped from an early frost. Russet apples delayed Johnny and Rebecca. They perched on stone walls and imitated the chickadee as they ate. It was growing dark for the days had shortened.

"Come, we should make haste!" Rebecca pulled Johnny's hand at last.

"Wait," he said. "Listen, did you ever hear so bold a bird? He answers my call nearer and nearer."

They heard it again, the sharp *chickadee-de-de-ee*. It was just ahead of them as they jumped down from the wall and started toward the sound. But their way was blocked by a gaudy savage so tall and silent that he might have been painted on a backdrop of the woods that lay between them and the forge. He raised his bow signaling them to stop. He took an arrow from his quiver and fitted it leisurely into the bow.

Johnny gripped Rebecca's hand. "Don't run," he said.

She whimpered a little. "I don't know the Iroquois answers," she whispered. "We're as badly off as the Conestogas."

As they stood there, the trees, each one, disclosed its savage. Some dropped down from the branches. Others stepped from the shelter of the tree trunks. The Iroquois in front of them shot his arrow over their heads and one leaf, pierced in the exact center, dropped at Johnny's feet. The boy's thoughts raced.

Something his father had once said flashed into his mind. "It is wise to barter with a savage. Fear makes them what they are. Friendliness with the Indians is our only hope of peace."

Johnny drew his precious hunting knife from his belt. He held it out to the Iroquois. Not to be outdone, Rebecca pulled off her string of beads and offered that too.

The Indian advanced slowly, took the gifts and lowered his head in thanks. He gestured to the savages behind and they were again secreted, shadows in the colored forest. Johnny and Rebecca walked safely through the lane of terror, but when they were a safe distance, how they ran! Panting, they sped on until a blazing light showed them the open door of the smithy. Inside there was warmth and safety.

The Coventry forge on the edge of the forest was a place apart from the village. In the daytime the beating of its hammers chimed like bells. At night the flames from the forge made a company of weird shadows that moved and changed in a pattern of mystery. Within, it was completely given over to the work that had to be done. The forge was of stone built in the form of a pyramid that stretched up to the chimney, foursquare and having the great leather bellows at the

side. It took strength to work the bellows. In the hills of Pennsylvania there were deposits of ore that would never give out. The forests gave the smith all the fuel he needed. Waiting for the fire to heat a pig of iron, Mordecai Lincoln sat on a bench, his Bible spread open on his leather apron. The boy started to pour out their story but his father motioned to him to wait. He read the end of his selection aloud:

> The smith also, sitting by the anvil and considering the ironwork; the vapor of the fire wasteth his flesh and he fighteth with the heat of the furnace; the noise of the hammer and the anvil is ever in his ear, and his eyes look still upon the pattern of the thing that he maketh, he settleth his mind to finish his work and watcheth to polish it perfectly.

He closed the Bible, looking up at the children. "Thus Ecclesiastes speaks to the Coventry smith," he said. "I'll warrant that the pearly gates needed some iron hinges to support them. It is good to see you, Rebecca. And how good your basket smells!"

Rebecca was still trembling. Johnny put a kind arm about her shoulders. "Rebecca was alone, her parents being in Philadelphia. She was doing her week's baking and has brought you some goodies for your supper. I told her that you were here in the smithy."

Rebecca found her tongue then. "The Iroquois are abroad. We met a scouting party. Johnny is a brave boy. He shielded me and gave the chief his hunting knife."

"Shall we close and bolt the door, sir?" Johnny asked, looking furtively over his shoulder.

"Not we Lincolns," Master Mordecai told them. "Sit you down on that bench and watch me. I have a mind to forge a bit before I eat this fine supper."

From the bench in a corner of the smithy, they could see only the shop. It always delighted boys and girls alike with its deeply glowing fire, the great leather bellows that went puff, puff, creak, as the smith blew up the coals to white heat. There, close at hand, were all the needed tools; hammers, tongs, swages, fullers. The anvil was hollowed from years of hammer blows. Johnny had learned something of his father's art; how he must have first of all a drawn design for the finished piece, then take the molten pig carefully from the fire and lay it on the anvil, and hammer at once with stubborn, well-planned blows. One blow on top meant flattening the iron on the under side. Chisel marks in the cooling iron made decorations. The work with the tongs and hammers must be done at arm's length for results that could, if he were skillful, be as clear cut as a piece of jewelry.

Fascinated, they watched the colors in the heating iron as Master Mordecai pumped the bellows. The pig became first a blood red, then darker, and finally a full red like the glow of the brightest ruby. Presently it changed to a lighter red, to a yellow heat, and at last the lemon yellow that showed it to be ready for forging.

Master Mordecai glanced over their heads into the path outside, to which their backs were turned. One at a time, silently, he saw a line of savages file headed north. The first one was holding with great pride Johnny's hunting knife.

He lifted the iron from the forge and laid it on the anvil. A spray of bright sparks arose as he beat it, turned it, beat it again, flattened it.

"What are you making, Master Mordecai?" Rebecca came as close as she dared.

"A present for a brave lass," he told her.

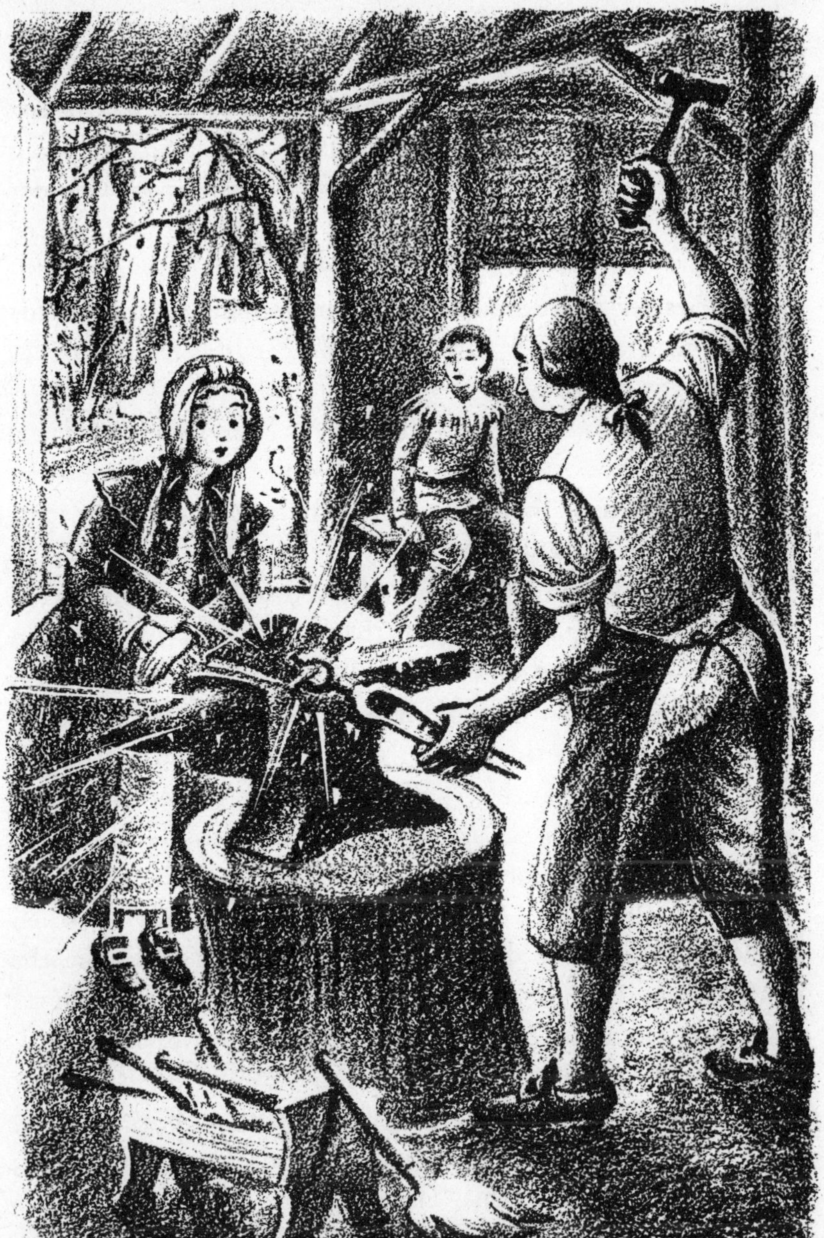

Bang, bang, the blows beat a tattoo of courage as the ringing of the Coventry anvil echoed through the clear air. The iron became a thin sheet. The smith molded and clipped it swiftly with his tools. It was as if the metal really felt and had a desire to conform itself to the will of the artist. Slender lines and curves appeared. The iron took shape and figure.

"Johnny, see!" Rebecca leaned above the anvil in excitement. "Master Mordecai has made an Indian! It has a head-dress of feathers and a bow and arrow. It is as thin as paper but wrought of iron."

The smith stood back, arms folded, as he looked with pride at his work. The figure would cool soon. Then it would be ready for whatever wind or storms the years beat against it. Master Mordecai explained.

"A weathervane for Rebecca's barn to tell the Indians that tribute has been paid to them, that her family may live in peace for all time. Any savage will respect it. I have an eye for a pretty weathervane, designed as a cock, a pine tree, or an arrow head. But this savage, with his bow pointed toward whatever wind he meets, will delight our red enemies and temper their actions as the fire tempers iron. It will be a covenant of safety for the household, its guests, flocks and herds. Now, let us eat, for the Iroquois have gone. And when we have finished we shall take Rebecca home and raise the weathervane as a surprise for her parents, and a token of friendship with our enemy."

The fire in the Coventry forge burned to embers. Outside the door of the smithy the road to Philadelphia stretched, widened, and became a busy thoroughfare. Through the years Master Mordecai's ironware traveled along it, together with that of other skilled artisans from all the old Philadelphia forges. There never was such beautiful hand-wrought iron as theirs. But as decoration began to supersede utility, iron in their hands, as well as on the anvils of the smiths of New England and of the South, Baltimore, Charleston, Savannah, New Orleans, Mobile took on new grace. Lacelike iron balconies were spread across the Spanish and French homes of Louisiana like fragile veils that concealed the beauty of some lovely Creole. Walled gardens of the North showed their color and spread their perfume through iron-wrought gates of twining vines, in lyre designs to catch the breezes, in patterns of tulips, lilies and flowery rosettes. The wooden picket fences of Boston and New York were replaced by iron railing in pleasing patterns. New houses were given iron stair rails, door and window grilles that we may see today in their ancient lovely designs.

Presently when the forges were torn down to be replaced by smoke stacks of Pennsylvania smelting furnaces, the casting of fine iron designs came in. Molds held the parts of a balcony rail, an especially graceful gate or grille that was later welded together. That was a pity for the hand-wrought iron with its chisel marks and other tool prints had a message of its own in tune with the chorus of all the anvils of our ancestors. It was that new word spread by Master Mordecai Lincoln and his neighbors, telling how art had come to our country, born of work and growing through faith.

Rebecca Flowers and Johnny Lincoln grew up with that song in their hearts and after a while they joined the pioneers who were taking their tools and their courage West. Master Mordecai lived out his days in his new house at Exeter, a well-thought-of man. The house had a desk and mirrors but he treasured in it his tongs and hammers, chisels and the designs he drew for weathervanes, hearth utensils, and lanterns. He treasured most of all his belief that even iron may hold beauty in its core. And we know that the strength of Master Mordecai Lincoln, blacksmith and artist of long ago, survived in his great-great-grandson Abraham Lincoln.

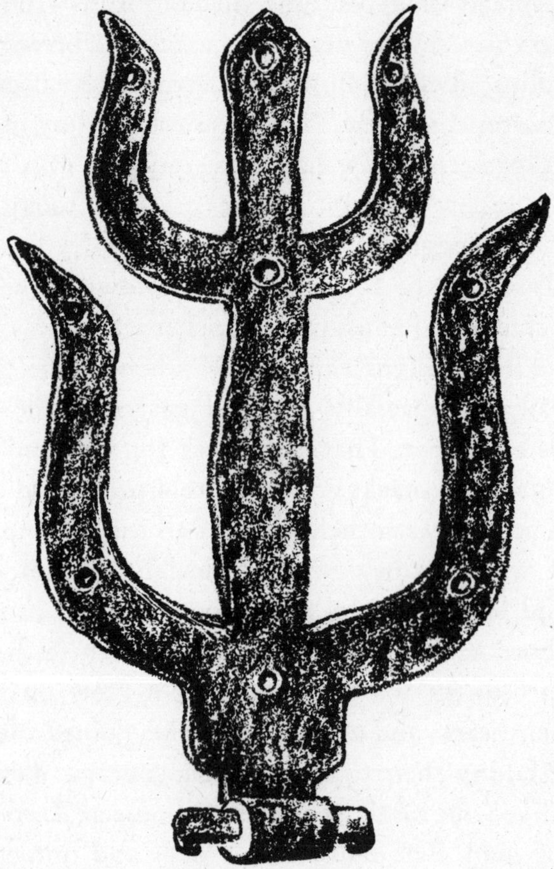

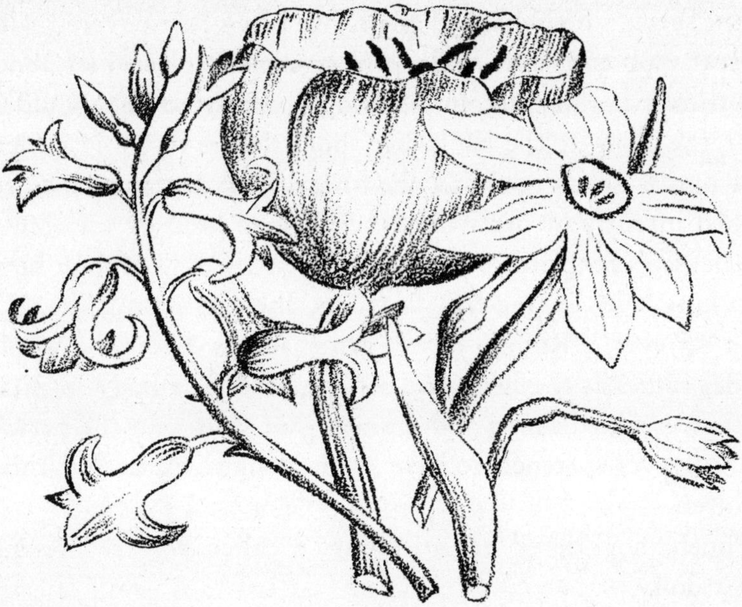

THE WAX DOLL

PHOEBE WRIGHT looked up from her sewing at their mother, whose fingers were shaping a wax head. Her sister, Elizabeth, was trying to brew the tea for supper. The kettle bubbled over the kitchen fire, but nearly all the hearth was taken up with the wax-pot. The pungent perfume of melting wax, turpentine, pitch, and fat filled the kitchen. Joe, the eldest, was grinding dry colors with a mortar and pestle into fine powder for tinting the wax that their mother molded into the most lifelike sculpture in all the American colonies. But their house in old New York was something like the tea kettle, crowded out of its business of homemaking because of the Wax Woman's art.

She sat in a high-backed chair, her black hair covered with a great mob cap with ruffles and streamers, a kerchief about her throat, her dress train reaching down from her shoulders over the chair at the back, her short sleeves stylishly frilled, and a great apron covering the finery. Her piercing dark eyes looked intently at her work, the life-size head of a Colonial gentleman complete with a periwig tied with a ribbon bow. Working with incredible swiftness, she was giving the face deep-set eyes, a Roman nose, even shadows. Later she would model ruffles at the neck and set the head on a body in small clothes, buckled shoes, and dignity that waited in the parlor. But her eyes softened to love as she looked up at her three children.

Phoebe considered her stitching, a calico flowered basque for a doll.

"It fits but poorly," she sighed. "A rag doll has no proper waist, and however I pull her in, she flops. I saw a doll displayed at Mistress Twitchell's millinery shop this morning that had come from London. It had a paper hoop skirt, hair of real flax, a muff and gilt earrings. Mistress Twitchell tells me that the children of London have very fine toys now, china doll babies dressed in lace and lawn, wooden mannikins of soldiers, sailors, bakers and the like. She says that she expects to import some beautiful wax dolls."

"You are thirteen years old, Phoebe," her mother said. "It is time that you stitched your own gowns instead of making dolls' clothes."

Joe stirred a little of his flesh-tinted color into a bowl of melted wax cooling on the kitchen table. "This color is so true that I had an argument with a boy yesterday about the Reverend Whitefield who stands near our parlor window.

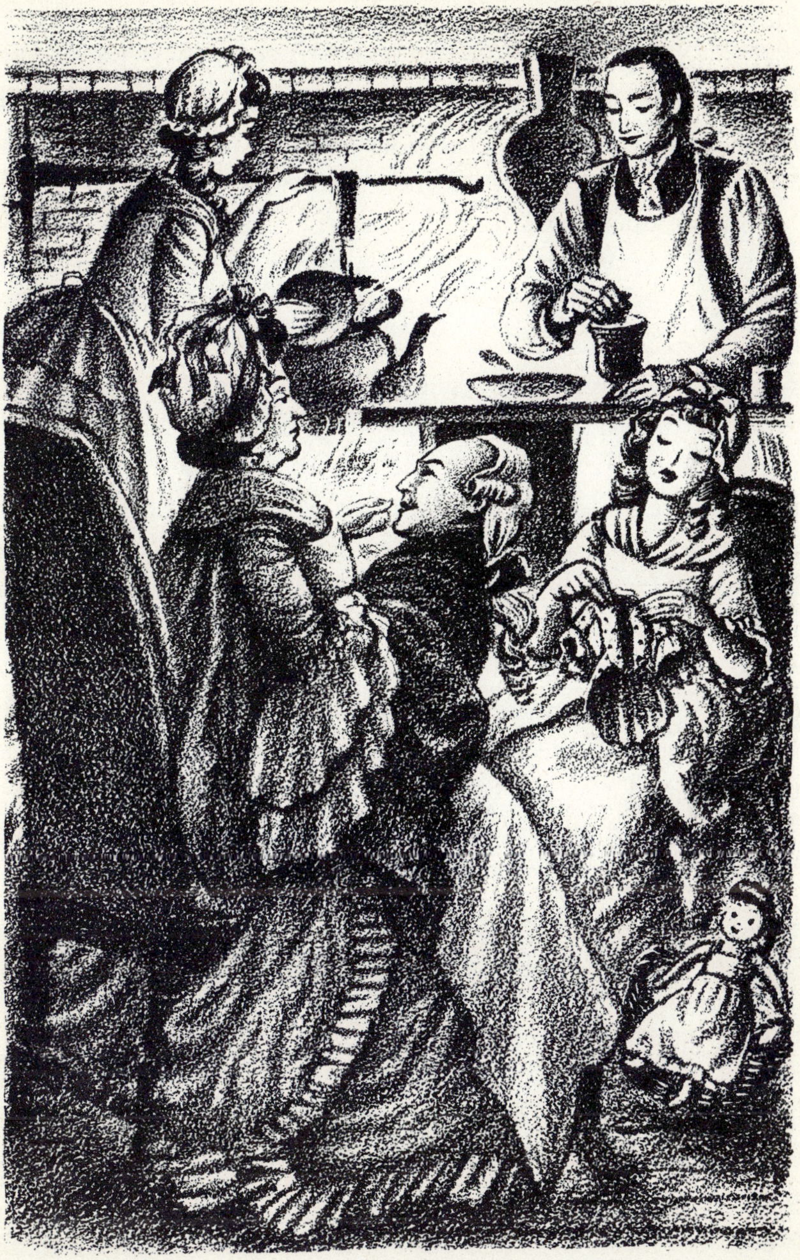

He believed that the great preacher is visiting us and would disapprove of our playing marbles in the street. I brought him into the house to feel of the gentleman's robe and cold hands. He left in haste," Joe chuckled. "My friend said he wouldn't enjoy living with such great waxen ghosts as ours."

"Shame upon you, Joe!" His mother smiled, though, with pride in her work. "I trust you showed your friend the Pennsylvania Farmer who stands beside the Reverend Whitefield, in his field smock and homespun, a model of industry, for all city boys? The Pennsylvania Farmer is as high an example to you as is the Reverend Whitefield."

Elizabeth left the hearth and leaned over the low rocking chair where Phoebe sat. She put her arms around the younger girl, comforting her. Naturally Phoebe wanted a wax doll. New York was trying to pattern after London in style and luxury. Along their street were shops of the feather makers, the drapers, and the milliners who were so clever in the fashioning of bonnets and cloaks, caps and tippets. The cobbled street rang with the wheels of brightly painted coaches, and the clatter of runners carrying the sedan chairs of the rich. The Wax Woman was celebrated in England as well as New York; she ranked among the greatest artists in wax of the period. And young Phoebe was trying to give a rag doll a waist line!

"Don't mourn, Phoebe," Elizabeth whispered. "Mother, tell us again about when you were a little Quaker girl, Patience Lovell, in Bordentown, New Jersey."

Without stopping her modeling, the Wax Woman took up the story. "Where images and pictures were considered wicked. But when I was much younger than our Phoebe I began making dolls and portraits of the neighbors in putty and even with bits of dough when I was kneading bread. I wore a long apron and I used to work on my figures underneath it, secretly. One day I was almost caught in my sin. I had molded a dough doll and hid it to harden under an apple tree. It rained, and the doll swelled until it was plainly to be seen. I fed it to the hens just in time. I should have been called before the elders of the meeting house if my parents had known of my wrong doing."

"It wasn't wrong," Joe declared. "You turned your fingers to making wax figures of our times that image the people themselves."

"It was always said that I had the makings of a witch," she continued. "My eye still penetrates the person I look upon, and I can foretell coming events. But I would rather shape a lump of wax than do anything else. I can give it life. It records my slightest touch."

Then her expression changed. That was their mother's charm for the three. Nearly all the time an artist, she would suddenly soften and her heart melt in her love for them and appreciation of their care of the house and of her, too.

"Phoebe shall have the most beautiful wax doll in all the Colonies," she said. "Tomorrow I will begin it. It shall be large, with moving arms and legs on wire. Its wig shall be made by a New York wig maker, its hoops by a milliner. It shall have furs for winter and lace for summer. There will be no such doll in America or England. This evening after supper I will go out and buy special wax for shaping Phoebe's doll."

The apothecary around the corner kept a supply of the white wax that Patience Wright used. It was an evening in June, warm and with a lingering sunset over the water that they could see from the parlor window. New York was stepping out toward the north, but the Wrights lived downtown not far from Battery Park. A fresh breeze from the sea blew the parlor curtains as Phoebe opened the window to wave good-by to her mother.

The Wax Woman waved back. "I won't be long. Be good children until I come home."

Elizabeth and Joe came into the parlor after the supper dishes were washed. It was a finely furnished room, but crowded with great wax figures. A pair of legs here, a headless body there, a finished wax lady in pearls and rich silk on the sofa. Delicately molded wax masks and portrait medallions lay on the center table and the mantelpiece. It was still too light for candles although the dusk began creeping down the street as soon as the crimson sun slipped into the horizon of the Jersey shore. Elizabeth tinkled out a small tune on the harpsichord to which Phoebe sang. It was a popular tune brought over to New York from London, but hardly approved of by the Quakers:

"Let your gown be a sacque, blue, yellow or green,
And frizzle your elbows with ruffles, sixteen—"

Joe stood beside the brass-railed grate which it was his work to polish and fill with coals on a chilly day.

"Cease your piping," he said. "I like not what the people in the street say of Mother."

"What, for instance?" Elizabeth asked.

"Nothing one can truly deny," he told her. "That she has a witch's cleverness in seeing character and bringing it to life in wax. That she has the body of an Indian, so tall and straight, and an Indian's piercing eyes. That she talks too much and knows more than she should about the intrigues being carried on between our Colonies and England. One day when she was delivering a bust to a purchaser, carefully wrapped up in a white cloth, it was rumored that she was carrying a dead man's head."

"Fiddlesticks!" Elizabeth laughed. "Mr. Benjamin Franklin thinks highly of Mother, and General Washington has commissioned her to mold his portrait when he is free to sit for it."

"A wax doll with a wig of real hair and arms and legs that will move!" young Phoebe was talking to herself. "She shall have a straw hat with ribbon ties, a frock for every day in the week, and a silk mantilla."

"Vanity, all is vanity saith the preacher."

Phoebe turned pale. Then she giggled. Joe had the gift of mimicry, and when their mother was not there to disapprove he often spoke for the great wax figure of the Reverend George Whitefield, that famous preacher, who stood in the parlor in his own wig and band and robe. Phoebe took one of the candlesticks from the mantel above the parlor grate, lighted it, and went over to the stuff curtain in the corner that made a little anteroom for the reverend gentleman beside the figure of the Pennsylvania Farmer.

"Did you speak, reverend sir?"

She pulled aside the curtain, holding the candle close to see the deep-set eyes, the delicately shaped fingers. Her wax doll would be molded with the same delicacy.

"Phoebe, have a care!" Elizabeth cried. But she was too late.

Joe snatched the candle, snuffing the flame and burning his hand. He tore down the curtain and tried to toss it out of the window. But they were both too late. The window curtain flared. Its edges curled, and the flame moved swiftly upward. The breeze pushed the blazing cloth into the center of the room where the table cover took fire and the waxworks began to droop their melting heads. Phoebe, terrified, ran out of the house shrieking, "Fire!"

Sedan carriers, coach drivers and street hawkers of fruit and muffins who called their wares until lantern-lighting time took up the cry. The Wax Woman sauntering home with a great cake of wax in her arms was not able to push through the crowd that gathered instantly.

She thought, "How safe I am with my three good housekeepers. Nothing can happen to our house."

Then she saw! She was almost run down as New York's new red fire engine drawn by two prancing white horses came rattling down the street. It was followed by firemen with leather water buckets. The engine smoked and puffed with burning coals that sent a trail of sparks behind; it was small for fire-fighting but efficient. As it passed, puffing and smoking, the crowd opened, making a lane through which the Wax Woman met an amazing procession. Heading it was Joe carrying the Reverend George Whitefield and behind him was Elizabeth, helped by willing hands as she tugged along the Pennsylvania Farmer. Phoebe, weeping, was carried by a fireman.

"I'm all right, Mother," she sobbed, "but I do not deserve a new doll for I set the house on fire."

"There, there, my lamb," her mother dropped her burden and gathered Phoebe and the great wax figure of the preacher into her arms.

Austere and magic-working though she was, Patience

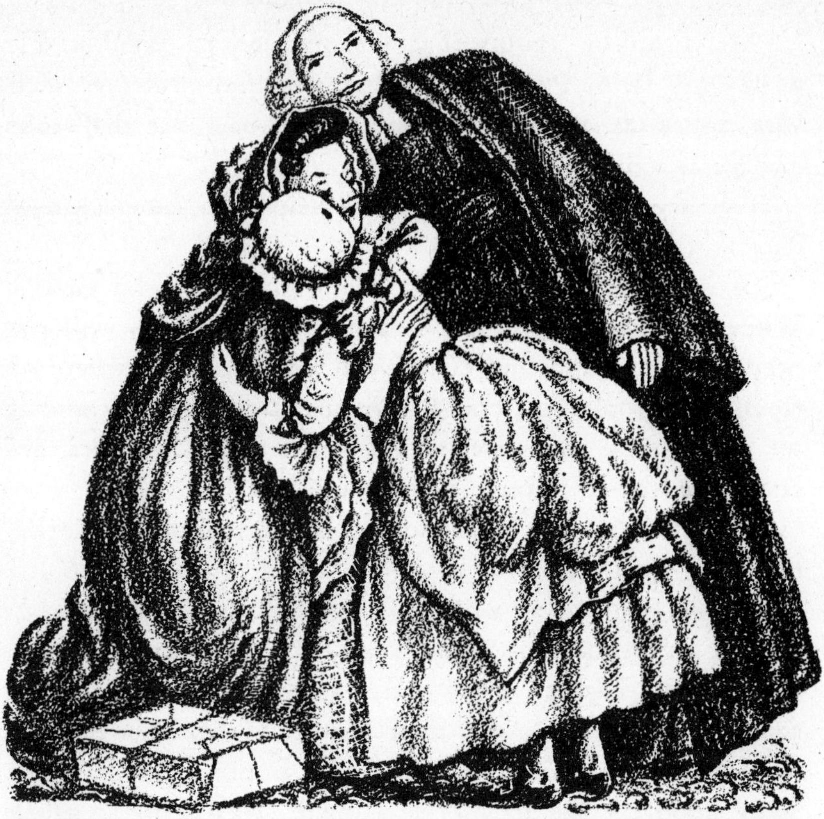

Wright, the Wax Woman, became only their mother. The strange family, human and wax, rested at last on the curbing. The street was roped off but they could presently see that the fire was out. Phoebe's quick alarm and the courage of the New York firemen, odd fighters in their scarlet uniforms and great hats, had got it under control. But most of the waxworks had melted and were quite useless for remodeling because the soot had spoiled the wax. The children were more discouraged than their mother as they talked over their future at a neighbor's house. The Wax Woman already had a cheerful plan.

"Mr. Franklin thinks that I should go to London. He writes me from Philadelphia that England preserves such wax figures as mine in Westminster Abbey. We shall take passage as soon as I can arrange matters here."

"I shall give up doll dressing and help with our packing," Phoebe smiled through tears.

Joe had a great idea. "Take along the Reverend George Whitefield," he urged, "and the Farmer too. They will not need passports and one chaise will do for us all when we reach Liverpool. You could never pack them safely and if we carry them the vessel may give us better quarters, accompanied by so notable a company."

"I can keep house in London as well as in New York," Elizabeth decided.

So it happened that in the year 1772 the Wright family, loaded with baskets, bags, and waxworks, set sail for the shores of England to try their fortunes in a strange land. Wherever they went, the great wax figures were couriers. They stood for the art of the moment, wax being so subtle and exquisite a medium for making likenesses of kings and queens, lords and ladies. Patience Wright's figures were even more human than those of the London waxworkers.

Her patrons often insisted that the waxen figures be dressed in their own garments, their gay silks and velvets, cocked hats, broadcloth knee breeches and embroidered waistcoats. But she could reproduce small-clothes, fine wigs, or a lady's Paris coiffure, lawn ruffles, a string of pearls, or the fine lettering on a book held by a waxen scholar.

At Liverpool, they were met by a special post-chaise through whose windows the two wax gentlemen stared with mild curiosity at the new scene. At the inns where they stopped no board was charged for them. England knew the great Methodist preacher who had visited and exhorted there. In fact, Patience Wright and her three young ones were given special inn rates because of the chance they gave other guests of meeting the waxworks.

They found a small house on Cockspur Street in London, not so different from their home in New York. Almost at once the Wax Woman received an order for modeling the famous Lord Chatfield, and she executed it well.

Draped in the robes he wore when he made his last speech in the House of Lords, the great statesman reposed in a glass case in Islip Chapel of Westminster, opposite Edward the Confessor.

Joe began doing wax sculpture himself. Later he was to model a bust of George Washington from which his mother made a beautiful medallion. That likeness may be seen today, the epaulettes, stock, and military buttons exact and subtly modeled.

Elizabeth slipped easily into her new housekeeping. Cockspur Street was a narrow cobbled lane, filled with delightful little brick buildings; chocolate shops, the makers of artificial flowers, sweets bakers, gold- and silversmiths, book stalls, and fruit and vegetable vendors. She grew to know the little maid-servants of London and mingled with them as they did their marketing. Even the vendors of prawns, trundling their barrows along Cockspur Street, smiled at Elizabeth, or chatted when filling their water buckets at the street pumps.

Phoebe Wright made a new friend in London, a very nice boy named John Hoppner, who brought his paint box to Cockspur Street and taught her how to mix the colors and lay them on. But it was Elizabeth who kept the house comfortable and saw that the family were fed.

Their mother had adventures. The three young Wrights thought her a most exciting person with whom to live. Benjamin Franklin came to London from Paris, took a dish of tea with them, complimented her, and came again. The wax image of the Reverend Whitefield was given a place among the great in Westminster Abbey. Patience Wright met Royalty in London. She became so well acquainted with England's king and queen that she called them George and Charlotte, and she scolded King George sharply for allowing the American Revolution.

"It is a great mistake," she told him. "Our two countries are so much alike, you should not allow any misunderstanding to separate us."

The years passed until the differences between England and the Colonies were settled. At last the Wrights, all but Phoebe, went home again. Phoebe had given up her dream of a wax doll and was to become Hoppner's most loved model and his wife as he painted her and their graceful children on canvases that glow today.

They found that they were remembered at home. The *Boston News Letter*, an important sheet, had printed the story of their fire:

On Monday evening, June 10, 1771, a fire was discovered in the house of Mrs. Wright, the ingenious artist in Wax Work, and proprietor of the figures so nearly resembling the life, which for sometime past have been exhibited in this city to general satisfaction. The accident happened when Mrs. Wright was away and only the children were home, and was occasioned by one of them accidentally setting fire to a curtain enclosing some of the figures which soon communicated to the clothes and the wax. Neighbors assembled and removed household goods. Fire engines played. The curious piece of the Reverend George Whitefield and that of the Pennsylvania Farmer were saved . . .

Although Phoebe Wright went without a waxen doll, her children and grandchildren played with them, fragile, beautiful creatures with cheeks like rose petals and blue glass eyes over which wax eyelids drooped. Presently wax puppets went traveling. Dressed in broadcloth and gilt braid, bright silks and satins as soldiers, dancers, and harlequins, they performed atop the music boxes and hand organs that toured our countryside. Their finery grew dusty and their complexions faded but the prepared wax made them live for years.

With the coming of home decoration that we call Victorian, no parlor table or mantelpiece was complete without a bouquet of wax flowers under a glass dome, or a bowl of wax-modeled fruit on the dining-room table. With delicate wooden tools, bristle brushes, and scissors, with dry color in the wax or surface painting, bright centerpieces were copied from beloved gardens and orchards. Lily-of-the-valley faintly cream-colored, lilacs, scarlet poppies, golden jonquils, roses of many tints, and blue and pink convolvus were molded by the artists in wax with a perfection that made them almost perfumed. Sometimes real flower and fruit leaves were dipped in wax, delicately veined with wire and added to the bouquet. Old stone jugs for pouring out the melted wax and hand-carved wooden molds were used for modeling apples, peaches, lemons and oranges, plums, pears and even a handsome tomato, just come into favor and called a love apple. These fruits were made of tinted wax and painted to show the sun's markings and the bloom of a peach or a bunch of purple grapes.

Joe Wright became almost as famous as his mother in this art in our country and Elizabeth, too, carried it on. Wax-works exquisite and fragile were cherished for a century. George Washington and Martha, life-size figures, went on the road with the showmen. Mr. P. T. Barnum opened a wax-work show before he started his circus. Museums still display wax portraits of our heroes. An attic here and there shelters a yellowing wax doll or a wreath of wax flowers, reminding us of the days when homespun art began.

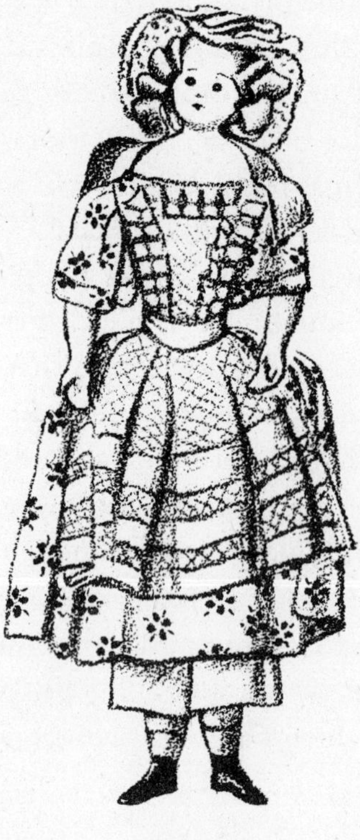

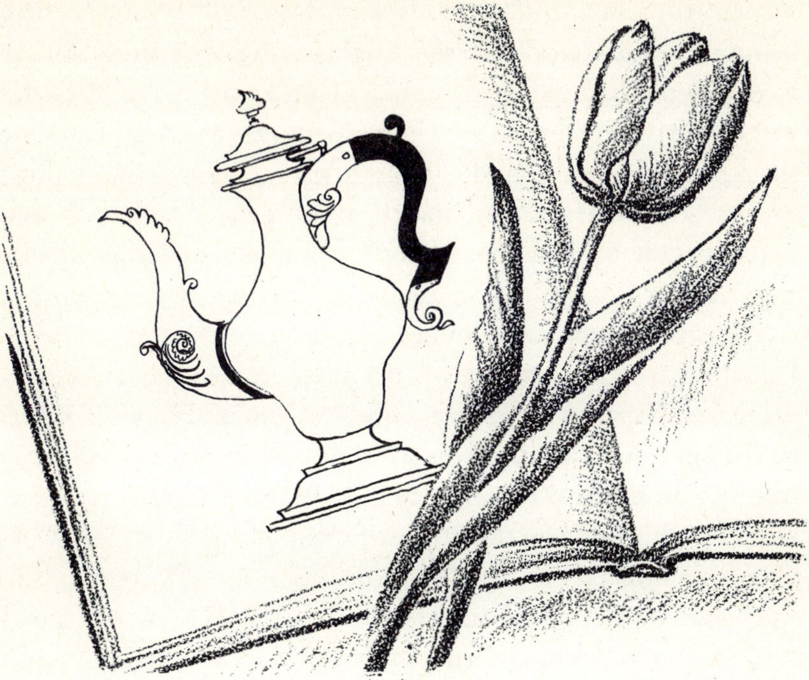

THE SILVER TEAPOT

On his way to the waterfront Charles stopped at The Sign of the Silver Coffee Pot to greet Thomas Sparrow. They were old friends. Thomas had been his father's assistant for some years and now had his own silversmith shop. He was successful although Charles did not hold with such industry. He was not much older than Charles who was fifteen, through school, and sure that the last thing he wanted to do was to settle down in Annapolis for the rest of his life. The day was brisk if warm for late autumn. The thrilling scent of a sea wind, salty and alluring as the Severn brought it shoreward, came to Charles. It was the year 1779 and a brig bringing some notables from farther south for their winter in Annapolis had weighed anchor down at the wharf. Charles was on his way there to see the unloading, the cargo, and the strangers. Visitors would fill the town's narrow streets until spring with their sedan chairs, their clattering top-heavy swords, wide brocade coats, and crinoline that billowed like sails. Annapolis was a fashionable winter resort for even the neighboring plantation owners.

But Charles, having grown up in the town, had a mind to go to sea. There was a large family at home. He would not, he thought, be missed. There were his sisters Nancy and Abigail, his brothers William, older, and young Hiram now ten years old. Hiram was the apple of their father's eye and William his namesake. As for the girls, they were always giggling and sharing whispered secrets about new ribbons and bonnets, boys and parties. Charles felt aloof from these boys and girls. Why there was even a Faris baby, St. John.

The tinkle of Tom Sparrow's hammers, the glint of the sun on his silverware, the small anvil and his row of shining tools had attracted Charles. He stopped by the open door. Tom called to him.

"Come in, Charles Faris. How is it that you are out strolling when the rest of us must work?" As he spoke, Tom held up a gleaming silver porringer upon which he was welding a delicately designed leaf handle with a thumb-hold on which he had engraved the owner's monogram.

Charles lounged against the doorway. "I've done my chores for the day," he told Tom. "Milked the red and white cow, wound the musical clock that stands in the hall. Also I have copied out the week's bills; five shillings for a silver thimble, one pound twelve shillings for six spoons. If I go home now I may have to water and curry the horses. We expect guests today."

Tom laid his porringer gently on a bench and began stirring the silver shillings and pence that were melting in his skillet. He consulted a drawing of a silver teapot he had made, pear-shaped to hold the heat, slender at the top for beauty, decorated with chased garlands and having a beaded rat-tail for a better grip on the handle. Every new piece of silverware at that time was an adventure to the maker, who studied its use and then combined the shape and the decorations for achieving its purpose. And Thomas Sparrow had benefited by his training. Master Faris, Charles' father, ranked as one of the greatest artists in silver in Maryland.

"Jealous, eh, Charles?" he asked smugly. "Wish you could do as fine work as this?"

Charles kicked the door. "Yes?" he scoffed. "After reading up on navigation with the Reverend Jonathan Boucher here at his school, you would have me apprentice myself to Master Faris, one of the hardest taskmasters in Annapolis! You know the oath of the apprentice. Seven years' work with only board and clothing for pay. Moral supervision! The apprentice obeys and keeps the master's secrets."

"But the silversmith ranks with the best of artists," Tom reminded him. "The term of apprenticeship is worth it. Think shame on yourself, Charles Faris, for repudiating your father."

"I would be twenty-two years old!" Charles sighed. "Let William or Hy learn silversmithing. I'm for adventure. I might take passage for the Canaries this very day as cabin boy."

He turned, but a shadow fell across the threshold of the shop. A foreign scent of musk mingled with the sea breeze. A softer voice than the harshly reproving one of Thomas Sparrow drifted over the silence.

"I beg of you not to take ship hastily, young man," the voice urged him, "unless your stomach is stronger than the ordinary. I assure you that the voyage between the Islands and Maryland is a test of one's digestion."

Looking at the stranger, a girl close to his own age but stylish where Nancy and Abigail were sober in dress, black of eye and hair but with the darkness of dusk that gives promise of stars, Charles suddenly felt alien. His stock, he remembered, was not clean. His corduroy breeches had oil spots from his house to house care of his father's clocks. His tongue felt thick. But the girl came to his rescue.

"My name is Judith and my father is the captain of the brig *Mary Lee*, this morning anchored. I have no mother and have been learning French and the social arts in New Orleans. Our ship is laid up here in the Severn for repairs and my father and I shall stay at an inn of whose fine hospitality we have heard, The Sign of the Crown and Dial. I precede the captain to see if I like that inn. My luggage is outside in a barrow. But may I seat myself? I still feel the rolling of the brig." The little lady took Charles' perspiring hand and seated herself on a chair in the shop.

But her indisposition was short. She pierced the shop's glittering store with eager eyes. She moved from one piece of silver to another, exclaiming, holding them up to the light.

"A baby's rattle with two little bells in the shape of bluebells. A creamer so delicate in shape that it puts to shame the rich cream it will hold. A comfit dish with a pattern of flowers the bee loves and trailing vines for the handle. A standing salt with hooks for napkins and legs that it may stand firm in the middle of the table for hospitality." But Judith stood in admiration before a massive teapot.

"If I might have that teapot with a creamer, sugar bowl, and tongs to match, I would be the envy of every young lady in New Orleans," she exclaimed.

"I am sorry, Miss, but my stock is all ordered and paid for," Thomas Sparrow said. "I weighed the silver shillings and sixpence that went into that teapot, melted them down, designed and wrought the service for a resident of our town."

"Then make the resident of this little country town another tea service."

Judith stamped one foot in its scarlet morocco slipper and the long plume on her bonnet trembled with rage. Charles looked admiringly at Judith. He felt a desire to impress her.

He interrupted the explanation Thomas started. "Come home with me," he invited. "My father taught this young man everything he knows. My father keeps the inn at The Sign of the Crown and Dial and will give you excellent accommodations. I," Charles finished with a flourish, "myself, will make you such a silver tea service as Annapolis, or New Orleans either, has never seen." He motioned for Judith to follow him, pretending not to see Thomas Sparrow's smug grin.

Outside Charles gave directions to the sailor who waited with the wheelbarrow that held Judith's hide trunk studded with brass nails and her gay hat box. The air was still sweet with late roses in the gardens and the perfume of the box hedges. The red brick of the houses, the blue water, and the life along the narrow streets, Chancery Lane, Carroll Alley, and the others that radiated like the hubs of a wheel from the ancient grounds of old Saint Anne's church, entranced Judith. They jostled wealth and fashion; gentlemen whose curling hair fell over their shoulders so that they carried their plumed hats under their arms for vanity, ladies with pyramids of hair surmounted by feathers and billowing brocades filled the lanes.

"My father is an all-round man," Charles explained, concerned lest Judith ask him what his own training in silversmithing had been. "He is expert in the making of musical clocks. He designs and builds furniture. He grows rare tulips, he keeps the inn well, and he pulls teeth."

Judith gasped but not at Charles' words. Coming toward them was an odd figure of a man. He stopped, here at a gateway, there at an open door, gossiping with the neighbors, peering into the coaches that brought the winter visitors to Annapolis. A ring of great jingling clock keys in his hand showed that he was making the rounds of those homes where his timepieces chimed and tinkled, but the news of the morning, as always, delayed him. As a sign that he was a Quaker by faith, he wore no wig and his braided powdered queue, tied with a black bow, swung along his back like one of his pendulums. His worn brown coat and short clothes were faded, but a row of big silver buttons decorated the coat and the buckles on his shoes were of finely chased silver. The spectacles tilted down over his sharp nose had silver bows.

"Who is that odd little man?" Judith asked.

The man now stopped in front of them, greeting Charles and looking at his companion with interest.

"That," said Charles, reddening at the remembrance of his promise to Judith, "is Pa."

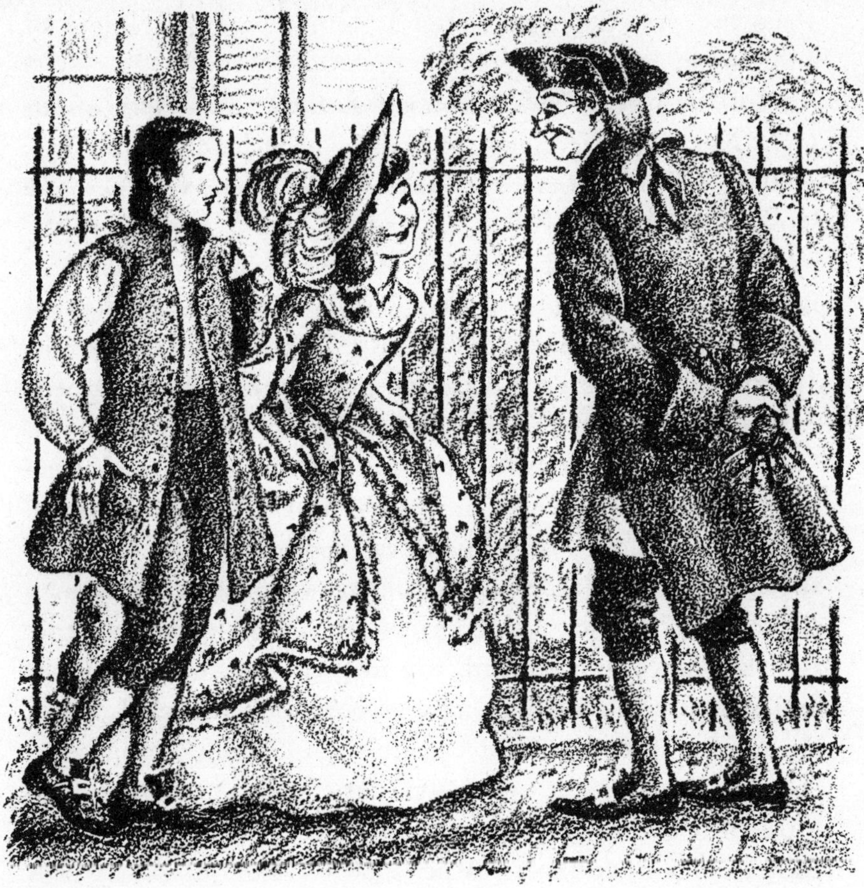

Judith curtsied. "Your son here is going to settle my father and myself for a few weeks at your home, sir. My father is laying up his brig, the *Mary Lee*, at the careenage here for repairs. I shall make the acquaintance of the Annapolis young ladies. Your son will employ his time until we leave in the making of a silver tea service which I shall take down to New Orleans as a souvenir of my visit."

Charles felt cold sweat beneath his stock. His father's eyes were two sword points aimed at him. Finally, wrinkles of amusement began to soften his face.

"So!" he agreed. "Well, you will find two lively girls of our own, Nancy and Abigail, to make you welcome at the inn. And I doubt not that my eldest son William will take you strolling while our skilled silversmith here is putting in the time necessary for the making of your silverware. Come, it is time I were home. We have a reputation at The Sign of the Crown and Dial for hospitality. The best entertainment and the kindest usage. Gentlefolk meet with polite treatment and hay and oats for their horses. And here we are!"

Charles was silent as Master Faris led them into the garden of the home, shop, and inn near the church. Foursquare, shaded by a grove of holly trees trimmed in the shape of sugar loaves, the garden still in bloom with wall flowers, snap dragon, and phlox, the comfort of it charmed sea-faring Judith. Nancy and Abigail, gay in their bright print frocks and ribbon-trimmed mob caps, greeted the stranger. Indoors, the neat common room of the inn with its long dining table, the tall clock made by Master Faris to play the hours in music, the comfortable rooms for herself and her father with chintz curtains and soft feather ticks on the four-poster beds pleased Judith.

"Make yourself at home," Master Faris told her. "When you have changed your finery for a plainer dress, the girls will let you share their preparations for Thanksgiving. They are sugaring the comfits and stoning the fruit. Each tenth raisin goes into a cook's mouth."

"Thanksgiving?" Judith looked surprised.

"A fortnight hence," Master Faris told her. "Not the day set apart by law for church-going such as they decree in New

England, but our Southern day of willing thankfulness for whatever good has come to us during the past year. Our first Thanksgiving was in 1698 when the governor of Maryland decreed a day of thankfulness for the end of the plague that had come upon our people that year. Since then, we keep Thanksgiving when and as we like."

"I could now get the gammon of bacon Mother needs. She spoke of it this morning," Charles suggested, putting off his moment of doom.

"Ah, no," his father said. "You will need all your spare time for making that tea service for our guest. Go you into the shop and begin at once. Mistress Judith will drop in from time to time no doubt to see your progress." His father's glance was cynical. Charles dragged his feet for shame as he entered the shop of the most skilled silversmith of the Colonies.

It was understandable that Thomas Sparrow had served there. A piece of hand-wrought silver at that time was both art and craftsmanship. Master Faris' book of skillfully drawn designs lay on his bench in the shop. The flowers he used in the designs had been pressed and they marked the drawings as Charles turned the pages. There were designs for a silver coffee pot, a tankard, some tea cans, a tea kettle, teapot, a widely curving bowl, a soup ladle. He had favored the tulips he raised in making the designs, but the classic lines of the acanthus leaf and such fancy touches as little animals, a sheep or a dog for thumb-holds, an acorn or pineapple for a cover knob, pear, melon, and apple shapes for teapots showed his versatility as an artist.

The shop, whose windows looked out toward the garden and let in the pleasant twitterings of pigeons and martins, had the best supply of tools in all Maryland. Charles touched them; the small anvils, the melting-skillets, the specially formed vise, punches, scales, hammers of all kinds, tongs, wood-sinking blocks, and shears. Some of the silver was engraved. Other pieces had hammered patterns. Charles sat down on the bench at last, his hands idle in his lap. The tools, the gleaming metal, or some unexplained impulse had given him the ambition to be a silversmith. Whether it was for Judith's sake or for the sake of his father, he could not have explained. But there were seven years of training ahead of him and Judith would not be in Annapolis very long.

There was a lure for any boy in the sheen of the blocks of silver, the power of the delicate tools and the grace of the finished silverware. Master Faris could give a silver inkstand lion feet, mount a necklace with coral, make a tiny silver service for Abigail's doll. He copied in silver the designs of the flowered cottons that ships brought to the Colony from the Indies. He worked for the sake of beauty. And Charles could not even draw. His head drooped into his hands. From the kitchen came Judith's gay laughter. He did not know it, but her desire for a silver tea service was changed to a taste for candied citron and chocolate. Judith was a butterfly of a girl.

But as Charles grew more and more discouraged, a shadow crossed the threshold. His father touched his shoulder.

"Have a hope, Charlie," he said. "There is a piece of work waiting for you that I find tedious in spite of its pretty results." He brought from a cupboard a silver bowl, deep and wide, smooth and unadorned.

"Place it so in this block," he said, "and beat it with this small hammer."

Charles began the tedious work. The silver was tough and the hammer marks almost too small to be seen at first. But as he beat the surface day after day, Charles saw a transformation. The hammered silver began to reflect the light. As a diamond glitters with its facets, absorbing and sending forth rays, so the bowl became radiant. It brightened the shop. It needed no other decoration than that the hammer gave it. It would shine as brightly by candlelight as in the sunshine of the shop.

Almost every day Judith, wearing one of Nancy's aprons, looked in on the young silversmith. She clasped her hands in front of the bowl, her breath coming in gasps.

"Beautiful, Charles!" she said. "It shall hold the fruits in the center of the Thanksgiving table. I can see it filled with apples and pears, grapes, and persimmons. Such a dinner as we are planning; wild turkey and sugar-cured ham, terrapin, duck, and venison, plum pudding, preserves, blanc-mange, fruit cake, nuts, and comfits. And perhaps you will give me your silver bowl when I leave. It would cheer my father on his long voyages, standing on the mess table of the brig."

"I was decorating it for you," Charles said, the idea having just come to him.

"Yes, Judith," his father agreed. "Charles has the makings of a fine silversmith in his hands. We shall see. We shall see."

There was plenty on that long-ago Thanksgiving board of Maryland. The table in the common room of The Crown and Dial glittered with silver; hand-wrought spoons and knives, the soup tureen, the tea service, the great standing salt, the gravy boat and ladle, the silver mugs. At the head of the table Master Faris glowed with pride in his handwork. At the foot, Mistress Faris wore the silver lace he had made for her. Up and down the sides of the table the Faris boys and girls, Judith and the guests ate for two hours, their good food tasting better for the beauty of the service.

"We have a special cause for thankfulness," Master Faris announced when the blazing plum pudding was brought in. He pointed to the center of the table and the glowing silver bowl of fruit. "We have a second silversmith in the Faris family. Stand up, Charles, and take a bow. Not all workers can hammer so well."

Judith was the loudest in the hand-clapping for Charles. The silver bowl would go to sea with Judith, but the touch of the silver remained with Charles. It had fired his heart. After all, it was the Faris baby, St. John, who went to sea. Charles and following him, Hiram, learned Master Faris' art. The Metropolitan Museum in New York shows us Charles' handsome silverware. In a Baltimore museum we may see a delicately curved creamer with three well-balanced legs and a sauce boat with a design of shells that Master William Faris wrought. A Baltimore home treasures the bit of silver lace he wrought. And Master Faris' yellowing book of designs for silver, the only one that has come down to us, opens its pages to the dried tulip markers he put in. For the old art of the silversmith was also an adventure and the Thanksgiving of Charles Faris' apprenticeship to beauty a very special day for being thankful.

There were many skilled silversmiths in our early days. As finer living took the place of toil the Colonies had time for creating beauty. As tea, coffee, and chocolate reached our shores, pots were designed for serving them. In lantern shape or formed like fruits, some of them rounded to imitate

Chinese porcelain, the Massachusetts silversmiths designed them. Ornamented with trailing vines, flowers, and wild berries, the creamer, sugar bowl, and tray matching, they were graceful and elegant. Silver cake baskets, sweetmeat dishes, standing salts, and service plates soon followed. New England silversmiths also designed church silver, baptismal fonts, and contribution plates.

The silver of Dutch New York was solid and useful like its artists. The Dutch silversmiths wrought heavy bowls, porringers whose thumb-holds were big enough for fat fingers and some of the plates so massive that they could be engraved with scenes from the Bible. There were more tiny sets of silverware for dolls made by the Dutch than by the other Colonists. They liked to attach bells to their large spoons as well as those for the babies. And no sleigh bells rang with such merry tunes as the silver strings wrought by the Dutch.

But the South has given us the richest work of the old silversmith. Perhaps that is because the settlers of Maryland and Virginia brought some English and French silver when they came. A few apprentices arrived with these settlers, and some books of design were brought. The rich soil and warm sunshine of the South left more leisure for practicing the arts. No old home of our South today is complete without a sideboard on which stand a shining silver tea service, bowls, beakers, candlesticks, and plates made by some artist-craftsman. And the fine silverware of the present is copied from the designs of Master Charles Faris, Paul Revere, and those other artists of the past who wrought for beauty as well as use, and whose hands made silver reflect the light and design of past days.

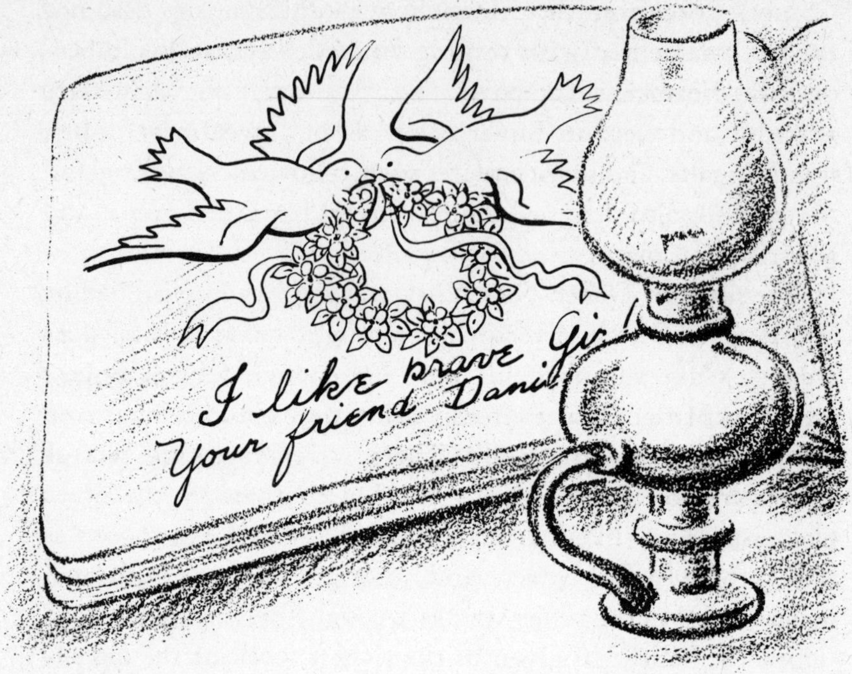

THE SPARKING LAMP

THE new round table in Captain Holcomb's sitting-room enclosed a bright circle of fancy work. A March evening there in New Hampshire had dropped a curtain of early darkness and all the candles were lighted. Even the old brass lantern from the barn had come inside for the evening and shone in the center of the green baize that covered the table, surrounded by wide-based tin candlesticks.

The table was built of mahogany with claw legs, and was large enough to seat the four girls and their parents. It had been brought by waterway and coach from New York. Captain Holcomb was one of the town's richest men and could afford the gilt-trimmed Franklin stove that sent a warm glow about the room. He had thought nothing of the cost of the table, but he held to the town's simple ways. As each one of his family bent over her work, he knew what was in her mind. Which girl, Betsy, Hepzibah, Hannah, or Polly, would be the one to bring home the cows? It was already past their milking time and the Holcomb cows had a liking for a wild pasture that lay a quarter of a mile from home, where the mountains shared their loneliness with the forest, and a creek, clear and cold, ran down to the valley. One of his girls, each night, found and drove the cows home. No modern art, encouraged by the space of the round table, was allowed to interfere with this duty.

"We need better light," their mother said as she laid another pheasant's feather on the wreath she was designing to frame and hang on the parlor wall. The wreath was made entirely of colored feathers from fowl and game birds. Hawks, grouse, whippoor-will, turkeys, and pheasants had all given their plumage to make the wreath. The feathers were fastened to a backing of heavy paper with tiny drops of sealing wax. When the gay circlet was finished it would be put under glass, framed in gilded wood and there might be a party to celebrate its hanging. As she held a stick of red sealing wax to a candle flame to melt, their mother sighed.

"Much more light, if we are ever to become artists. Over at Robert Hughes' glassworks they are making all kinds of oil lamps. Round and square, urn, balloon, and Gothic-window shape. He is putting in cork holders for the wicks that let them drop deep into the oil and give a steadier light. One of Robert Hughes' glass lamps would look well in the center of our table."

Captain Holcomb, oiling his boots beside the stove, sniffed. "A seafaring man over at Portsmouth spoke to me of lamps recently. He says that a woman is more beholden to the whale than to any other creature under the sun. It gives her stays, perfume, and lamplight. If candles do not suffice you, my dear, give up your art work."

Betsy, the eldest, looked up from the bead purse she was netting, embroidering a pattern of roses and pinks in tiny glass beads upon a crocheted foundation of gray silk. The purse would go well with her spring frock of gray silk, the blue polonaise, and the flowers on her bonnet.

"Well," she said, "not even Captain Holcomb's family may count on having one of Robert Hughes' glass lamps. It is said that even Boston must wait for the peddlers' carts that stock lamps from his Temple factory. He has none to spare for our townsmen."

"I can't see to place my stitches," Hepzibah complained.

On the backing of an old flour bag Hepzibah was embroidering a chair cover in needlepoint. It glowed with the colors that New England in that year of grace, 1782, was hungering for; cherry red and apple crimson, pumpkin gold, and the orange of marigolds, made the flower design in the center. The background would be madder. The years would fade but only mellow the colors.

"I, too, could do with more light. The girls are hogging the candles," nine-year-old Polly said.

She was splashing away with bits of tinsel, flour paste, a

colored picture or two, and her box of paints as she decorated a cardboard lampshade. They could be bought plain at the village store waiting for artistic touches to be put on at home.

"Here's the shade, but where is the lamp?"

Hannah, fourteen, was silent. Her forehead wrinkled, her tongue stuck out, as she worked by herself a little outside of the circle at the table. She was occupied, as she had been for many evenings, in the making of her autograph album.

Although farm chores were still done by the daughters of the town, life was becoming more of a pastime for them. Their houses were brighter, too. The Holcombs' new frame house was touched with color in the cherry and yellow pine of the furniture, the painted floors, the gilt-framed mirrors with scenes painted on the upper part of the glass. Green and ruby glassware in the corner cupboard reflected the light.

There was time now for their fancy work. Their mother had in mind the decorating of her parlor as she made wreaths, either of feathers, hair, or colored grains and berries to frame and hang upon the new scenic wallpaper. Betsy's art was for her own adornment when she walked out in floating skirts, her dark eyes peeping out from beneath a ruffled silk sunshade. Hepzibah's needlepoint would grace her own home one day. Polly had just changed from paper dolls to ornamenting lampshades. Hannah, in-between her sisters in age, had chosen the autograph album as her art expression. Within its pink, yellow, and blue pages she hoped to have a record of friendship that would enrich her whole life.

The cardboard covers of the album were neatly mounted with marbled paper upon which Hannah had inked in two doves holding in their bills a wreath of roses, with *Autographs* written in the center. Nearly all the pages that she had stitched in firmly with linen thread were of white paper, but there was a box factory in a near-by town that sold bits of colored paper, and one page in six of the album was of this. On the white pages she had drawn designs in pen-and-ink scroll work; a rose, a beehive to symbolize industry, a bird, a butterfly, a sketch of the country scene outside their front

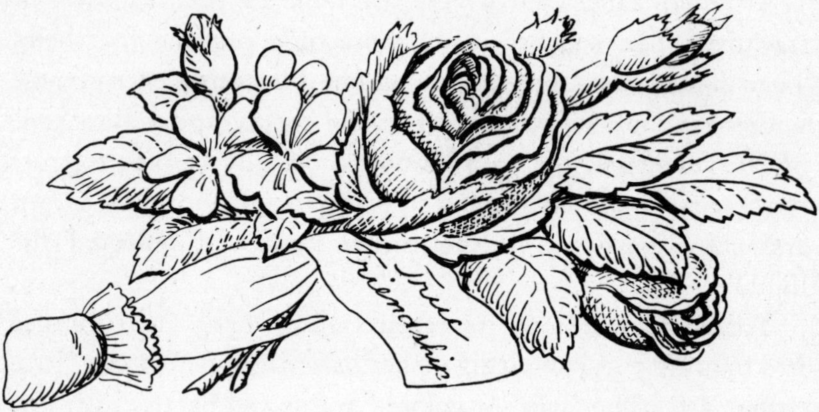

gate. As she drew, Hannah thought of the inscriptions her friends would write in the curling longhand they learned in school:

There would be of course the popular ditty,

> The rose is red, the violet blue,
> Sugar is sweet and so are you.

A daring boy might write on one page, "Oh, I don't know," which was a byword of the times. A serious-minded friend would inscribe,

Only a sigh on the sea of life,
Blending with yours in care and strife,
You see but the shadow of the fame
That might have been for this poor name.

Hannah's eyes grew dreamy with the sentiment that would fill the album. If she could have seen far enough she would have read on one page, in forthright script,

Yours truly,
Henry W. Longfellow.

Her father's voice interrupted her dreams.

"I hear that Daniel Searles has come home from college and is appointed surveyor. He's measuring the glassworks. The town wonders where Robert Hughes is getting his sand. It may be that he is encroaching on town land."

The girls were all attention. "His father plans that Dan should teach the school next year, being now seventeen. He's a likely looking lad," their mother said.

"And with money in the bank from his father's mills," Hepzibah added.

Polly sang in a teasing drone, her mouth partly full of paper clippings, "Danny Searles likes Hannah's curls."

Hannah was glad of her dim portion of the table that hid her flushed cheeks. Once Daniel had sparked her home from singing school.

Their father set down the boots and arose. "It is already late and I see that your fancy time-wasting has made you all forget the cows. If I am not mistaken it is young Hannah's turn to bring them home."

She was glad also of the darkness to cover her flaming cheeks and the cool night wind to still her beating heart.

Daniel Searles was almost a stranger now to Hannah, but she had admired his high marks in school. She had not been far behind him, having herself some skill in spelling and figuring. His father had built the first grist mill and a saw mill in town. Whenever anyone spoke of Daniel, it was in praise. He was known to have a superior mind. He must have grown up in his two years at college, Hannah thought, far aloof from his Temple schoolmates.

She stepped out briskly into the night. It was pitch dark but the trees had hatchet notches that marked the cattle walk down the hill and into the grasslands where the cows nibbled through the melting snow. She pulled her hooded cape close about her with one hand and felt of the tree trunks with the other. The night was full of undertones, a hooting owl, the far-off bark of a fox, the crackling of frozen branches as hawks stirred in their high nests.

Hannah had left the lantern at home. The family needed it. She thought, as she felt her way along, how wonderful it was that oil lamps had come in. Robert Hughes, the Boston gentleman who had built the Temple glass factory, was far-sighted in his business. He made green and yellow glass bottles, large and small, but his glass lamps were famed as far as the fishing banks to the north, and south to New York. They were in such demand that out-of-town dealers took up nearly all, leaving scant store for the townspeople. Well, Hannah thought, perhaps the family would sometime have a table lamp, a beacon in the sea of industry that the new center table made.

Because she was longing for the bright flame of an oil lamp, her eyes pierced the darkness for light. The days were still short. By supper time the forest that surrounded their hill was as black as near-by Tophet Swamp, than which there could be nothing blacker. A bounty of two dollars had been recently posted in the general store for a wildcat that had been eating town chickens boldly. Hannah knew the ways of these small, lithe, and cruel cats that haunted the mountains thereabouts, sliding down old trees, creeping along the ground as silently as a snake. Their eyes were their only warning, gleaming like yellow topazes in the night.

She had come so far from home that she was not quite sure where she was. In thinking of the glass factory, remembering the pleasant evening, its embroidering, decorating, and the like that she had left, Hannah had neglected to find some of the marked trees. Losing even one of the notches took her the wrong way. Before she realized it, she was staggering around in a circle of confusion. The cows were no help to her, for as soon as twilight dropped they found beds for themselves in the shelter of the deep pine groves. Still Hannah pushed on. When she could not find a single notched tree, she knew that she was lost. That was not only a calamity but a disgrace. Ever since they were small the town girls had brought home the cows. It was a chore in which they took pride.

Hannah was brave, but as she stumbled over unfamiliar ground, fell into a piece of soaked marsh, pulled herself out only to fall again over a gnarled stump, she began to feel afraid. The memory of the posted wildcat bounty came to her mind, made her heart pound.

"Cats are scarce around Temple," she had heard her father say, "but one never forgets the taste of a chicken. It will chase a man to get to a chicken yard."

"They see in the dark like a house cat," the boys of the town said.

Surely it was not her fear though that made Hannah catch the near-by crackle of dry branches, the rustle of bushes. Ahead of her she saw a small bright light moving here and there; a yellow flame-like flicker like a cat's eye. It was moving closer. She could not help the scream of terror that forced itself into the night as that moving eye approached and shone down on her.

"Why, it's young Hannah Holcomb!" A tall boy holding a lamp above his head spoke to her. "What are you doing out here alone, close to Tophet Swamp?"

"Daniel Searles!" Hannah gasped. "How do you come to be here with one of Master Hughes' new glass lamps? I am trying to find the cows, but where they are I know not. I was wool-gathering and lost my way. I thought your lamp spark was the eye of a wild cat."

"Poor little lass!" Daniel had grown tall since their school days. He had to bend down to take Hannah's hand. "I spent the day measuring town land and I found that Master Hughes is well within his rights in taking sand for his glass-blowing from the pit nigh to his factory. I stopped to sup with him and he showed me his broad swords. He is a master of sword play and teaches it to the young Boston gentlemen. He also showed me his parrots, chattering birds of gaudy plumage that he brought home with him from his sailing voyages to the Islands. He was pleased with my surveying for he is not of a mind to cheat the town. In gratitude he gave me this lamp ready filled with oil and having a long wick. I was trying it out on my way home. It burns as well as any lantern."

It was a low, bowl-shaped glass lamp with a handle

carefully shaped to fit the thumb and forefinger. It had the new patent cork holder for the wick and it was decorated on the bowl with the hobnail pattern of raised knobs that reflected the light. The glass chimney protected the clear flame. It was indeed a light in the darkness to lead a lost cowherd to the spot only a few yards ahead where the cows lazily roused and stumbled toward it.

"Coo, boss!" Hannah called, her courage renewed.

Daniel added his deeper tones to hers. The herd by instinct found the cattlewalk and went lazily on ahead, rubbing their heads against the trees. Daniel held Hannah's hand until they were well out of the woods and could see the lights of her home at the top of the hill.

"You've grown tall since I was in Cambridge," Daniel said. "I mind me of the time when you spelled me down in the district school, me a big gawk three classes ahead of you."

"You excelled me in figures, Daniel," she reassured him, but she glowed with pride.

"This lamp shines as bright as any lantern," Daniel said as they came to the door.

"So it does," Hannah opened the door and the lad followed her in. "We are hoping to buy a lamp one of these days," she added boldly.

The table still held its circle of workers. Daniel stood beside them, watching.

"Good evening, sir. It is good to be home, where I have a Temple." Captain Holcomb took his hand.

"Good evening, sir. It is good to be home, where I have a mind to remain." He praised the wreath, the beadwork, and the lampshade. Then Daniel took the autograph album, turning its blank pages. "Is this the work of young Hannah? I remember that she cherished her friends in our school days together."

"A piece of frivolity," the Captain grunted, but he laid his hand on Hannah's yellow ringlets that her hair net would not keep smooth. "My womenfolks have gone daft over fancy work, but Hannah is a biddable girl. She left her occupation tonight to find the cows. Why, if you would believe it, Daniel, my family wants a table lamp."

"Have you a quill, young Hannah?" the lad asked. He took it from her and finding a pink page of the album he deftly drew two doves holding a wreath in their crossed bills. Beneath the drawing he wrote in flowing script,

I like brave girls.
Your friend, Daniel Searles,

Then he placed the sparking lamp in the center of the table. "This lamp was a gift to me from Robert Hughes, and it is my pleasure to give it to Hannah to light your evening work."

What a gift! They were breathlessly silent at first. Then Hannah spoke. "We thank you, Daniel. It is beyond our dreams."

"Come to supper on the coming Sabbath beneath its flame," their mother invited.

"Sit down and rest yourself, Daniel," Captain Holcomb urged. "There are doughnuts in the crock and buttermilk in the dairy."

As Daniel sat down beside Hannah a new splendor touched the lamp-lit art.

Daniel Searles was to become a member of the family and

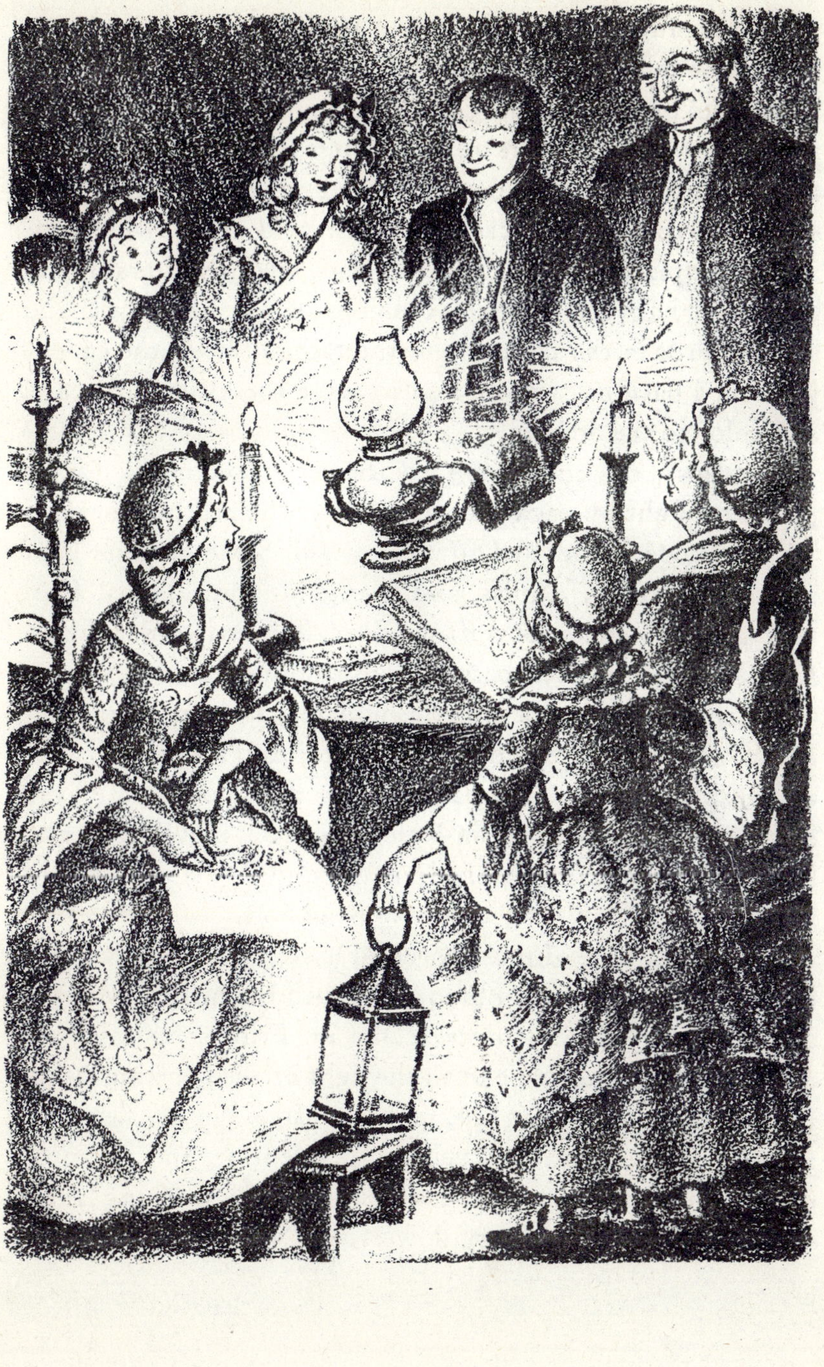

Hannah's autograph album filled itself with verse and pictures that tell us their story. The lamps that took the place of candles brought flashing colors to light, illumined brighter rooms with our ancestors' revolt against Puritanism. Pink luster china, gilt stenciling on cherry and pine chairs and settees, scenic mirrors, and clock faces with gold and scarlet, blue and green pictures painted on the glass, wreaths of grains and berries, of hair and feathers, cushions of gay beadwork, and stuffed birds in the parlor were the fashion. Even the calico-patterned barn cat was invited to share the kitchen fire and add color to the house.

Outdoors, red roofs mapped the gray landscape. Cactus plants brought by packet boat to Boston flashed in dooryards where Rhode Island Red fowls strutted. Some families kept a peacock. Salvia, zinnias, and marigolds flamed until frost fell. Glass sunbursts above front doors illuminated dark halls. Knockers and foot scrapers were of shining brass.

Cut-paper designs became fashionable; lacy for heart valentines, cut-out urns and flowers that decorated the pages of autograph albums. Card patterns for the squares of woven bedspreads were designed in Rose of Sharon, clover-leaf, and ladies'-plaid patterns, carefully marked with the numbers of the loom levers and loaned among neighbors.

That was a time of more cheerful living. Its art grew cumbersome at last as the lambrequin draped the mantel, and the crocheted tidy for furniture came in. Fringe, tatting, and crocheted lace tangled beneath the light of the sparking lamp. But we were happier at last, more carefree. Fingers flew and a faded feather wreath, a yellowing valentine, and an autograph album in an attic tell us the story of the sparking lamp, of the evenings when fancy flowered in New England.

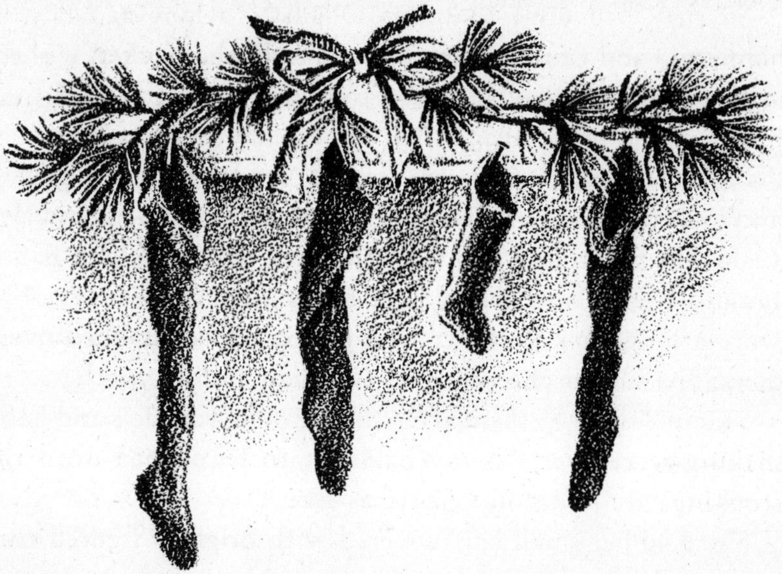

HANG UP THE CHRISTMAS STOCKINGS

THE stage, creaking on its winter runners, stopped at the Whitinville general store and left Gretje, Obadiah Whiting's Christmas-tide company from New York, and a letter for Obadiah's father. Gretje had been invited to take the long trip by packet boat to Boston, then by stage to the little village of Whitinville in old Vermont because her father was a business friend of Mr. Whiting, shipping him the calicoes, tea, and chinaware needed in the store.

"Mr. Ver Planck gives good value in cottons," Obadiah's father had said a month before. "Let us show our appreciation by asking him to send his daughter to us for a country Christmas."

So they had done that but Obadiah, a long-ago boy in homespun and fur cap, high boots, and leather jacket, wished, as the stage unloaded and then took its slow way toward the hills and the next village, that his holiday guest, Gretje Ver Planck, had been a boy. He stuffed the letter in his pocket and looked at the girl. She appeared to be his own age, twelve years. She was round and rosy-cheeked, with two long flaxen braids hanging on either side of her quilted scarlet hood. She wore a long dark green traveling cloak and fur-lined overshoes. She smiled cheerfully at Obadiah and his mother.

"Here," she told them after the how-do-you-do's and hand shaking were over, "is my bag, not to be opened until the stockings are hung on Christmas Eve."

She held her small bag, covered with brightly figured carpeting, closely. "It holds gifts from New York to put in your stockings. I shall miss Christmas in New York with my grandfather dressed as Saint Nicholas, the Christmas tree trimmed with sugar toys and gingerbread figures, and the carol-singing in the Bouerie. But this is nice," she added, looking around at the pleasant store interior, warmed by a big wood stove and scented with cheese and tea, apples and hams. Gretje darted toward a pile of hand-knitted stockings that lay on the dry goods counter. She pointed to a long one, indigo blue and well-shaped. "That," she exclaimed, "shall be for this boy, Obadiah. I shall fill it myself, for I hear that the good Saint Nicholas who came in the ship with us Dutch folk to New York, has not yet found his way to your New England."

Mr. Whiting, seated on the high stool at his counting desk, turned and looked sternly over his spectacles at enthusiastic Gretje. "No, you are right, Gretje, in that. We have no Saint

Nicholas here. Nor do we of New England indulge in the pagan fashion of hanging up stockings at Christmas. You will enjoy the hymn singing at church and you and Obadiah may help stir the Christmas pudding. But this unnecessary custom of making and receiving presents other than useful ones is frowned upon. We wear our stockings for comfort and work, having none to spare for packing with gimcracks."

Obadiah came to Gretje's rescue, seeing her sudden look of surprise and dismay. "You'll have a good time here, Gretje," he promised. "My old skates should fit you and I made a new sled this winter. It is big enough for two." He bravely swallowed his shame at the thought of what the other boys would say at seeing him coasting with a girl, and a Dutch girl at that.

Mistress Whiting put a kind arm around Gretje's shoulder. "Come and eat a bowl of hot porridge and maple syrup," she said. "Then unpack from your bag only those things you will need. Keep its secrets tightly shut. You and Obadiah shall crack walnuts for a boiling of molasses taffy and there are raisins to stone and sample for the Christmas pudding."

His father smiled, trying to soften the hurt he had felt obliged to give Gretje. "We welcome you, my child. Christmas for us of this cold hill country is not the festival of which the Dutch make it, but you will have a happy time. No letter, Obadiah?"

Ah; Obadiah had forgotten it! The letter in the boy's pocket felt like scorching coals. He should have given it to his father the very first thing. That was the rule. Mail was slow in coming by stage. Sometimes for a month at a time none was received. And mail addressed to his father, the Whitinville storekeeper, Obadiah knew, was always important.

Better, he thought, to wait and lay the letter on the counting desk after supper than confess that, in the arrival of Gretje, he had forgotten it.

"I helped Gretje down from the stage," he said avoiding a direct answer.

His father sighed. "Thomas, the stage driver, is more and more careless," he said. "I expected a letter following my reply to that amazing one I received six weeks ago; the inquiry from the selectman in New Hampshire."

Obadiah tried to cover his chagrin by explaining to Gretje. "A stranger, who seemed to be an important man in New Hampshire, wrote asking if my father had taught school in Greenville in that state ever so many years ago; he asked if he had been that schoolmaster named Whiting? Well, father wrote him that he had been the Greenville schoolmaster, but we have all been puzzled as to why a stranger should have written asking that."

"Mr. Whiting was a New Hampshire schoolmaster, and a good one, in his young days," Obadiah's mother said.

"Oh, yes, a very good one," Obadiah hastened to add remembering his father's earnest tutoring of his son in the tables and spelling, his exasperation with mistakes.

"I hoped for a reply to my letter by this stage," his father said, turning back to the figures of his ledger.

Before he went to bed that night, Obadiah looked at the postmark on the letter. Concord, New Hampshire, he read just above the red sealing wax. Yes, it was probably from the stranger who had written to his father. Those words, "I hoped for a reply by this stage," repeated themselves in Obadiah's mind and kept him from going to sleep. He postponed putting the letter on his father's desk. He kept it under his pillow and in his pocket in the daytime. It seemed to burn a hole in his pocket but although he planned every day to confess his negligence, he found this difficult. His father was kind indeed, but strict so far as truthfulness was concerned. Obadiah knew that he had been dishonest in deed, more so every day that he concealed the letter. The thought spoiled that week before Christmas when there was no school, when Goose Pond was bright with the mufflers, hoods, caps and mittens of boy and girl skaters, and the Whitinville hills were alive with coasters.

But no care kept Gretje from having a good time. Her joy made up for Obadiah's gloom. Almost at once she showed their playfellows that she could cut figure-eights and pigeon wings wearing Obadiah's old skates on Goose Pond. She was so

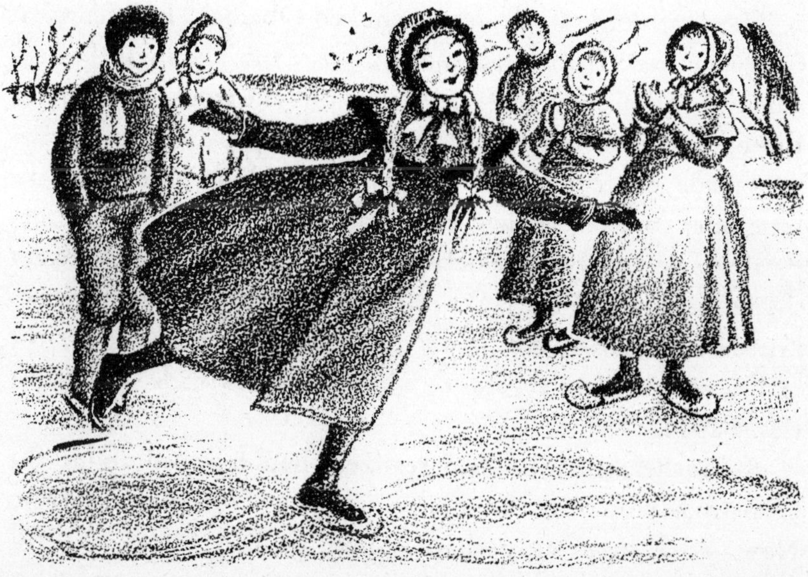

fearless a coaster, learned to steer a sled so skillfully, that the boys allowed her to ride with them. It was real Christmas weather, icy cold but dry, with snow that held a light crust and warm sun in the middle of the day. Indoors, there was so much activity in the kitchens, chopping mince meat, blending the fruits, sugar, and suet for the Christmas pudding, baking holiday cakes, that no one admitted any lack in the New England celebration of the season. Only Gretje, covered with a gay apron splashed with a pattern of tulips, mixing and baking Dutch cookies and crullers with sugar icing, remembered.

"How well these would fill the toe of a stocking!" she sighed as she shaped her cookies like chickens, hearts, and figures of Saint Nicholas. "Here, scatter your frowns, Obadiah," she laughed as she thrust a warm ball of the fried cruller dough into his mouth. "One would think that you dreaded Christmas instead of loving it as I do."

The toothsome treat almost choked Obadiah. Indeed, what Gretje said was true. He dreaded Christmas. The night before, when he had been helping his father put the stock in order for the extra customers who crowded the store for the Christmas trade, he had picked up one of the long stockings, the blue one, that Gretje had exclaimed over the day of her arrival. As he felt of it, he detected a bulge in the toe, the exact shape and size of a big jackknife. Obadiah wanted a new jackknife more than anything else just then. He needed it for the spring season when tops were whittled, boats made, and whistles shaped.

His father, Obadiah had realized, had relented about the Christmas stockings. In honor of their Dutch guest from New York, he was perhaps going to hang stockings for

Obadiah and Gretje. And there in Obadiah's pocket, the neglected letter from New Hampshire was still hidden. Every day, every hour made the boy more ashamed.

Three days before Christmas, his father got out the first letter from the stranger and re-read part of it aloud as Obadiah swept the store.

"My object in writing to you," he read, "is to ask if you are the person who taught school in Mason, New Hampshire, about the winter of 1787? If you will inform me of this by mail, I will then inform you of my object in asking this question—"

"I informed him," Obadiah's father said to the boy who had stopped sweeping to listen, "but he has not even thanked me for writing."

Suddenly, Obadiah felt a great courage surging up within his spirit. No matter what happened to him, he must be fair to his father who had always, if strict, been completely fair with him.

"Here's the letter, sir," he gasped, pulling it from his pocket and holding it out. "I forgot to give it to you the day Gretje came and afterwards I was afraid to. I beg your pardon, sir." He laid the letter down on the counting desk.

His father was too surprised, too curious, to do more than break the sealing wax, unfold the letter and read it:

"You were my teacher, sir, I discover from your letter. All passed pleasantly between us until one day in the last term of my schooling when, about an hour before the school closed in the afternoon, you called me up and ordered me to stand there for whispering, depriving me of my reading and spelling. You did not say a word to me the rest of the day, which I considered a great insult. I was about eleven years old at that time.

"I remained until you and all the scholars, except a boy named

Samuel who took care of the schoolhouse, had left. I then decided upon revenge and collected your books, inkstand, quill pens, and ruler with the intent to burn them. But before I could effect this object, Samuel saw what I contemplated and saved all except the inkstand, ruler, and a small book or two, say to the value of from three to six shillings. Samuel said that I would be jailed for life which brought me to my senses, I then resolved to leave the town.

"I had an uncle who lived in Concord and I was off for that town in a day or two. So I escaped the punishment I so truly deserved. I apprenticed myself in a trade and finally, in manhood, became a selectman of the town. But I have always regretted my fault and have intended if ever I could find you to make an apology and give you satisfaction, though, perhaps, you had forgotten the transaction.

"I now, sir, enclose to you five dollars to pay debt and interest which I hope you will receive with the same kind feelings that I have in sending it to you; and wish you to consider my extreme youth when the error was committed—

Respectfully yours,

"Here it is, sir. The note fell on the floor!" Obadiah snatched up the five-dollar note from the floor beneath the desk where it had slipped out from the folds of the letter. He gave it to his father.

"I had forgotten," his father said. "Who would have thought that the wild freak of a boy of eleven years, in attempting to escape punishment for a pardonable fault in school, would lead him to forsake his father's house, all the love of home and family, and his young friends? And that this event would be his first step toward making a place of honor for himself; would lead him toward discharging what he terms a debt and interest to me!

"But you, sir! Untruthful in deed and word, for it is as

evil to conceal the truth as deny it. A birching is in order."

Obadiah hung his head.

"But I doubt if the rod is as severe a punishment as you deserve. There is this matter of celebrating Christmas in the New York way," his father went on. "I doubt if there is any great harm in hanging a stocking above the fireplace. Customs, even here in New England, are changing. In fact, I had such a plan in mind, since we have the spirited and domestic Gretje in our midst." He turned to Obadiah. "Two dollars and a half of this amount shall be spent for gimcracks to put in your mother's and Gretje's Christmas stockings. You may go into town and buy presents by tomorrow's stage," he said. "The remainder of the money shall be given as a Christmas offering to the church."

"A ribbon and a bottle of scent for Gretje, sir?" Obadiah asked. "And a gilt brooch for Mother?" There was no doubt in his mind as to the nature of his punishment. Only two stockings would be hung.

The door between the store and the sitting-room was open and Gretje, knitting beside the fire, had heard the conversation. After bedtime, when the house was still, a blanket-wrapped figure crept downstairs, entered the store where Master Whiting still sat at his ledgers. But the New Hampshire letter lay on a page, covering the figures. Instead of addition he saw a blue stocking with a jackknife in the toe. He started as Gretje touched his arm.

"The New York boys are all wearing nickel watches on tortoise-shell chains. I brought Obadiah such a watch. I should admire to put it in his stocking Christmas Eve."

Mr. Whiting pulled Gretje's long braids and smiled. "We

shall see," he conceded. "Now get you to bed for I must write our thanks to this good friend and ask him to visit us if his travels ever bring him as far as Vermont."

Obadiah felt as if he were walking on stilts the remaining days. He would have a great disappointment but he felt at peace with himself, having turned over the letter. And the whole household seemed full of cheer. His father was affable. His mother was making richer cake than ever before. And Gretje went about with a secret laughter in all her ways and speech. He felt the holiday spirit even if his fair punishment was that of depriving him of hanging a Christmas stocking. On the Eve they hung two stockings above the fireplace and while Gretje blinded her eyes, Obadiah filled her stocking. Then he went to bed, as Gretje urged. "I want to fill your mother's stocking," she explained. "I promise not even to feel of mine."

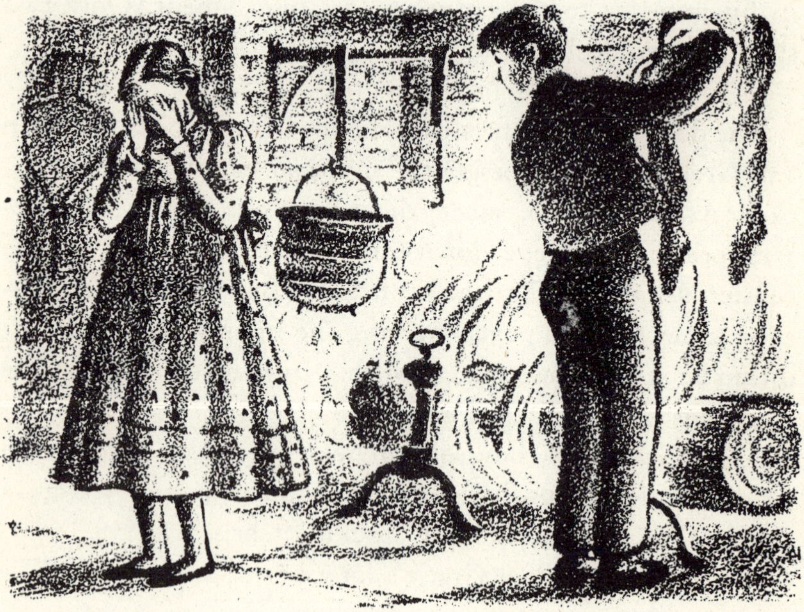

After a Christmas breakfast of chicken pie and griddle cakes with syrup, they sat on the hearth and feasted their eyes. A plump red stocking for Gretje. A plump white stocking for Mistress Whiting. A bulging blue stocking; that was Obadiah's!

In addition to Gretje's ribbon and a little crystal bottle of lavender perfume, she found treasures; one of the new and beautiful wax dolls—she still made the excuse of her fine sewing for dressing dolls—some shining new knitting needles, a thread and needle case that Mistress Whiting had stitched from scarlet leather, apples and Christmas cakes to fill the empty places. Mistress Whiting found her brooch and a beaded bag. Obadiah's stocking held his shining watch that ticked almost as loudly as did their tall kitchen clock. His jackknife was the best in the village, with good steel in the blade and his initials on the polished wood handle. His father had written on the paper wrapping, "For a boy of good intentions." And Gretje had brought fur-lined kid gloves for the entire family.

"What a Christmas!" Obadiah shouted.

"All because a boy ran away from your father's school ever so long ago!" Gretje reminded him.

Obadiah paused a second from winding his watch. "Well, I wouldn't say that exactly, Gretje," he said. "I'd say, because that boy was honest and paid my father 'debt and interest!' You know that line we have to write in our copy book about honesty being the best policy?" Gretje smiled mischievously. But it was Christmas. She did not remind Obadiah how close he had come to forgetting that proverb.

So Dutch New York and New England came together in

our first keeping of Christmas. Fireplaces that had held only iron pots on their swinging cranes decorated their overmantels with rows of colored bulging stockings. The evergreens from ancient forests beyond the farms twined themselves to weave Christmas wreaths. Pine, spruce, the ground pine that grows close to checkerberries, Southern holly and mistletoe came as far as home doors and graced windows. Then, since greenery had begun to celebrate Christmas in our land, whole trees began marching to town from the woods, at first on sledges, later by freight train and truck. The Christmas trees trimmed their boughs with frosted gingerbread figures, strings of snowy pop-corn, and cranberries, shimmering balls and birds blown by the early glass-makers, clear barley-sugar toys red and yellow. The candles that had lighted only duties shrank and colored themselves to light the Christmas tree. Bayberry candles matched the green of the holiday season and shone in farmhouse windows.

It was only a step from Christmas at home to Christmas in church. We walked to church without fear; muskets had been left at home. So the arms of church-goers were filled with wreaths and ropes of evergreen to decorate bare rafters and hard pews, to festoon walls.

When we moved from a village to a town, and then to a great city, we set up great lighted Christmas trees on lawns, in parks, and even churchyards in remembrance of beloved woods and Christmas on the farm. Curtains were drawn aside in the evening to show the lighted trees inside. Wreaths of holly and evergreen hung on the outside of doors. Small crèches, lighted, could be seen in windows.

Many nations of Americans helped keep Christmas here. Saint Nicholas and gingerbread figures were the gifts of

Dutch New York and Pennsylvania. Marzipan, the colored candy fruits that Italians make with great skill; toys from Germany and Russia; Christmas pudding, pantomimes, and carols from England; candle-lighting from France combined in a merry Christmas. Our Christmas grew beautiful as artists designed and painted greeting cards, our forests, neighbors, music, and story-tellers re-created Bethlehem.

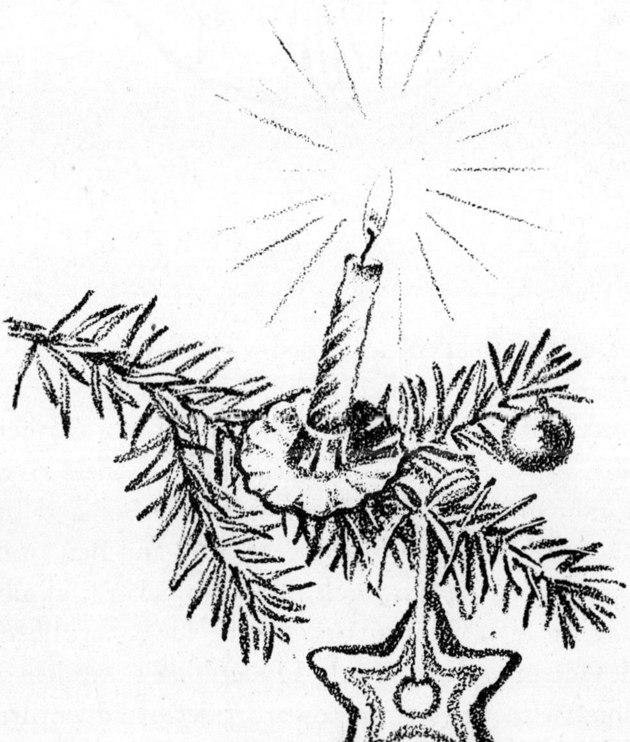

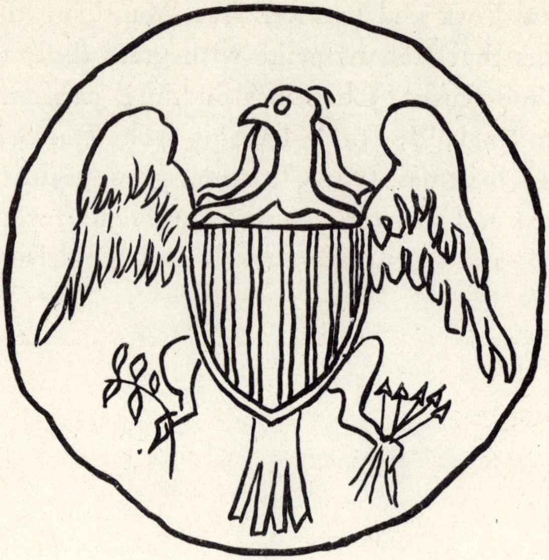

AMERICAN-EAGLE PORTRAIT

BENJAMIN ONDERDONK listened with only half of his mind to the talk that circled the breakfast table, accompanied by the rattle of clam shells dropping on brown earthenware plates. His heart thrilled to the rippling of their river. He could hear it on its way to Hempstead Harbor and the sea. It was an April Saturday of the year 1790 and Benjamin was day dreaming, eating hardtack instead of clams, climbing a ship's rigging instead of sitting at the long, scrubbed pine table in Goodman Heindrick Onderdonk's kitchen as he sailed along with the stream toward tides of adventure.

One of the hired men hummed as he opened the shells with his jackknife:

"If fresh meat is wanting to fill up your dish,
We've carrots and pumpkins and turnips and sich.
And if there is mind for a delicate dish,
We haste to the clam banks and there we catch fish."

Fish! Benjamin wished that he need never sniff it again. Out beyond the town limits, at Mosquito Cove, he went clamming and digging oysters nearly every day after school, for the whole family worked and fourteen-year-old Benjamin did his share. But weathered sails dipping into the wind always drew his eyes from the beach.

"This spring air gives me an appetite." His older brother William helped himself to the largest olekoke of the big bowl.

"A good day for airing the quilts," Phebe said.

"And loosening the earth around the tulips," added Sister Maria.

"The house-cleaning shall begin this day," Phebe's pride in their home gave her words emphasis.

His father was silent, thinking of business matters.

It was a handsome house, one and a half stories high with dormer windows and two chimneys. Looking about the kitchen where bright rag rugs and pots of flowers on window sills brightened the room, Benjamin admitted that his father was doing well. The big fireplace had andirons wrought by hand in the shape of a Continental soldier. The great hand-hewn beams above were festooned with bunches of thyme, catnip, and sage. Bags of flax waiting for the spinning wheel filled one corner. There were other comfortable rooms beyond and above. From a chamber came the *creak-creak* of screwing up the corded beds. A maid who started work at sun-up was using a wrench to tighten the bed cords. It was a mammoth four-poster with curtains of flowered chintz. Another maid was pounding samp in a big mortar, ready for mixing a pudding stuffed with dried fruits for dinner. The ladder-backed kitchen chairs had patchwork cushions for comfort. These Long Island Onderdonks, like their Dutch neighbors, believed in comfort. Hanging to some of the chairs were the girls' calico knitting bags. The sun was bright and strong, lighting the tulip beds out in the garden.

"I have a mind to go to sea today," the wandering half of his mind tempted Benjamin. "There is a ship going to New York for cargo this afternoon and from there to the Indies. There is always need for an extra cabin boy."

"A fine day to get on with that order for white letter paper," said his brother William, shoving his chair back from the table and swallowing a last clam whole, and with gusto. "That peddler from Philadelphia brought a big load of linen rags last week and they are already in the pulp vat. Come on, young Benjamin. You can help dip and couch."

Suddenly the whole of Benjamin's brain began to work in revolt. He made a great clatter as he banged down his plate and tipped over his chair in rising. He hated the paper mill. What if it was the first paper mill in the North? What if his father destined him to learn the business from that of vat-man to coucher? What if, already, their family had one of the finest houses in Hempstead, with its two chimneys and a stoep, near the clock tower, the Common, and the Duck Pond? Benjamin smelled in distaste the mass of pounded wet rags and lye that made the steaming paper pulp in the vats. He remembered his backache from dipping and shaking the molds as he tried to keep from falling from the slimy platform into the vat. Paper was becoming ever so important.

Our country was writing as never before; writing letters, the records of our great beginnings, and even books. But, young Benjamin Onderdonk thought, let some other boy work in their paper mill.

"I have a mind to take this Saturday for my own affairs."

At this announcement silence, for a moment, surrounded Benjamin with despair. Then they spoke.

"Think shame on you, Benjy!"

"Are you not allowed your schooling, when other boys are put out as apprentices at thirteen?"

"Look at the fine blue breeks you are wearing, and the leather shoes! A boy so well dressed should do his bit toward keeping the mill going."

"Do you not know that there will be a monster round of beef for dinner tomorrow? Those who eat should work for their victuals."

So the family reproached Benjamin. He was a cheery lad usually, if his dreams did often take him beyond the mill. Now he hung his head. Red-cheeked, tow-haired, his home-spun shirt matching his eyes, wearing a pair of embroidered suspenders over his shirt, he looked the Dutch boy of New York that he was.

"I was going down to the Cove," he protested. "If I do a few hours dipping this morning, may I have the afternoon off?" The ship would wait for the tide to run out. He might still get aboard.

There was no question in anyone's mind what his father's answer would be, but at that moment the pound of approaching hoof beats on the hard road through the Common drummed into the discord of talk. A shadow touched the threshold of the opened half-door. They had a glimpse of a scarlet uniform, a glint of gold on epaulets that caught the sunshine. A galloping horseman stopped to call out,

"George Washington, the President, is passing through Long Island. He spent the night at Goodman Young's at Oyster Bay and is even now nearing Mosquito Cove."

Benjamin's behavior was forgotten in the excitement of the Onderdonk household. Gathering their clam shells in their aprons, the girls disposed of this evidence of an humble meal. In a trice a fair hand-woven linen cloth was laid upon the table and Phebe set out the East Indian china teapot with its silver band and the gold and white cup and saucer, the solid silver spoons and the silver cream jug. From the cellar they brought rich preserves, quince, plum and gooseberry, the last of the year's goodness from the garden. Maria, always skillful with her broom, scattered white sea sand over the kitchen floor and swept it into a pattern of flowing swirls and whorls. Hardly were these preparations made when a sound of wheels, a snapping of whips, then the grinding of brakes, announced that the President's coach and his outriders had arrived.

Goodman Onderdonk's house stood out in the village, neat and attractive with its early flowers, the straight maples and pines in front, the ivy-hung eaves, and the two settles on the sides of the stoep. What wonder then that the yellow coach and the horsemen should come to a stop before it, that President Washington should step out and stand, waiting a welcome, on the threshold of the Onderdonk home!

"Come in, Mr. President. I beg of you, honor our household by drinking a cup of tea." Goodman Onderdonk opened the doors and bowed almost to the floor. The girls curtsied low. Benjamin pulled out the chair at the head of the table.

"Thank you, Goodman. I have been on the road since

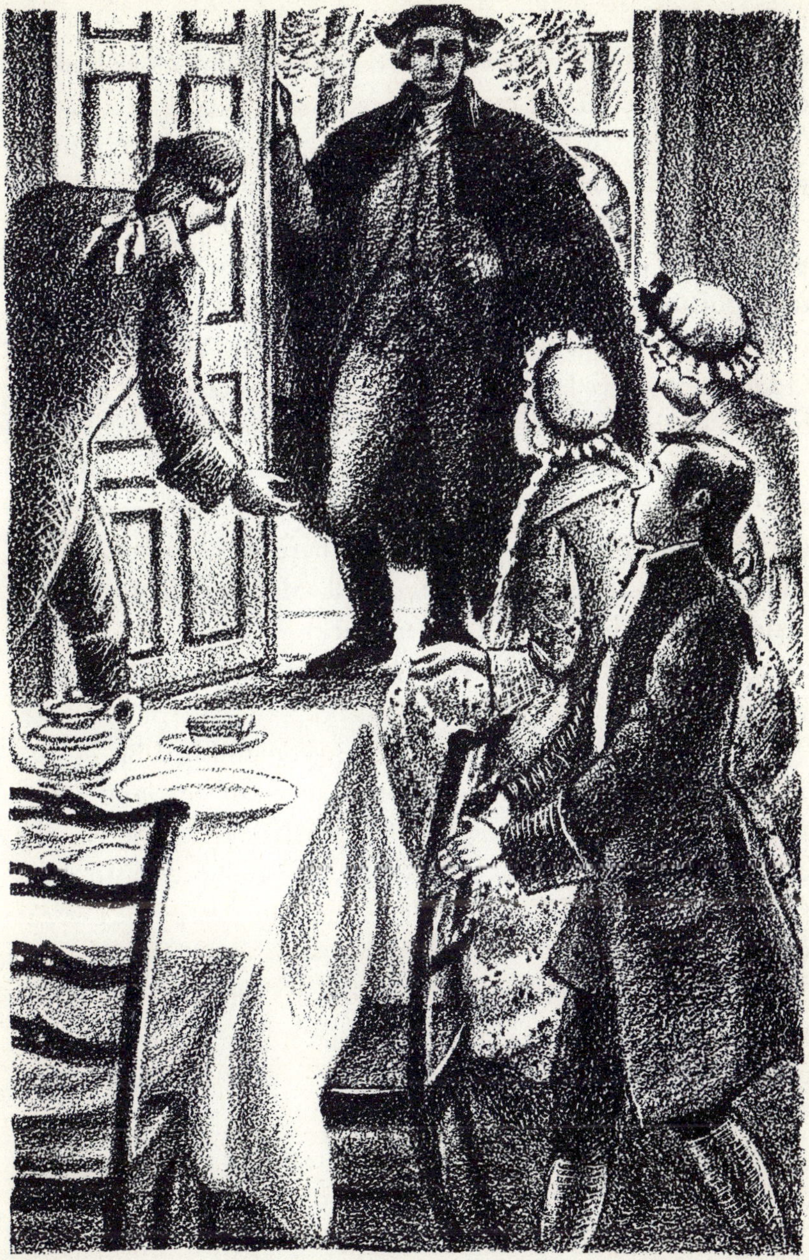

before sunrise." President Washington stooped that his tall figure might enter, threw off his dusty traveling cloak and sat down, pulling off his travel-stained boots.

"Ah, China tea!" He poured the fragrant brew from the pot to his cup, then into his saucer, daintily sipping it. "I am touring Long Island in the interest of agriculture," he explained. "We of the South have much to learn from you of fruit culture and the raising of tubers. Also, I hear that your town may provide a site for a fortification. You, Goodman Onderdonk, have land on the river, I hear. You could perhaps help us in this matter."

"I have two grist mills and a paper mill, Mr. President," the Goodman explained. "The land on which my paper mill stands would be an excellent site." There was a tone of wistfulness in his reply. "It is a fine mill, Mr. President. We are designing and imprinting water marks on our paper, as well designed, as fancy, as any you could import from England or France."

"A paper mill!" President Washington finished his Dutch doughnuts and preserves, a second saucer of tea, and arose. "I am reminded of the saving of worn frocks and shirts, the gathering of bark and acorns, even, for pounding with ashes from your fireplaces and water to make paper pulp. Let me visit your mill."

"Benjy! Son Benjamin!" Goodman Onderdonk fairly shouted. "Come and bring the bootjack. Help the President pull on his boots. He will do us the honor of visiting the mill."

But Benjamin was gone. At the President's words he had dashed out of the house and was out of sight.

William, the older brother, whispered aside to his father.

"The vatman is ailing. The mill is under-staffed and will make a poor showing."

But he stooped and tugged at George Washington's fashionably tight boots, at last pulling them up over his hand-knitted socks.

There was nothing to do about the vatman. Led by the President and Master Onderdonk the party started out, Master Onderdonk explaining as he went.

"It is difficult, Mr. President, to keep our workmen. The heat of the pulp kettles, then the strain of the dipping exhausts the best of them. Our molds are about the size of a square pie tin. They must be dipped, turned, faced upward, then carefully lifted out of the pulp vat, evenly covered. Next, we shake them, right, left, front and back, difficult and arduous work, in order to cross and mat the fibers and shake off the water. Then the coucher takes the mold, holding the thin moist sheet against the draining board. When the sheet is solid and lustrous we overturn the mold and the sheet is laid on a piece of felting for the last drying. So the vatman and the coucher work together skillfully and without stopping until a quire of paper, one hundred and forty-four sheets, are finished."

"Very interesting." President Washington had listened intently. "Now if you please, describe the processing of these water marks of which you speak. I understand that our best artists are turning their skill into designs, laurel leaves, stars, flowers, and other fancy pictures that may be imprinted on our American paper to make it beautiful."

"Ah, yes," Goodman Onderdonk explained. "The design is outlined with fine wire on the couching felt. When the sheet dries, there it is, imprinted."

He was about to expand on the method but they had reached the stone mill and through the door he saw, in amazement, Benjamin. His heart pounded with dread. Usually Benjy's work in the mill was that of stirring the pulp or passing the molds from vatman to coucher. But there he was, balanced on the slimy platform of the pulp vat, dipping molds with wild energy, shaking them and passing them to a terrified coucher. He stopped, a dripping mold in hand, and bowed as the President entered.

"My youngest son, Benjamin." Goodman Onderdonk murmured, motioning to Benjy to get down.

But President Washington stepped upon the platform beside the boy. The President took an empty mold and held it over the vat.

"Show me the method, my lad," he begged. "I have a desire to make a sheet of paper."

In an awesome ring about the vat, Master Onderdonk and the President's staff watched. Washington dipped his mold, laden with the white fibrous liquid, lifted it out, shook it in the four directions, stepped down, and couched it. As he did so, the coucher slipped a small piece of paper between the sheets.

Benjamin watched, directed, even criticized. "You need practice, Mr. President," he suggested.

"Young whipper-snapper!" his father spluttered. "A smart birching you shall have for your disrespect!"

But the President shook his head, patted Benjy's tow head.

"Very well spoken," he said. "The lad is right, for in all things practice makes perfect. I am persuaded that your paper mill, Goodman, is of greater importance to the country than a fort. I shall leave my poorly executed piece of paper as a souvenir of my visit, wishing you all good fortune and peace upon your house and business. But," he turned over a pile of the snowy sheets stacked in a corner of the mill waiting for shipment, "those hidden pictures, the water marks, will they last?"

Goodman Onderdonk took Benjy by his coat collar and stood him in a corner. In this last piece of work he was not going to be superseded by a boy. He showed the President how deeply the designs were imbedded, couched on the damp paper and deeply impressed. When the sheets were dry, there they were, lasting and picturing America on our first paper. A bird, an anchor, a flax flower, a tree, a leaf, one of these had been carefully drawn and reproduced in the upper part of each sheet.

Benjamin watched, then he could not endure being out of the scene. He joined the others, pushed his way into the group.

"Look, here is the best water mark of all in my opinion." He thumbed through the pile of paper, found the sheet he wanted, and held it up. "Mr. President," Benjy held the sheet between Washington and the light, "Look at this water mark; a noble bird, well drawn and in full flight, the eagle."

The President took the fair sheet of paper with a gesture of reverence. The American eagle, one of our first American-designed water marks, was already, on land and sea, a winged symbol of our freedom.

"Not a fort, but a mill, shall stand here, my friends," the President said as he motioned for his staff and took his departure.

That night, by the light of a candle, President Washington wrote as was his custom in his diary:

April 24, 1790

I left Mr. Young's at Oyster Bay before six o'clock on Saturday a.m. and, passing through Mosquito Cove, breakfasted at a Mr. Onderdonk's at the head of a little bay where we were kindly received and well entertained. This gentleman works a grist mill and a paper mill, the last of which I visited. He seems to carry it on with spirit and profit.

On their way home, Benjamin walked a little behind his father, respectfully and fearfully.

"That vatman feigned illness, I think, this being Saturday and good fishing weather," he ventured. "I knew you would want the mill properly staffed for the President's visit, so I took over the dipping."

"Enough!" His father was gruff but his face wrinkled into a smile. "Vatman Benjamin Onderdonk, you fancied yourself, the lad who tried to beg off work this day with, I know not what, adventure in mind!"

Benjamin ran forward, grasped the Goodman's hand. "I was minded to run away, sir," he said. "I thought of shipping as a cabin boy but now—"

"Now?" his father asked, taking Benjamin's hand.

"I have decided to be a vatman," Benjamin announced.

Where New York's first paper mill stood, today only a great tree stands, firmly rooted among old foundation stones. Through its wind-blown branches there is whispered the story of President Washington and a yellowed sheet of paper, delicately water-marked and preserved for generations at the Onderdonk mill. Unevenly dipped and dried, it showed George Washington's interest in the occupations of peace.

Hempstead, on Long Island, did its share in manufacturing

useful things for our growing country, thimbles, jugs, butter firkins, and pie plates. But Heindrick Onderdonk and his sons and daughters, especially young Benjamin, flourished, grew wealthy, and developed papermaking there. They made paper money, delicately traced with crimson silk threads, for the Government. They became land owners, town officers, and preachers. But, best of all, they made in America as beautiful writing paper as any that we had previously imported from France and England.

From town to village, from mansion to cottage, went the old rag peddlers, bartering their bright tinware and pewter for hand-spun and woven cotton and linen that was needed for pulp kettles. Girls wore calico, boys, their work shirts on the Sabbath day, that the paper mill might be supplied with pulp. Benjamin was not always the vatman he had aspired to be after Washington's visit, but he served his country as a good Dutch burgher and philanthropist. The paper we made at that time bore the stamp of beauty. Water marks, fine in design and drawn from the everyday beauty of everyday things, were couched on each sheet. And the eagle-stamped paper, that they covered with the fine writing of old quill pens, was popular with the Washington family. Upon it were written mighty adventures in the story of our country.

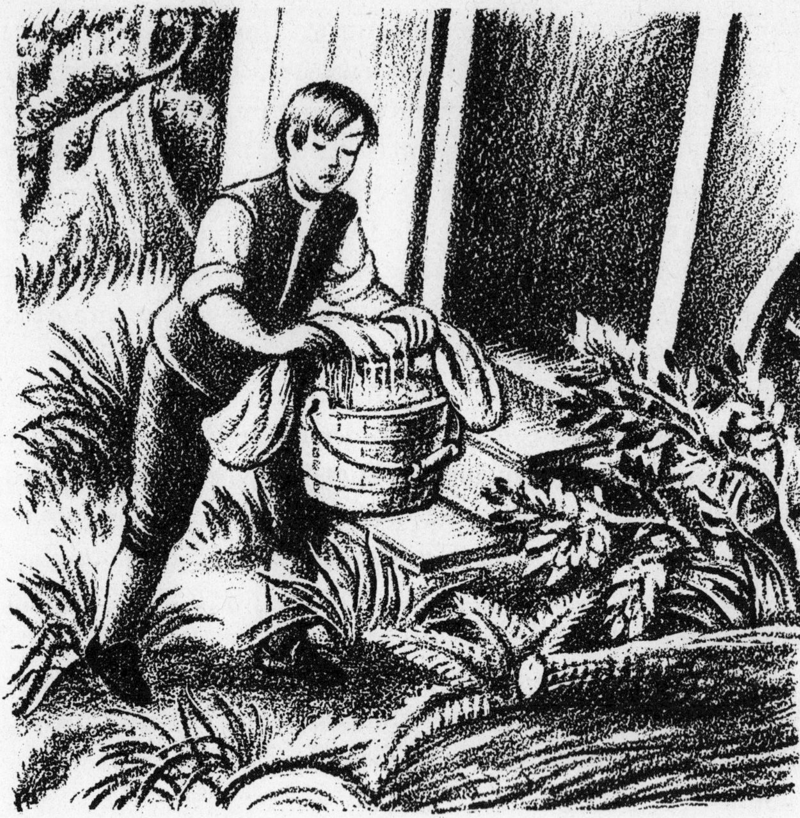

FIDDLIN' FOOL

AS HE SCRUBBED soft soap into his hunting shirt, doing their washing in a bucket set on the wagon steps, Jesse Weems could scarcely believe that they were only a week from home. Inside the wagon he heard his father rustling about among the books, talking to himself, humming as he arranged them, jingling the money they had taken in that day.

"God prosper well our noble state,
In wisdom, wealth and peace,
And grant that reading, all too rare,
May day by day increase."

Jesse had no need to look within to see his father, buxom, rosy-cheeked, wearing the black clothes and stock of a cleric, an ink horn decorating the lapel of his coat and a quill pen stuck behind his ear. Lovable, completely a peddler, and born for the road, was Parson Weems. There was scarcely anything else, except his fiddle, for which he cared.

He had begun his travels before Jesse was born, starting out with a pack of books on his back and walking from Baltimore to Philadelphia. Then had come the wagon days, when Parson Weems had followed the Potomac Path south, until he knew every mile of the tidewater land with its lure of birds and flowers, its dangers from freshets and wilderness.

There he was, again talking to himself, "My heart will be on books when my strength has failed."

His father showed no sign of failing strength, Jesse remembered as he soused flannels and linens in the amber-colored swamp water. He sighed as he looked back to the day a week ago when he, his mother and the girls, his sisters, had packed the jersey wagon at home, Belle-Ayr Plantation in Virginia, for this spring book-selling trip. Belle-Ayr stood foursquare, built of rosy brick, one end guarded by a great chimney, on the highlands of Dumfries. Before the great living room fireplace that was large enough to roast a whole ox, spread out on the parlor floor, covering it, had been Parson Weems' spring book stock. Ever so many Bibles, bound brightly in crimson leather with gold trimmings, made the highest pile.

"A Bible should not frighten people," his father had said as he piled them. "This is an alluring edition."

His *Life of George Washington* came next, another good-sized pile.

"My story of Washington will sell better than any other book of its size," Parson Weems assured them.

That was true, Jesse thought. Thousands of Bibles had been sold from the back of the wagon, but the *Life* was a close second. They had helped pack books that were also popular: *Robinson Crusoe, Toy Books, The Child's First Book, Animated Nature, The American Primer, Morse's Geography, Pilgrim's Progress.* Maps that unfolded the panorama of their

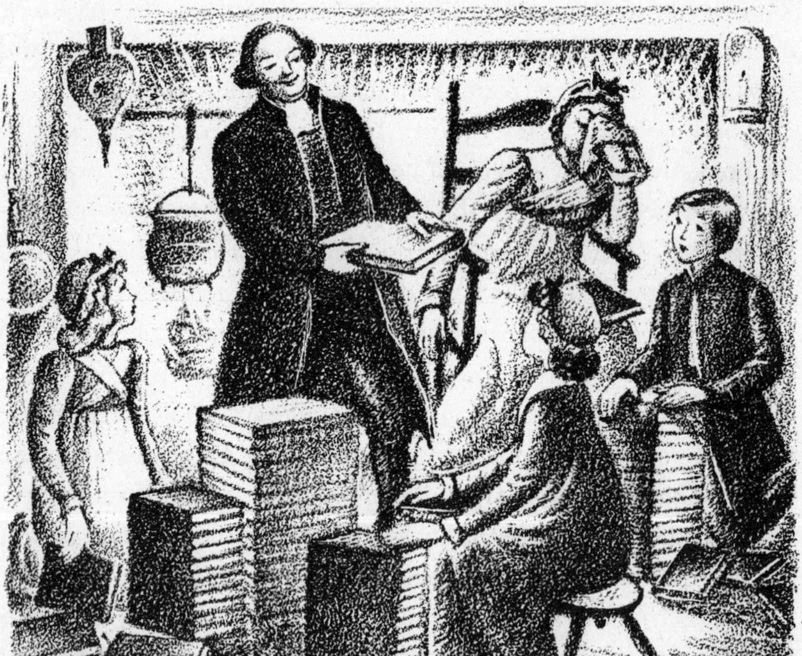

growing countryside. His mother had worked with tears, remembering long days alone on the plantation. But Parson Weems whistled to cheer them all.

Finally he had put on his wide-brimmed hat and stepped through the door, holding his fiddle wrapped in a bit of old silk damask tenderly. "There is nothing like fiddle music for bringing out villagers," he said. As the wagon creaked its way toward the road, the family stood on the wide portico of Belle-Ayr and waved good-by.

"Good-by. Keep well and happy," he called back. "I shall send home money soon."

Then the wagon had rolled on. The greening fields of Belle-Ayr had arisen to meet the downs. Then, before they knew it, they had rolled down to the tidewater land.

"I aim to establish book stores in all the hills and valleys hereabouts," Parson Weems declared.

And that plan would take them up and down the whole South before they came home again. The villages were far apart. Sometimes they stopped on a village green, where the sight of so gay a parson and the merry scraping of his fiddle called the people to stand enchanted about the wagon. Again, they drew up beside a lonely cabin on the edge of the swamp where likely as not, there was hot journey cake for them and a tune from the fiddle in payment. They lived like gypsies, eating at inns, farmhouses, but in the forest mainly where they learned its wisdom and lore.

Their days were all right, Jesse thought, but too short. Already the pale April sun was dropping behind the tangle of juniper and cypress trees that made a crisscross above the forest where they must spend the night. Small noises sounded ominous to the boy. The far-off whimper of a wolf, the echoed bark of a fox, the slinking rustle in the leaves and moss that might be a copper-head. Jesse splashed to drown his homesickness. He would give his precious hunting knife for a glimpse of the candlelighted windows of Belle-Ayr. As if he had known his son's timorous thoughts, Parson Weems came out of the wagon, and sat down on a log beside the eleven-year-old boy.

Jesse hung his washing on the back of the open door and sat down too. It was chilly for April and he wrapped his fringed cape closer about him, was glad of his warm moccasins.

"Cease your housewifely duty and listen with me to the croaking of these Dutch nightingales," his father urged, throwing an arm about the boy's shoulders.

"But the frogs sound so doleful," Jesse protested.

"That depends upon the way we listen to them. A frog is handicapped by having but one string to his bow. Now, my music . . ."

Jesse interrupted him. "Yes, I know. There isn't a hawker anywhere about the land like you, so ready with a fiddle tune that suits the place and hour. That puppeteer for instance." He tried to drum up his courage, keep faith in his father.

"Ssh!" Parson Weems looked about as if the forest had human ears. "You know that I like a good Punch and Judy show, but it would have appeared unseemly for a parson to play for one."

"But the puppeteer's fiddler was ill."

"Yes, and so I played for Punch's antics behind a screen on the village common."

"And the screen fell down and there you were, in your black coat."

"Which so pleased the villagers that they bought books to a man." Parson Weems chuckled, forgot his impulse toward secrecy.

Jesse started at a crunching sound in the marsh grass close by.

"Only the nag, gnawing her supper," his father reassured him. "She must take her ease at the end of the day while I order the book shelves and you do your chores. We are three partners. I said to the printer in Philadelphia last winter, 'If you will finance me to the extent of a jersey wagon and a new horse, I shall take my little son with me on the spring trip for help and company! A fine lad,' I wrote thus in my letter."

"And the nag has behaved badly; such jumping and kicking, straddling the traces, falling on the poles, lying down and rolling!"

"All due to the britch-band that irked her tail," Parson Weems chuckled.

"Why didn't you harness her carefully?" Jesse was moved to say but kept his peace.

Why should he blame his father, the most energetic bookseller of the countryside, the only one who was bringing fiddle music to commons, church thresholds, and homes where it was lacking. From a psalm tune to "Charlie Over the Water," from "Columbia the Gem of the Ocean" to music for a reel on the village green, Parson Weems' bow flew daily. It was a privilege to go along with the wagon, Jesse knew, but they had come such a long way from home. Here they sat at a swampside, listening to a chorus of frogs. And Jesse decided that he must tomorrow take upon himself the added duty of harnessing in order that it might be done properly.

"Such stalling of wagons and sweeping away of stages as we have seen! Such heavy rains and deep roads." Jesse watched the last watery rays of the sun trickling down through the ceiling of branches and interlacing vines.

His father gave him a rousing back slap. "Come, come, my good lad," he urged. "When I was a little shaver I never could believe as you seem to that life was short and full of misery. Surely my favorite son is not of that belief. Also, remember the clinking of our money bag. It is filling with dollars. My *Life of Washington* is so popular that I am considering writing some new stories for another edition of the book. And how the red Bibles take! I expect to set a mark in sales before I am done."

Jesse was silent, reflecting. He loved his father but since he was now going on twelve the faintest shadow of questioning had settled like one of those evening clouds over that love. He saw again their fine plantation house. It was one of the most spacious in Virginia, three-storied, with gables and a porch with pillars that rose to touch the gently sloping roof. Within, there was usually plenty; at least they fared well when Parson Weems sent home money. Belle-Ayr had a Washington room, set aside for visits from that family. Jesse's Uncle Ewell had been President Washington's doctor. Parson Weems had preached in the Virginia church that the President attended. Belle-Ayr was riding distance to Mount Vernon. Why, Jesse wondered, had his father given up all this respectability for his peddling way of life?

"Fiddlin' fool!" a bystander had sneered that morning as the wagon halted and Parson Weems seated himself on the store steps and tucked his violin under his chin.

But the instant that the golden notes touched the air the

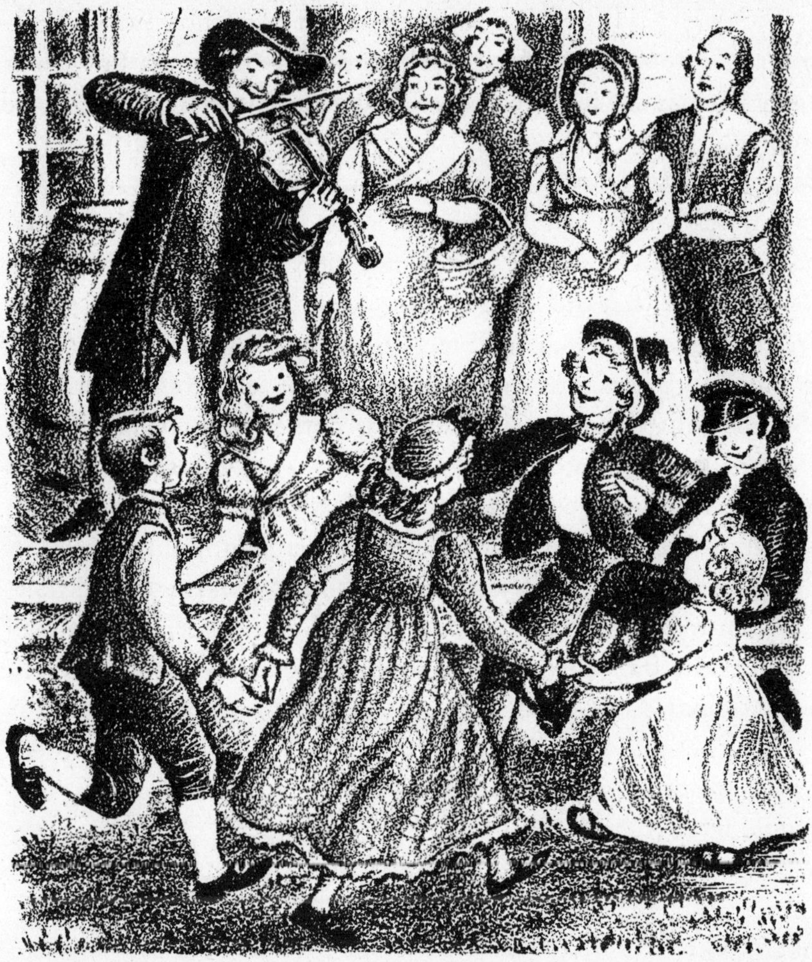

store had emptied. Burdened men and women had laid down their tools and baskets. A ring of boys and girls had clasped hands for a game. Music was a new language for these hard-working settlers. In the North, even then, the year 1810, music was discouraged. Parson Weems was carrying it like a banner for courage and comfort.

But what a life this one of the road was! His father was merrily disposed, cheerful, and fond of movement, but they never knew where they were going to spend the night. It might be in the shelter of a barn snuggled close in the sweetly fragrant hay. They might shake down in the wagon or, if the night was warm, find beds in the moss under the stars. It was supper time. His father had gone inside the wagon again and Jesse knew that he would forget all about preparing the meal. He, too, returned, wringing out his damp washing and hanging it on a branch nearby. It would never dry in that dew. He rattled around among his pots in the wagon where Parson Weems had lighted candles and was again sorting books, clinking the money in his leather bag. Its ring echoed through the forest. The week had been a prosperous one.

Jesse sliced side meat with his hunting knife, mixed a skillet of corn meal and water, hung the lighted lantern where the clothes line had been on the wagon door. His father smiled in anticipation of food.

"Mother may have baked a pound cake today," Jesse mused as he placed forked sticks from which to hang the tea kettle.

"We should rather give thanks for peace and a hoe cake in a cabin than cakes ambrosial in a palace," his father observed.

Jesse sighed. He must take a short trip, perhaps a long one, to gather dry fuel for his fire. Deeper in the forest where the swamp dampness had not penetrated, he would be able to find peat and moss, dry sticks and bits of bark. He wrapped his traveling cloak close, wishing that his warm linsey-woolsey shirt were dry. The lantern was a beacon as he made his way through the maze of bushes, in and out among the great trees whose low-hanging branches caught him like great arms. The vines hanging from the trees were an entanglement. His moccasins sank deep into the moss and ooze held him. Before he realized it, he was trudging around in circles. Looking back, he thought he saw the wagon light; then he realized that it was a flickering will-o'-the-wisp, glimmering faintly and leading him on toward confusion. He fancied that he heard footsteps.

There were not many Indians hereabouts but the backwoodsmen were desperate marauders, his father had said.

"They are not many years removed from savages," he had warned Jesse, "living in the tidewater wilderness by their wits rather than their trade. That is one reason why I endeavor to spread the Gospel here in the wilderness. I shall not cease my wanderings until there is a Bible in every settlement, a bright red one, I hope."

Jesse had seen one or two of these dark tidewater marauders. They wore hunters' leather, were unshaven and shaggy of hair. They carried long rifles and slunk like cats in and out of the swampland. He was reminded of them as an especially human-looking tree arose in his path and caught him with a fist-like branch under his chin. His cloak was clumsy for the errand of gathering sticks, tripping him and making him drop the few fagots he had been able to pick up.

But there was the lantern at last, twinkling to show Jesse the way. He was close to the wagon at last. Under his arm were dry sticks, gathered in the fold of his cloak were bark and moss. In a few minutes there would be a crackling fire underneath the kettle and the skillet would begin sizzling. His father would come out and sit on the wagon steps beside him, telling him a story about young George Washington as they supped.

But the trees still moved and stretched in the evening breezes. Jesse fancied that they whispered together. It almost seemed as if they were creeping ahead of him and would reach the wagon first. Their roots took the shape of great boots, their branches seemed crooked over rifles. Slowly, softly, with caution, the juniper and cypress took their dark way before the lad. He hesitated, rubbed his eyes to wipe away his fear. Then a shot pierced the quiet and at the same instant the light of the wagon lantern was blasted out. Jesse stumbled and fell, striking his head so hard that he was dizzy with the pain. He dropped his fagots as he fell and sank into darkness.

But presently the darkness felt friendly and the ground as soft as one of the Belle-Ayr feather beds. The trees echoed to the stars the thrilling notes of a fiddle, playing all the tunes of the new world his father knew and had taught him to understand. The solemn call to arms of the settlers. The gayer rhythms for spinning, for hoeing, and raising anchors, for wood-chopping, and for keeping time to the clacking of looms. The marching music of the minute men. The psalmody of the churches that raised their white spires from the north to the south. The reels and minuets of Belle-Ayr and Mount Vernon as tiny high heels tapped the time and silk and satin, lace and brocade swirled to the measures. Drum and fife, flute and fiddle, had each a rhythm for the work and play of their land, Jesse's father had told him. Music was a new word for a new world, even if it had to be carried by foot and horse. Lying there comfortably, Jesse saw the pageant of the music makers of America, weavers and harvesters, soldiers and sailors, preachers, leaders, and hawkers. He almost resented it when he felt himself moved, lifted up, up toward those singing stars.

"My brave little lad!" a candle flickered and showed Jesse his father's smiling face, looking into his.

One of the nag's blankets felt pleasantly warm and his father's arms were strong about the boy's shoulders. The music had ceased.

"What happened?" Jesse asked opening his eyes.

"Just a couple of thieves, or that is what they intended to be, who heard me unwisely counting our dollars and thought to have a share in them. These woodsmen are sure at a target. They shot out the lantern. I fancy it would have gone ill with us save for——"

"I fell down," Jesse interrupted. "I tripped myself and hit my head on a stump. Then I dreamed I heard you playing the fiddle."

"No dream." Parson Weems chuckled. "Music hath charms. Oft in the stilly night and so on, as the poets write. I was outnumbered and had no recourse save to try music on the marauders. I doubt if they had ever heard the tunes I know. They must have looked on me as some piping faun for they came no farther than the steps of the wagon, but sat there and listened as I played inside. When I thought my arm would drop off from weariness with pushing the bow, they slunk off into the dark."

"Will they return, do you think?" Jesse asked. His father had carried him all the way, and he stood unsteadily by the wagon.

"No . . . Look what they did in their gratitude."

Why, the supper fire was lighted. It burned with a bright

hot flame. His father brought out the side meat and hoe cake. Supper would be late, but more than welcome.

"Fiddlin' fool, indeed!" Jesse repeated softly to the forest. He felt great pride in being the son of Parson Weems.

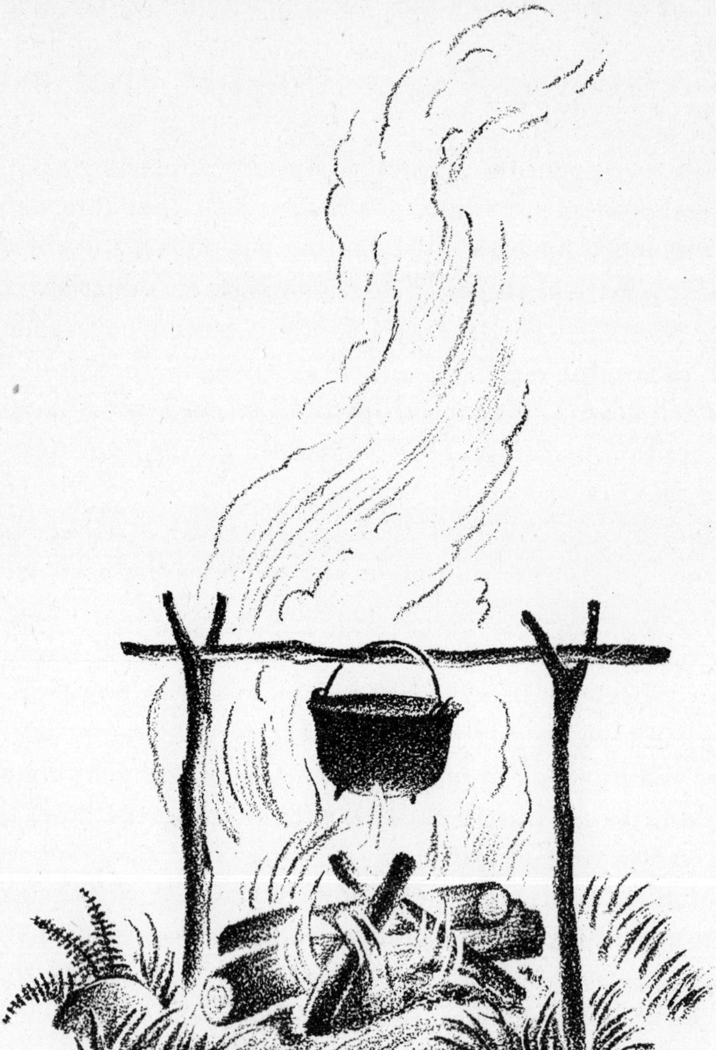

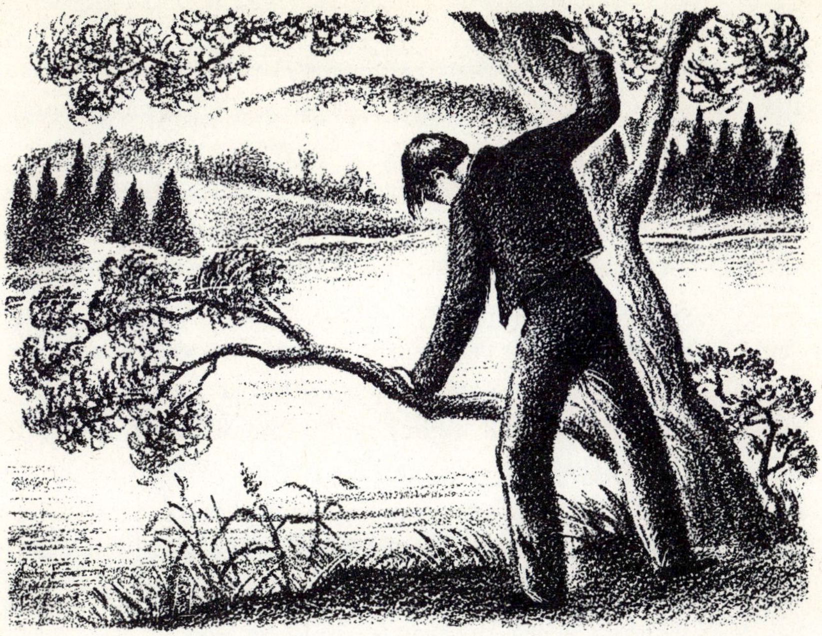

A NEW SHAWL FOR ELIZA

As she put the teacher's desk in order for the last time, Eliza felt close to tears. Frank had done the best he could, she thought, considering his nature and his farm work before and after his teaching hours. And he was only a few years older, at nineteen, than she and the others of his advanced class.

The kaleidoscope was gone from his desk. Frank had taken that and his one brush and colors when he said good-by to the classes that afternoon. Frank had been late again that morning, having lingered beside Wyndham Pond to watch the light and shadows play on a big perch. Then he had painted a likeness of that perch on the pine boards of the school-room wall, as lifelike as if he had caught and used it for a model. It had happened that the selectmen had decided upon this day to visit the school and put the children through an examination.

Eliza, called upon to recite arithmetic tables, stood on tiptoe in front of the desecrated boards, spreading her calico skirt in an attempt to cover the painting. But the rows of stern selectmen, wearing their black frock coats and spectacles, had seen it. The children did none too well with their recitations, and only Eliza's father, fond of this boy whom the neighbors considered flighty and of no account, spoke of the wall painting.

"I do not hold with decorating the inside of a building. Paint is for the protection of a barn or house. But I will say that this perch is lifelike. If I were to hang a real one beside it, I doubt if the difference could be seen."

Eliza felt grateful for her father's kindness, but a chorus of sniffs had been his only response as the selectmen filed out of the school.

It was early September, of the year 1819, and a good time for the village to hire another teacher. Frank knew, without being dismissed, that his services would be needed no longer.

"It was not fair," Eliza thought. Frank had worked without pay on his father's Connecticut farm until his hands were calloused, his shoulders untimely bent, and his bare feet sore. But he had the eyes, the fingers of an artist. He had taught his pupils to draw.

Frank Alexander was Eliza's neighbor. He sometimes walked beside her through the Connecticut fields and lanes to the one-room schoolhouse there in Killingsby, Wyndham County. Oftener, though, he had been late. And he had charmed the pupils with his colors and brush, making pictures on copy-book pages of their green countryside, instead of teaching spelling, or telling them how he was experimenting with mixing colors and skim milk into a kind of paint that had a special smoothness.

Frank was ever so poor, Eliza knew, but forward-looking. He had extravagantly spent part of his forty-four dollars yearly salary for the kaleidoscope, a delightful new invention. When the school had been especially industrious, he took the kaleidoscope out of his desk drawer and allowed the children to look at the bits of rainbow glass through its telescope end, turning it until the colors dazzled their eyes, and flowed together in sparkling designs.

Eliza brushed her eyes of tears as she put on her bonnet and shawl. Suddenly she heard a clear whistle outside the window, the call of a thrush; their own signal, hers and Frank's. She ran outside. There he was, tall, thin, smiling. He had a bundle under his arm.

"Sit down beside me here on the steps, Eliza," he said. "I may not see you again for a year or more."

"Where are you going, Frank?"

"I shall catch the bus at New Haven," he told her. "Captain Bunker's steamboat there, the *Connecticut,* exchanges passengers for the *Fulton* that goes down the Hudson to New York."

"Can you pay your way, study painting in that great city?"

"I haven't a doubt of it," he assured her. "I have what is left of my teaching wages, and I know that I can draw a figure well. Haven't I copied our cattle and pigs, the pheasants, fish, and birds ever since I was small? I can paint scenery and people, too. New York must be kind to me, Eliza. I will work for my chance. Think what a new day we are living in. A steamboat has crossed the Atlantic for the first time, going from New York to Liverpool in only twenty-six days! We have some new states in the Union, Mississippi, Alabama, Illinois, and Maine. I have bought one of those newly invented brushes for cleaning the teeth. The world is moving on, Eliza. I am going along with it."

"Shall you return?" Eliza's voice trembled a little.

"That depends upon circumstances," he said loftily. "Perhaps I shall board that ocean-going steamboat, the *Savannah*, for further study in Europe."

"Oh, Frank!"

His rashness frightened her. She knew that he had never seen a body of water larger than Wyndham Pond. He wore new shoes and a cap with a visor, but his tow suit was sleazy for the chill of autumn that had touched them early that year.

"Take my shawl!" she begged, laying its checkered wool comfort over his bowed shoulders. "The boat deck will be cold." Her instinct told her that he could not afford a cabin.

Frank looked at his girl friend gratefully. He would miss Eliza. In winter they had been the best skaters, able to do a polka on the ice of the pond. In summer they had gone berrying, paddled a canoe, listened to the wood thrush. He had known that there was little he could teach Eliza, and she had been his severest critic, telling him those tints and shades that best colored a landscape, assuring him that he would be a great artist sometime. It had never entered his mind that Eliza would miss him so much. That shawl was her winter protection. She was going to New York with him through her comfort and encouragement.

"Thank you, I'll bring it back sometime," he told her.

He drew the folds of the shawl closer. "Good-by, Eliza. Don't forget me."

He had a shy impulse to kiss Eliza's cheek, but the bonnet was turned away from him hiding her face. She did not want her tears to dim the beginning of Frank's great adventure. And as he started toward the east, walking the long wintry road, planning to sleep in some barn on his way to New Haven, as long as he could see her, Eliza sat there on the school steps.

It was a bleak September. The *Fulton,* one of the new Hudson River steam packets that paddled their slow way down to New York, charged seven dollars for the cold bed afforded by the deck, and the steward demanded a rake-off for reserving Frank's deck space. Food, too, was costly on the boat. His few dollars shrank daily. It was one hundred and fifty miles of discouraging travel. As the *Fulton* steamed along, overtaking and passing sloops and schooners as if they were at anchor, the frigid river wind pierced Eliza's shawl, Frank's only coverlet. But the light of the stars kindled the fires of his spirit. Each bitter night, each lonely day, were like peeps into the glittering colored glass of his precious kaleidoscope. That bright toy was a sign of the turn of the century. Color and change were coming to the drab life of New England, and Frank felt that he was bound to have a place in the panorama of the beginning nineteenth century.

New York in the young century! The life, the activity, the vividness dazed the eyes of a boy used only to rocks and stumps, briers and thistles. Along the esplanade of the Battery where he walked when his hours of drawing at Mr. Robertson's studio were over, he saw wonders. Handsome houses of brick with fancy ironwork balconies, Wall Street where the great merchants had their counting houses, Battery Park itself with a grand view of blue water and islands, sunsets and the green line of the Jersey shore. A pageant of fashion as New York ladies in crinoline, silk shawls and hoops; gentlemen in cutaway coats, loose trousers in colors, yellow kid gloves, and swinging ivory-topped canes paraded. Fraunce's tavern, celebrated from the days of General Washington, where dinners included chops, steak, and a roast, fish, pastries, ices, and for a sweet the new orange fritters. Street hawkers calling their nuts, tropical fruits, coconuts, and hot chocolate, the popular drink. Luxuries and strangers passed the country boy whose money was gone.

Eliza had questioned how far forty dollars would go in New York. Now he knew. Why, it hardly fed him those brief six weeks. The New York artist, Robertson, had taken pity on the boy and allowed him to copy some landscapes in pencil and India ink, but Frank's heart was aglow with the passing scene and its colors. Battery Park and the water, the people in styles from across the Atlantic, shifted and painted themselves upon his mind. All he needed, he knew, was a canvas and paints. All he had left was the necessity of working his way home to the farm.

Eliza went to the post office every day but there was no letter for her. Frank wanted to write of his success, not failure. That fall, her father bought a house in Canterbury, quite a distance from their prosperous farm beside Wyndham Pond. It was ever so thrilling to help settle in. Her family also had moved on with the times. There was much red in the new house, vermilion-stenciled chests and chairs, a red plush album on the parlor table. Pumpkin pine, warmly

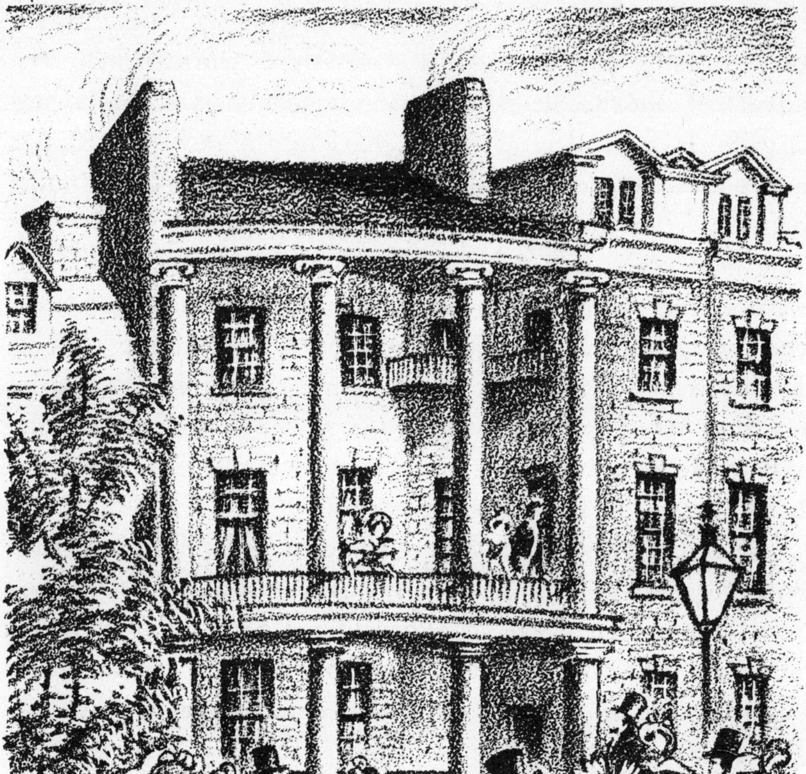

bright, paneled the walls. Scenery mirrors had gilt frames. Gay worsted-embroidered flowers were worked into the covers of the needle-point chairs in the parlor. In corner cupboards of the dining room canary and pink luster teacups and plates replaced the old blue and white ware. Upon floors painted yellow, hooked rugs repeated the pattern of flowers. The new house was enclosed by a neat white picket fence with a green gate. Eliza's father was well-to-do but even so, the Canterbury house was something to talk about back in Killingsby. When Frank came home from New York he heard about it, but he did not get in touch with Eliza. She was too fine for him now, he thought. Yet all winter he wore her shawl for he had no warm jacket.

After the farm chores were done he experimented again with his skim-milk paint. There was plenty of beautiful pigment for it right at hand. The old red barn paint was rich in effect, and the lime it contained made it permanent. It became, through Frank's careful mixing, a real Indian red. Indigo, rose-madder, and the colored clays and roots from their own earth combined with oil, turpentine, and a few powdered colors from the apothecary's gave Frank all he needed.

He worked out a plan for wall painting: "Strike a line around the room breast-high for the horizon line. Paint the wall from top to six inches of the horizon line blue, using whiting mixed with indigo. Do the space from the horizon line to the blue, red, made from whiting and yellow ochre. For clouds, strike the horizon-red upon the blue. Change the sky-blue two shades and paint your river, ocean or lake. Mix the sky-blue with forest-green, this green made from ship-blue and chrome-yellow, for the mountains and highlands, and shade with blue heightened with white. The trees may be heightened with sulphur green and shaded with blue-black."

His mother was sure that he would be successful and she let him paint the old plastered walls of the farm house. How those old walls glowed! For a century it had been considered sinful to decorate one's house. But Frank Alexander's wall paintings of the Killingsby farm, with the farm animals carefully drawn and colored, his village scenes in which the neighbors in bonnets and calico, overalls and Sunday tow, seemed alive, became the wonder of a half-mile radius. The kitchen was filled with admiring folk. Frank wished that Eliza might surprise him by coming over from Canterbury one day. It was not far away and her father had a fine horse and buggy. But Eliza never came. And although the wall paintings were exclaimed about, none gave Frank an order. Not for several months did his skill begin to pay him.

For her part, Eliza too remembered constantly. The Canterbury house, two stories high and so grandly furnished, was a pride but she often wished for the Killingsby days, Frank's companionship and the country school. Eliza attended a young ladies' seminary at New Haven, being sixteen and a young lady. Once she wrote a letter to Frank. Frank did not know that she was away at school. She would tell him about it.

Then she thought, "Frank is probably a young man about town in New York and has forgotten all about me." She tore up the letter.

When Eliza came home that spring for a holiday she found the parlor at Canterbury closed. "It is a surprise. Your father is having some fancy decorating done," her mother told her.

"Also, the workman prefers to be alone."

There were keyholes in the new house, for latches had been replaced by glass doorknobs. Eliza peered through the parlor keyhole, but all she could see was the back of the workman perched upon a step ladder that covered the marble mantel. The secret in the parlor was something to wonder about. It served to take Eliza's mind away from her homesickness for country ways. It was indeed a great day when the parlor door was opened and she and her parents crossed the threshold to find—a painting on the wall above the mantel, and Frank standing with quite reasonable pride beneath it.

"These wall paintings are the fashion now," her father said, "and the news of Frank's skill came to us, so I engaged him. And he thought that a picture he remembered from New York would be admired."

There it was, as clear as if cut from colored paper, in blue and green, sepia and red. Among elm trees with round tops and drooping branches and primly-shaped cedars, were white houses with red roofs, a church with a tall steeple, a stretch of blue water on which a ship lay and beyond that a lighthouse. People in fashionable clothes strolled along, but Eliza's eyes were caught and held by one of the well-painted young ladies. Although her hoops were as wide, her bonnet as blooming as any of the other New York gentlewomen, she wore a country shoulder shawl, its red and gray checks and red fringe making a spot of glowing color in the center of the painted panel.

Frank's eyes glowed too, and his face broke into a smile as he led Eliza over to her portrait.

"There you are!" he said. "I meant to return the shawl, but you never wrote to me. When your folks asked me to do this wall painting, I thought here's my chance. I didn't stay in New York very long, Eliza. You were right about a man needing a lot of money to live there, but your shawl kept me warm while I did stay."

Eliza's homesickness was lost as she entered into the pleasant painted scene. "It's grand, Frank," she said. "It is the Killingsby Green, and I dare say, the water scene at New York. The shawl looks fashionable on the young lady. You painted it in graceful folds."

"Your shoulders, and yourself in a New York bonnet," Frank explained. "Although you do not need a Paris headdress, I thought you would fancy a French bonnet. I am glad that the picture pleases you, Eliza."

Canterbury, Brooklyn, and Cheshire in old Connecticut boasted soon of Francis Alexander's wall paintings. A Garden of Eden, in which lifelike forest animals, even a panther with a long tail crouched on a tree limb, decorates a wall of the ancient Allen house and is credited to him. Another village green with its church, people and horse carriages, may be seen in a wall painting of Cheshire. Francis was soon able to study again in New York and later, when he had learned to be a skilled portrait painter of his time, he painted Daniel Webster's portrait, one of Charles Dickens, and many of the important families of Boston and near-by towns. The great Gilbert Stuart was his friend and it is said that Francis Alexander's portraiture was almost as popular for a time as Stuart's. We may see his portraits in museums today, but we like to remember him as a boy who taught school, who struggled for his art education, and who began the art of decorating ancient walls with pictures of his home and his girl friend.

Plymouth and Marlboro in Vermont; Saco, Maine; Hancock, New Hampshire; Washington and Old Lyme in Connecticut have cleaned old walls and discovered beneath the dust and layers of wall paper, the homely scenes within which our ancestors built our nation. Hand-ground and hand-mixed pigments, green, blue, red, buff, and moonlight-gray color panels and frescoes in wall paintings so large in their design that they often spill over their space. Mural painting in our country began with Francis Alexander and his fellow artists. Like the limners, they traveled the countryside, bringing to life the American landscape as the limners did its folk. Sailing ships and steam packets, village scenes, our flag, and the American eagle were the subjects they liked best. Today's murals have the same background of life, workers, national scenes, patriotism, history, but the old wall paintings tell the story of our nation's beginnings, brave, and handmade.

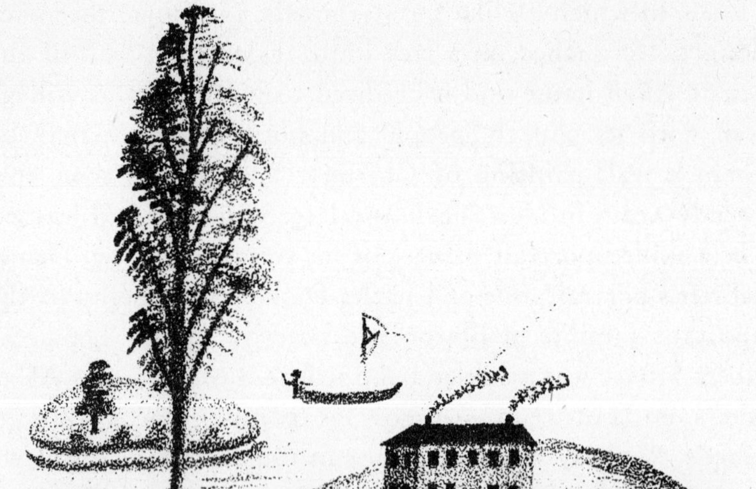

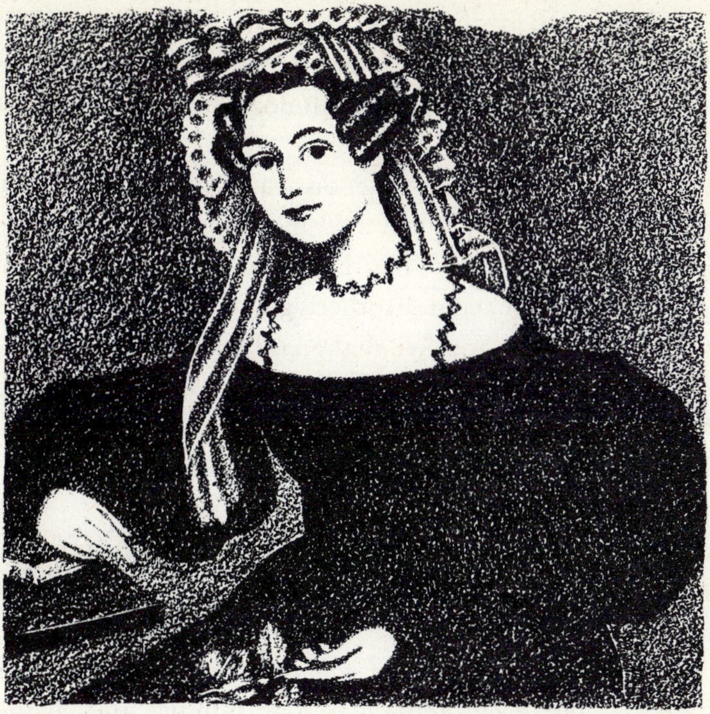

A CAP FOR MOTHER

THERE was hardly anything about the house that Charlie could not do. The family had need of him, for there were many weeks, especially when spring was coming to old Salem beside the sea, when they were alone. Their father was an important man, going about the countryside mending umbrellas, a skilled occupation and a necessary one as well. Umbrellas were fairly new, expensive and constantly breaking. So it was helpful to have a tinker arrive at a farmhouse with his tools and a supply of new ribs. But spring meant plowing the Salem vegetable garden, house-cleaning, and planting. Ever since Charlie, with a mysterious bundle under his arm, had rapped at the kitchen door, he had made himself useful.

It was a custom of the time, our early nineteenth century, to practice hospitality when a stranger of the road asked for food and shelter. Charlie had begun at once to repay them. He seemed like an older brother, going fishing with young John, helping their mother make and patch pants for John, mixing colors for Betsy to paint her paper dolls' dresses, cutting finer quill pens than the schoolmaster could for writing letters to their father. Best of all, Charlie told the three, Betsy, Emma, and John, good stories.

He had come to them almost a year before, and in the room beneath the gables which they had offered him, he had stored his bundle. If the family wondered about it, they did not question Charlie. He was reserved. In all his tales of adventures, he never explained that bundle, and he never tried to earn any money as even young John did.

It was a large flat bundle securely tied, and their mother said that Charlie kept it underneath his bed. They all wondered about it, and also why Charlie got up at sunrise but never came down until almost too late for breakfast. And he often kept his lamp lit long after the others had gone to bed. The watchman said that on many evenings he saw a tall shadow beside the lighted gable window, busily mixing magic in an apothecary's mortar.

Salem witches were only ghosts, but the town still believed in magic, and whispered about the stranger in the umbrella-man's house. Nobody knew where he had come from or why.

But the family had grown to love the quiet young man. If he did keep to himself part of each day, he was dependable the rest of the time.

"Charlie more than earns his keep," their father said.

"I don't know what I should do without Charlie, especially his help with the spring tailoring," their mother said.

"Tell us about your travels," the girls asked one evening when the supper dishes were washed.

They needed diversion for their mother had just told them that there would be no new frocks that year. Charlie had tailored a new suit for the umbrella-mender that he might make a prosperous appearance on his spring route. The girls were to wear their old green merinos, washed and pressed, to church on Easter Sunday.

"Well," Charlie began, "I started carving ships' heads round about here when I was a lad. Then I bought some dry colors and ground them for painting pictures on coaches and signs for inns. I could always get a week's lodging and food at a house or an inn while I was painting. Shops, too, wanted signs drawn and colored; a sheaf of yellow wheat for a baker, a pair of smart boots for the shoemaker, a well-drawn hand for the glovemaker, a cap with flowers for the milliner."

Emma sighed, pushing back her brown pigtails. "A cap with flowers. I believe everybody we know will have something new to wear this spring. Mother has a desire that she keeps secret, for a new cap."

"I would gladly give up Father's new suit if Mother could have a fancy cap," Betsy flung her blue gingham apron on a chair, "and for myself a string of coral beads."

"Who are you to question a new suit for Father?" young John reminded her. "Should an umbrella-mender look like an old-fashioned peddler? And so on?" he urged Charlie.

"Oh, on to the road again," Charlie's blue eyes were looking through the kitchen door, beyond the cobbled road.

"Did they pay you a great deal for the ships' figureheads, the pictures on coach doors and the signs?" practical Betsy asked.

"Why, no. I guess I never asked for wages. I just liked the work, and everybody was kind to me. For years I haven't lacked a lodging."

"If I were to say what I think, I'd blame you, Charlie, for being too impractical," Emma said. "Now for my part, if there were any way that I could earn money, I should buy finery. I am thirteen. Betsy is ten, and John is eight going on nine. I want black satin slippers, a blue silk dress cut low from the shoulders and having ruffles and puffed sleeves. A cameo pin such as the jewelry shops here in Salem stock from the packet boats, and a pair of pantalettes trimmed with tatting would also become me."

"A modest bill," Charlie suggested, but the others ignored him.

"I would like a yellow challie dress with a pattern of flowers." Betsy saw it in fancy. "With it I should wear new coral beads. My pantalettes would be longer than Emma's and trimmed with lace from Venice. My slippers would be laced with ribbons and I would have one curl down the middle of my forehead. So!" She coquetted in front of the kitchen looking glass.

"And could you pay heed to the parson's text, sitting beneath the pulpit in all that finery?" Charlie asked mildly.

But John broke in. "What I want is one of those big new dogs, a Newfoundland. Father says I may never have one as they eat too much. And I should not be averse to having a drum or a sword."

"Instead of star-gazing," their mother laughed as she looked in from the sitting-room, "how about studying your lessons for tomorrow? The lamp is lighted and we can all sit around the table, Charlie too," she added.

There had never been a better mother. They all had the same thought as they looked at the slender figure in the door. She and Emma looked like sisters. Her smooth brown hair was parted in the middle and folded itself back softly above the calm forehead. It was unadorned and her print dress with its long full skirt and trim basque were also without trimming. Mother looked all right to the children; patient and ready to understand dreams, skillful in cake baking and mending, clever at pumping tunes out of the parlor organ. But other Salem mothers, the wives of prosperous sea captains and ship builders, no matter how young they were, wore caps. Their lace caps were trimmed with gauzy ribbons of rainbow colors, so sheer that they seemed like bits of sea foam. Bows of ribbon, streamers and ties of ribbon, bunches of silk flowers, moss rosebuds, violets, and velvet pansies decorated these caps. The same thought captured each one of the children. Emma would give up her blue silk dress, Betsy her coral beads, John his drum if mother might have a cap for Easter.

As the five heads bent over the round table, the lamp in the center, mother with her mending basket, and the geographies opened, Charlie idly sketched with a newly cut quill pen on a scrap of paper. He studied the four through half-closed eyes as he drew: Betsy's perky little curl that would creep out from under the net that tried to hold her unruly brown curls in order. John's freckles, his crop of red hair and his steady hazel eyes. Emma's growing-up look that brought wisdom to her serious brow and longing to her blue eyes. The curve of their mother's face. Charlie's fingers were extraordinarily long and nimble. During the time that it took John to trace on his map the route of a packet boat from Philadelphia to Salem, their mother to weave a small darn, Charlie had finished these sketches and started on the head of a big dog with a coat of thick black hair and a kindly expression.

He folded his paper, got up, and from the parlor threshold said, "Good night, my friends."

"Good night!"

"Sleep well, Charlie."

But as soon as he had closed the door, John spoke. "He won't be going to bed."

"At school today, one of the girls told me that Charlie was seen down at the wharf, unloading cargo in return for some pieces of sail canvas."

"Although I frequently try to lift his latch, I never can," Betsy admitted. "He must fasten his latch with a nail."

"For shame, Betsy!" their mother chided.

But she sighed. They had great trust in their lodger but he was secretive about all but his adventures. How, she asked herself, did they truly know if his carving, sign-painting past were real? And he changed the talk when they asked him his last name.

"Isn't Charlie enough?" he answered, a look of impishness on his pointed face and an inscrutable smile baffling them.

Because it was a late spring, and the anchoring of the ships bringing spring cargoes was delayed by storms, the Easter season fairly burst upon the town. John tried to get work at the wharves but he was too small. The girls and their mother had no extra chicken and egg money to spend yet. So the children did only window shopping. It seemed to them that never before in Salem had such bright and desirable finery been offered; Paisley shawls like Oriental sunsets in their rich coloring, India lawns, ribbons that spread a rainbow wherever they were unrolled, gauze fans with painted designs and silk parasols with carved ivory handles. And, oh, the caps! Paris milliners competed to send them to our ports. They were fashioned of filmy lace and net. They draped and ruffled themselves above demure faces. They flaunted great ribbon bows. They tied themselves beneath chins that tried to hide girlish dimples. They cost ever so much.

"Now, look at that one." Emma pointed to a cap of cobweb patterned net displayed in a shop window on a wax dummy. "I can see Mother wearing it, with those rosettes over the ears and the wide ruffle at the back. It would become her."

Charlie, out walking with the children, looked over Emma's shoulder. He took out his ink horn and pen and busily sketched a few lines.

"Charlie isn't really interested in caps," Betsy said.

"Just in getting through his work and latching himself in his room to carry on his strange doings," John said. The gossip of the neighborhood was beginning to influence him.

"Ssh. He might hear you," Emma warned. But Charlie had left them. He strolled down the brick-paved street toward home.

"I heard him scraping and pounding last night when I

went up to bed," Betsy said. "As if he were mixing something with a mortar and pestle, as mother mixes spices."

"Such a pretty day!" Emma sighed. "Look how the sun shines on the brick walls coloring them rose."

"And we can't buy Easter clothes," Betsy added.

"Come on home," John urged. "You just wait and see. Tonight, I am going to find out what Charlie is up to."

They were not mischievous children, but the mystery had become too much for them. Added to their curiosity, Charlie shut himself away all that afternoon, although their mother needed help with the last of the house-cleaning. When their bedtime came, the three went willingly upstairs. But when the house was still, and only Charlie's light burned, three night-capped, night-gowned figures crept along the upper hall, stopped beside the door of the gable room and listened.

Inside there was a steady grinding sound. Then a long silence.

"Shall we rap boldly?" John whispered.

"Try the latch," Betsy spoke louder than she had intended.

The door was suddenly unlatched and the children almost sprawled on the threshold in the unexpected entrance they made.

"Come in, my friends," Charlie welcomed them. "I intended to send for you soon."

It was a homely little room with rag rugs, painted walls, and furniture; but now transformed by a crowd of occupants. Leaning against the walls, covering the four walls in fact, was a strange company.

The children were speechless, wondering, awed.

There they were huddled on the threshold of Charlie's room, their real everyday selves, in old cotton night things.

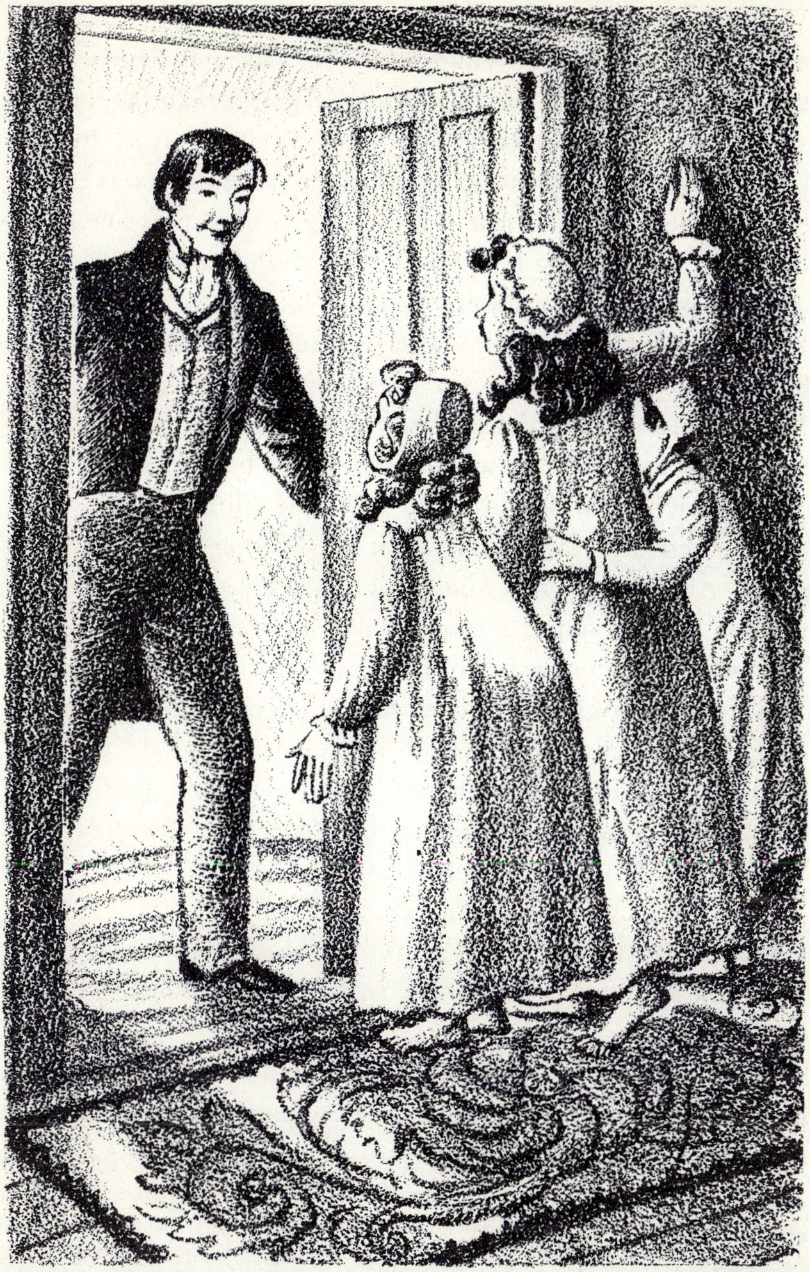

Within the room, in splendid array they saw their dream selves, the decked-out young folks of their spring wishes. Emma was dressed in the blue silk frock for which she longed, a rosy cameo pin ornamenting it and black satin slippers peeping from the folds of the full skirt. There too was Betsy, her curls let loose and one lying coquettishly upon her forehead. Rosy coral beads twined Betsy's neck and her yellow dress bloomed like a flower garden. John gasped as he saw the great black dog of his wish, stretched beside a boy like himself, its head resting on the drum in his lap. But, ah, Mother's lace cap! There she was, wearing a velvet dress, holding a bouquet and wearing the most beautiful and lacy of caps, ribbons fluttering, and frills enfolding—

But there was the sorcery of it all. Mother's cap enfolded space. All their figures and costumes were painted on canvases in bright colors, gamboge, ultramarine blue, vermilion, yellow, but not a member of the family had a head!

A sudden brighter light showed their mother in the hall, called from her evening's sewing by the sound of the unlatched door. She held the lamp high, its glittering glass prisms and bright flame throwing more splendor upon the scene. She too was spellbound. Then she spoke.

"Why, Charlie, is it possible that you are a portrait painter? Have we had the honor of housing a limner all winter? But we cannot pay ten dollars for a canvas to say nothing of four portraits."

Charlie smiled as if he were still enjoying his secret. "I aim, ma'am," he explained, "to combine the useful with the agreeable. The wood carving I did on ships' figureheads gave me a feeling for the human figure, and painting signs is excellent training in line and color."

He put some ivory white, with a dash of gamboge and vermilion in his porcelain mortar and began grinding, then diluting the paint drop by drop with oil.

"Tomorrow," he promised, "we shall begin sittings and put in your heads."

One at a time, with Mother first, they posed for the portraits as Charlie deftly gave each a head. Their dreams came true for Easter. But the best one of all was Mother's portrait in the cap she would never have bought for herself, the rich velvet gown, lace trimmed, that no Salem shopkeeper had been able to persuade her to afford. Betsy's head was painted a bit crooked above the coral necklace, but that only made her portrait more lifelike. And it seemed as if John's portrait dog would bark, step out of the canvas and go down to the wharves with him one day.

They had no words for thanking Charlie. Their portraits hung on the parlor wall gave them distinction in Salem.

"When Father returns, perhaps he can pay you," they told Charlie.

But one day Charlie left Salem as unexpectedly as he had come, his bundle of canvases and palette under his arm, his brushes and mortar in his pocket. He was lost to them, a nameless, kind, impractical artist, the family thought. But there they were mistaken.

Charlie wandered up and down New England roads, stopping for the winter at some farm or village home to paint handsome clothes and bits of landscape, bunches of flowers, a book, a spy glass, a toy rabbit, a doll, a drum, a beloved dog or other pet on his headless canvases; then shop for heads. He was one of the old-time company of limners whose paintings grace our art museums, and the homes of those today who love their ancestors. Charlie Purdy was at last successful enough to disclose his name. Beside him other limners trekked through dust and mud, storm and sunshine, burdened with canvas and palette. There was Chester Harding who journeyed into our West and persuaded old Daniel Boone to sit for his portrait; he had been a maker of excellent chairs before he took to limning. There were Vincent Canadé, the plasterer, John Kane, the carpenter, Joseph Badger, the Boston silversmith, Charles Peale whose training began with modeling coaches, and making clocks, and William Prior who kept bees to support his family while he painted. These were makers of history, for they painted New Englanders as they hoped to be when their hardships were ended. A few asked payment, but most of the limners worked for the love of their art.

Since there was little spare money for fashionable dress, these portrait painters often prepared their canvases in couples, a father and mother in broadcloth and satin, high starched stock and embroideries. The children, wise and industrious beyond their years, were given in these old paintings the toys and pets that everyday life had denied them. They wore the fancy frocks, the lockets and curls, the slippers and ruffles they preferred to tow and leather.

The limners painted truth too. The elders were painted with backgrounds of the land they loved, trees from their home acres, a bit of farm meadow, or the pillars of the new house they had built. The preacher and his wife held Bibles. The sea captain held his spy glass or his compass and there were stars and blue sea behind him. The lawyer wore his robes of office. The soldier carried his sword. The housewife stood beside one of her painted chairs, her feet set firmly upon a Brussels carpet of red and blue. The flowers they held in these portraits were precious to them, moss roses, forget-me-nots, lilies. Sometimes the family mouser was painted in also, looking as wise as her young mistress. But all these canvases were alike in being unfinished. Either the heads were lacking, or dress and accessories waited to be painted according to the wish of the sitter.

New England was growing up fast, but thrift and hard work were still habits. In these old portraits, mothers in rare lace, children in fragile slippers and gay frocks, fathers

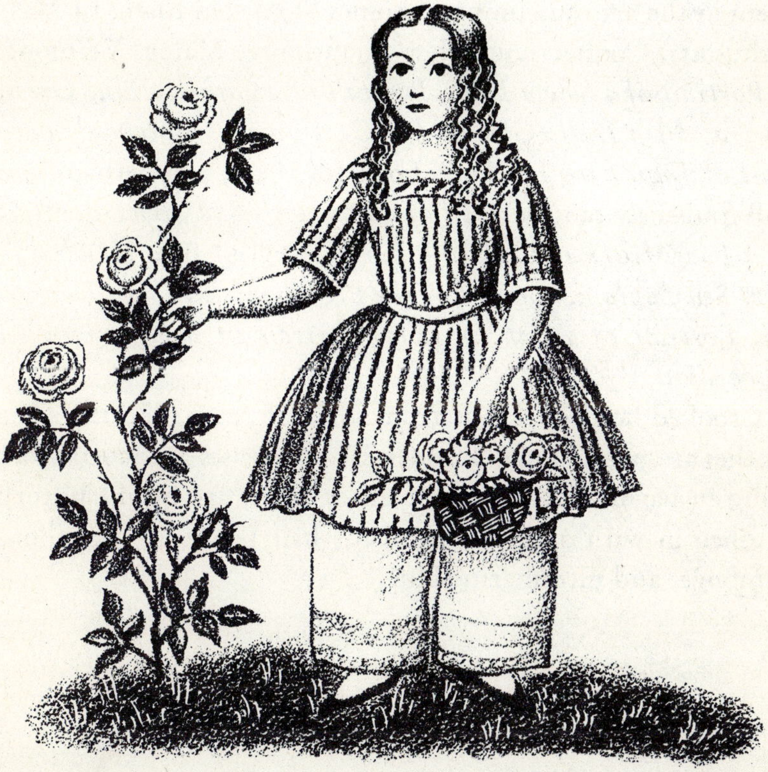

holding the symbols of their success, decorated the walls of the new houses that arose on the sites of log cabins. The limners drew and painted crudely, with vivid patches of contrasting color, but they preserved for us the wisdom of young faces placed upon the garments of dreams; the books, weapons, and tools that had brought prosperity to their elders.

Soon, for Charlie and his fellow limners were seers, these paintings set fashions. Presently trade with India and China, Paris and London, and the industry of New England made possible the prophecy of the old portrait. A lace cap for Mother, coral beads for Betsy, a blue silk frock for Emma, and a big Newfoundland dog for John became facts. We see them in the art museums and homes of the old towns of Massachusetts, Connecticut, New Hampshire, Maine, Vermont.

Portrait of a Salem Lady. Portrait of a Girl in a Blue Dress. Portrait of a Little Girl with a Curl on Her Forehead. Portrait of John with His Dog. Look for them, and perhaps you will find these too: *Portrait of a Boy with Red Shoes. Portrait of a Lady from an Outlying Farm. Portrait of a Newburyport Sea Captain. Portrait of the Lighthouse Keeper's Daughter. Portrait of Aunt Lucinda. Portrait of a Girl with an Accordion.*

Crooked heads look out from some of them, and the same clothes are painted in a number. The canvases are faded from lying in barns and attics, but all of them are bright history brushed in with quill pen and cat's-hair brush, in vermilion, gamboge, and ultramarine blue.

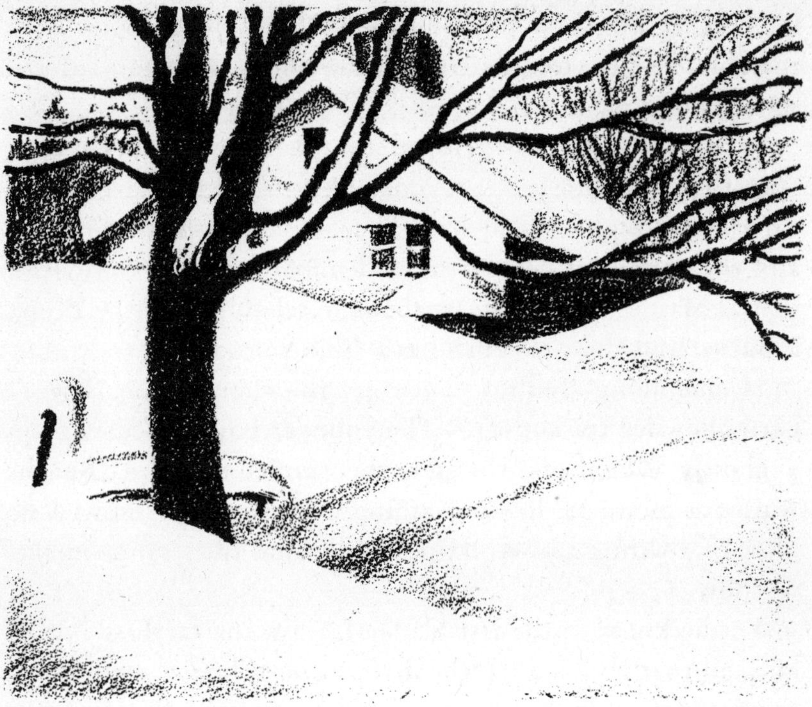

SNOW-BOUND

IT WAS the heaviest snow storm John could remember. In open weather no other roofs could be seen from the Whittier farm there in Haverhill. The faraway sound of bells and the roar of the waves combing Salisbury Beach drifted on the wind to mingle with the hum of bees in the orchard, the chirping of birds in the elms and oaks. It was a solitary place in summer. But now the snow had fallen softly, steadily for almost a week and transformed the familiar home place. As he stood at the entrance to the white tunnel that he and his brother Matthew had dug to the barn, John shook with the cold. Partly, too, he trembled with the unreality of the snow-bound scene.

"Look, Matty," he gripped his younger brother's arm. "See the old bridle-post; it looks like an old man wearing a cape and a high-cocked hat. The brush pile is a white hill and the corn crib has towers and minarets like the Moorish castles Master Coffin tells us about in school! Country Brook is buried and the well-curb has a Chinese roof!"

"Come along, Johnny. Let's get the chores done. There's corn chowder for supper." The younger boy's voice came in a ghostly echo back through the tunnel to John. But he waited a moment, looking at the gray sky that showed no glow of a winter sunset, fixing in his mind the strange images of snow.

Yet he knew to the last blade of grass, the farthest line of hills, all that lay beneath the drifts. The Whittier elm, eighteen feet around and casting a noon shadow of a hundred feet across, stood guarding the two-story farmhouse. Low green meadows and woods of pine and oak encircled their acres. Country Brook would again turn the wheel of the Haverhill grist mill. Yonder, invisible through the curtain of the snow, was Great Hill from whose top the Whittier boys and girls could count thirty towns on a clear day and on whose slopes huckleberries grew in thick tasty sweetness. The drifts only kept like a secret the picture of his homestead, John Whittier knew. He loved the countryside. At fifteen, he hadn't a wish to leave it as so many other boys of the town planned to do. If he could paint or draw it, just as it lay in white magic, he wished! That would be success enough.

"Hurry up, Johnny," Matthew called again. "The old

horned ram is stamping his feet for his supper and the cock crows on the barn rafter because he thinks it is morning."

John pulled his knitted cap down and tied his muffler tight to keep the snow from his ears. He wore no underwear; red flannel had not yet come into fashion, and his homespun suit, spun and woven, cut and stitched by his mother, let in the cold. The knitted spencer that was tied over his chest made poor shift for an overcoat.

He was a tall boy, and thin. You noticed first John Whittier's eyes, dark, far-seeing, deep-set and luminous. He went about the task of making the farm creatures comfortable for another stormy night. He and Matthew pulled down hay for the horse, for Buck and Old Buster, the oxen, and scattered feed for the hens. From the stalls where the seven cows waited patiently to be milked, there came soft lowing and their sweet breath lay frosted on the air. Last, the boys littered the creatures' stalls for warmth.

"We'll need to bring in more wood. Step along, Johnny," Matthew urged. "Brush and foresticks, light-wood and if we can manage it a few more big logs."

"Thee's energetic, Matty," John approved. "At ten thee's a better farmer than I at fifteen."

"Well, maybe." The younger boy threw an arm about his brother's bent shoulders as they started toward the woodshed, wading the fast thickening snow through which they had cut a path but a few hours before. "But thee was writing verses on thy slate at school at my age."

John took a deep breath of the icy air. He saw something familiar that the distance and the snow shut from sight, the district school and the young teacher, Joshua Coffin, who had begun his patient guidance of a seven-year-old boy and still inspired John with stories of faraway places, with fireside reading-aloud from Robert Burns' poems, and the pure phrasing of that other bard, Shakespeare. Lines of verse sang in John's mind, driving out sums and geography. But here was sculptured poetry outlined by the drifts.

Master Coffin lived in the Whittier home, a valued boarder. In the summer he took off his scholar's black, put on jeans and a peddler's pack and followed country roads as far as Boston. Master Coffin could tell tales of what was happening in New England towns, sagas of long sea voyages, of the arming of village militia, of the Greek and Roman gods who walked beside him whether he sold needles and thread, or sat in front of the Whittier's hearth telling stories. So, John thought, the world came to them at home, a pleasant prospect on a night like this. After supper they would draw their chairs in a half circle before the fireplace, all the family; his father reading his favorite book *The Farmers' Almanac*, his mother in her Quaker cap and long apron, the schoolmaster, their uncle, the older sister spinning, gentle Aunt Mercy knitting, Lizzie the little sister a patch of sunshine as she played with a rag doll on the blue and white braided mat, he and Matthew side by side on one of the settles. Home thrilled John, sang itself unwritten within his heart:

> Shut in from all the world without,
> We sat the clean-winged hearth about.

Matthew's warning brought him out of his dream. "Have a care, Johnny! Thee almost fell into a drift. I'm not the man to pull thee out by thy long legs. Here we are! Quick with the door or the wind will blow out the candles."

The Whittier kitchen was so wide that pools of darkness filled the corners in spite of candlelight. The sanded floor was swept in swirls by the turkey-wing brooms that also brushed clean the bricks of the hearth. The great fireplace, with its oven for baking bread and beans at one side behind an iron door, could hold a five-foot back-log easily beneath the swinging crane. Iron pots and kettles ranged the front and upon the over-mantel shone the pewter candlesticks. The old leather bellows for blowing up a tardy flame hung at one side. One the other side stood the spinning wheel that whirred and sang after supper with Mary Whittier's industry. The small panes of greenish glass at the windows were now white, while the wind cried down the great chimney. But it was warm and gay in the kitchen. It was the year 1822 in Haverhill, Massachusetts, when home bounded all of the family's loves and hopes.

John's mother sat sewing beside the hearth. Beside her was Goodman Whittier, his gnarled, horny hands turning the pages of the almanac. Joshua Coffin sat with them, sharpening lead plummets for his pupils to write with when the storm should be over and the roads broken to the schoolhouse. This was a large family, an uncle, an aunt, the schoolmaster, living too in the house. They all thought this the best hour of the day. After supper, John and Matthew made a little hollow in the warm ashes of the fireplace, laid on brush and lightwood, piled small logs and at last tugged the huge back-log into place on the andirons. The red Turks' heads that topped the andirons gleamed with a savage delight as the brush caught, a tiny spiral of smoke arose, the logs broke into sparks and sudden flames brought the whole circle of the family into one picture about the hearth.

Goodman Whittier thumbed the almanac pages, finding notes he had made:

"The year after thee was born, John, 1808, we built the new stone bridge there in Haverhill. The ice going out made the arches tremble but not a stone was displaced. That was a winter like this one. Haverhill has always been far-seeing if extravagant. In another two years we set up the Light Infantry with their standard made by Miss Polly Dow, the seamstress, and voted their allowance a princely ten dollars a month. It was an elegant flag and the Infantry had tents and all needed for a fatigue march if the occasion arose. Weather—"

He looked over his silver-bowed spectacles at the older children. "You should remember why I have made records here. One May 29 cakes of ice were seen coming down the Merrimac River. In the summer of but five years past frost killed the crops and a gale blew down Master Ladd Haseltine's chimney and killed his son Jonathan. Salt spray came inland on the gale that season. But a few years ago, we had a summer hail storm when I myself filled a bushel basket with hail stones. The following winter the snow was as deep as it is this week. Shoveling the Common we made a tunnel through which a man on horseback could ride without stooping."

Listening, John knew that the pleasantest part of the evening, the story-telling time, had begun. He sat, turning some sheets of brown paper stitched together to make a writing book.

Joshua Coffin, watching him, knew that those pages would bear scribbled verses instead of sums. John began to lose, as if he had dreamed it, his father's Haverhill history. Words of his hearthside content wove a closer reality:

And ere the early bedtime came,
The white drift piled the window frame,
And through the glass the clothes-line posts
Looked in like tall and sheeted ghosts.—

—the old, rude-fashioned room
Broke flower-like, into rosy bloom—

While red logs before us beat
The frost-line back with tropic heat—,

Singing words, hidden within his happy heart.

"The scalping story, Mother," Matthew begged.

She clicked her knitting needles and tapped her stout shoe in a tattoo of Indian drums, belying her Quaker peacefulness of speech.

The Indian hordes came down
At midnight on Cocheoco Town
My own great uncle bore
His cruel scalp mark to four-score.

I see once more your father ride
On Memphramagog's wooded side,
Sit down again to moose and samp
In trapper's hut and Indian camp.

His mother was telling the story in prose but her words came to John in rhymes of his own phrasing.

A creaking beam, the crack of a burned log falling apart, made the story circle start, move their straight-backed chairs closer. Their uncle spoke. He had no book-learning but whether he wandered the woods in summertime or heard the witch-grass singing in the autumn as withered hags on broomstick steeds stopped for rest, this uncle of the Whittier children knew magic.

"On a night like this," he told them, "wizards are out when man is indoors. Birds sing and the bare branches of the lilac tree bloom beside the house door for those with hearing ears and seeing eyes. Warlocks prowl, lighted by elf-candles, and headless men pass on mare-back carrying their heads under their arms. If you listen well you will hear, not the breaking of frozen branches in the wind but the clacking of the mill wheel as it is turned this very night by the goblins."

"Hush thee, brother." Their mother foresaw nightmares in the small chambers under the roof where the boys and girls slept. "Matthew, do thee fill up the basket with apples to roast and hickory nuts. It is time that John did his share for our evening's pleasure. Tell us a tale, Johnny."

John felt his cheeks flush with his shyness. "What have I to tell?" he asked. He was a silent boy, slow of speech and timid among his elders.

"Surely thee can at least try to do thy share in our evening's entertainment," she chided him.

Young Lizzie tossed her bright curls and came from the hearth rug to lean on her favorite brother's knee. "Tell about that wicked little city, Boston, Johnny," she urged. "How thee went there alone, wearing thy new coat of gray, long and with boughten buttons."

"Yes, son," his mother urged. "We never tire of hearing about thy trip to visit Cousin Nathaniel Green on Beacon Hill. A great man, Nathaniel, the Boston postmaster, and his good wife sets so grand a table."

"I never made so fine a Quaker hat as the one I stitched for thy Boston visit, John," Aunt Mercy spoke at last. "All stout cardboard cut to fit thy hair nicely and covered with gray cloth."

"We warned thee to have nothing to do with play-acting in Boston," his father said.

"And to eat what was set before thee, asking no questions," the elder sister said.

"A play actor had dinner with our John at Nathaniel Green's," Matthew grinned, remembering.

"She was a beautiful lady," John found his tongue at last. "As kind as mother and as righteous in her speech although not wearing Quaker dress. She told me what book to buy and study here at home. The shop windows in Boston are a rare sight, but the boys on Boston Common made sport of my Quaker garb. I bought a copy of Shakespeare's plays, but I came home sooner than I had planned, having found Boston less inviting than home."

Matthew, looking over John's shoulder, now gave a great shout. "Johnny's making up rhymes again. He has been writing them in his composition book." Matthew read aloud:

> "What matter how the night behaved?
> What matter how the night wind raved?
> Blow high, blow low, not all its snow
> Could quench our hearth fire's ruddy glow."—

His father arose to his great height. "Thee has not got over thy old tricks of setting down doggerel? Thee should have given it up with thy slate and A. B. C.'s." He started toward the offending book, motioned toward the blaze.

But Mistress Whittier laid a firm hand on his arm. "Stay thee, Mr. Whittier! John's a good boy. If he dreams, hears

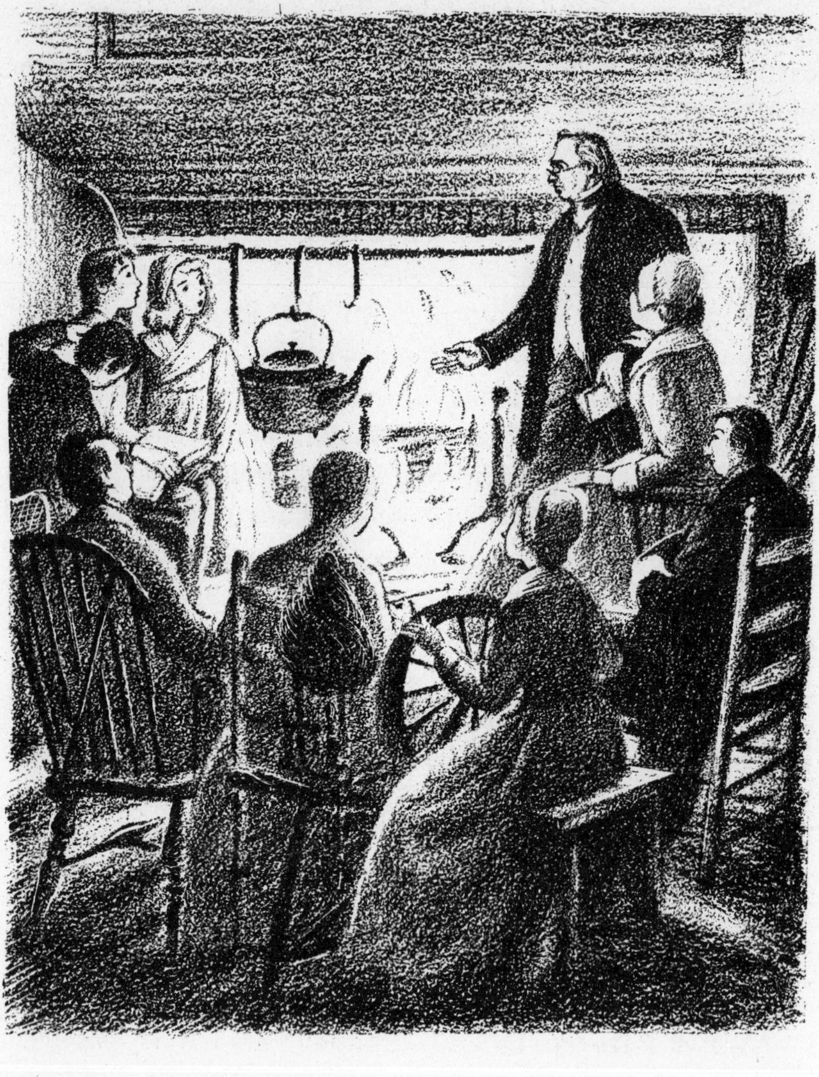

words sing instead of marching along as they do in the Testament in orderly fashion, he does his chores."

Joshua Coffin too spoke up. "The sonnets of Shakespeare that you all enjoy when I read aloud may not rank with those of our young poet here, but you respond to their spell." He gave the boy a friendly dig in the ribs, "Someday our John may be as much loved as is Bobbie Burns who wrote homely poems that sprang from his own hearthstone and his Scottish soil."

John felt hot tears close. His cheeks flamed. He was no boy prodigy but he could not help hearing rhymed phrases like a swarm of honey bees, humming among his everyday thoughts.

"I fear that I am but an indifferent good Quaker," he said.

His mother beckoned to him and he sat down on the hearth at her feet. His father still frowned but she smoothed his brown hair.

"Thee's our elder son and a biddable boy," she comforted him. "So long as thee does not neglect thy work I can see no harm if our home gives thee poetic feelings. There might, as Master Coffin suggests, be a poet born of New England."

Those Haverhill folks who passed the shoemaker's shop two years after the winter of the great snow saw a taller boy, his wrists and ankles outgrown from his clothes, sitting within at the bench. He was pegging stout soles on country shoes, stitching leather patches, and dreaming. The window of the shop through which John Whittier looked, as his hands moved blindly, so well had he learned his trade, opened upon the scene that grew more precious to him every year.

Barefoot boys, like the boy he used to be, passed whistling with fishing rods over their shoulders or overflowing berry baskets in their hands. The old schoolhouse was still there at the crossroads, ragged with climbing weeds and vines, but alight with sun. The breezes brought whiffs of sea air and memories of happy days of tenting on the beach. The banging of the Haverhill militia's drums as they maneuvered on the Common, the humming of bees in clover, the singing of the trees, the fancied piping of fauns in the woods beyond the fields—all these enchanted John. Now and then as he finished a boot and set it out ready for its owner, he reached into a box of papers underneath his desk and took out one. The box was crammed with all sorts of paper, foolscap, the backs of letters, brown paper, all covered with John's neatly slanting handwriting. He was still writing poetry. He had finished one hundred poems. But so far, although he persisted, worked alone in the shop by candlelight, the bench cluttered with wax and bristles, rosin, thread, and the paste-horn, not one of the poems suited him. Nor had one found its way into print. But he could not stop writing. His urge was irresistible to put his home scene and the New England soil, its legends, ways and folklore into singing words.

When he took an evening off, John walked down to the post-office. A vain trip for no one wrote to him. He was surprised one day of that, his seventeenth year, when a neighbor on horseback stopped at the door of the shop. The man pulled a letter from his pocket, one of the rare letters of that time, carefully folded so that it made its own envelope, then sealed with red wax.

"It's for you, John," the man said. He reined in his horse in curiosity. "Why don't you open it, see who it's from?" he urged for John only held the letter in his trembling hand, his face white.

"Want me to break the seal?" the man persisted.

Just then John's father came up, on his way to the village. "A letter, son?" he asked. "Maybe it's a mistake."

John was shocked into action. "No, it's for me. It says Mr.

John Greenleaf Whittier all right." He tore it open, read, speechless at first. Then his voice choked. "It's from William, from William Lloyd Garrison. You remember Willie, Father, just a little older than I but a man of parts. He's printing his weekly paper over at Newburyport and he writes that he sees promise in my poem, 'The Exile's Departure.' I mailed it to him for an opinion. He will print it in his paper."

"You don't say! John Whittier having a piece printed!" the horseman started on to tell the news.

Goodman Whittier said nothing. He looked at the green pastures, the hills folded in gold and blue, the smoke rising from the chimneys of village homes, then down at John's dark eyes, at his proudly lifted head. Perhaps, he thought, there was a special way of telling the world how much one loved one's acres, the seasons of snow and Mayflowers, of blueberries and pumpkins; the closeness of families, the warmth of hearthfires, and the delight of old stories told after supper. John had puzzled his father, a good lad as his mother always insisted, but concerned with writing, wanting to be a poet. But if John could put the humdrum into verses, if so coming a young printer and statesman as William Lloyd Garrison thought he was doing all right, who was he, Thomas Whittier, to censure the lad?

John still looked silently across the road, up to Great Hill. His father at last reached over to grasp his hand.

"Thee'll likely need a flock of pen points now, Son. Perhaps thee'll do a piece about the great snow. When thee does, thy mother and I've got a few coins saved in the blue china teapot on the kitchen mantelpiece. Help thyself."

When John Greenleaf Whittier's long poem "Snow-Bound"

was published in Boston in 1866 it became so cherished a word picture of loved acres and close-knit families that not only the United States but England read it. Soon it was translated into foreign languages. The ten thousand dollars that the first edition paid the poet was but a small recognition of what he had achieved. "Snow-Bound" tells the story of that long ago week in Haverhill when the Whittier family were shut in together, doing homely tasks, sharing pleasures and companionship. Howard Pyle and other great artists illustrated it. "Snow-Bound" is the most popular of our native poems, because it is true. It can never grow old.

The Quaker boy of Haverhill is known also as the poet of freedom for he lived to share in the struggle of the States, to write ringing poetry of patriotism. His manner of writing was so simple and truthful as to create unmatched phrasing. He wrote as Abraham Lincoln spoke, without affectation and with undying appeal.

With "Snow-Bound," we cherish John Greenleaf Whittier's "The Barefoot Boy," "In Schooldays," "My Playmate," "Maud Muller," "Telling the Bees," "The Sycamores," "Skipper Ireson's Ride," "Barbara Frietchie," "The Pipes at Lucknow," "The Garrison at Cape Ann," "The Swan Song of Parson Avery," "The Double-Headed Snake of Newbury," "Abraham Davenport," "The Eternal Goodness." Hundreds more!

We read them in the city and visit in dreams the countryside we long to see. We read them when we find the farmhouse among wide acres that waits for all city-dwellers. New England, in John Greenleaf Whittier, gave us a poet of hearth and hill, liberty and Americanism.

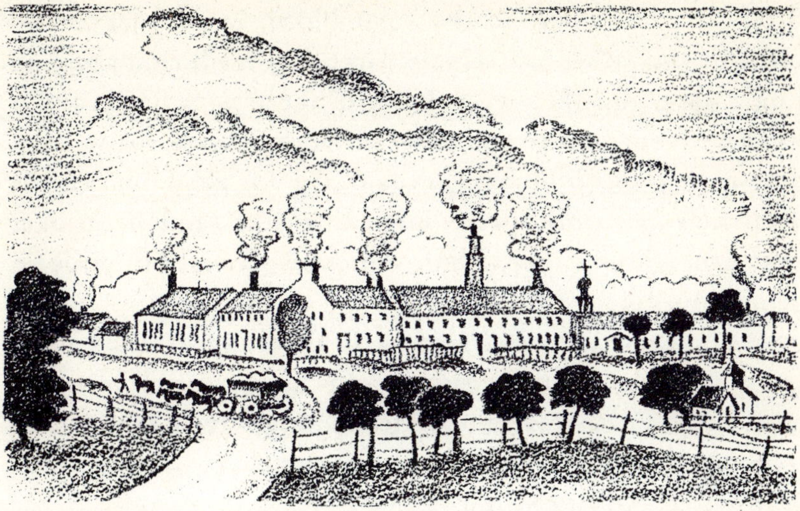

THE JEWELS OF SANDWICH

As he stood on the doorstep of the glassworks, James saw that Master Deming Jarvis was too busy to look out. School was over for the summer, and James, eight years old, found the works more interesting than play. But, truly, the colored glassware that his father and Uncle Samuel made and sometimes brought home was enough to rouse anybody's admiration. James' mother had a set of sapphire-blue plates for tea parties, and her Sunday frock boasted crystal buttons with a tiny glass rose imbedded in each. On his father's desk stood a glass paper weight in the shape of a gentleman's tall green hat. James had a set of glass whimseys given him by his Uncle Samuel and standing on the mantelpiece in the parlor; a rooster with colored feathers, a little bottle in the shape of a bear, and a striped glass cane. The glassmaking of

Sandwich Town was in the boy's blood. Master Jarvis had brought his father and Uncle Samuel from Birmingham in England because they were skilled in the art. He had brought workers from France and Belgium also. Because the sand of near-by Plymouth Beach was too coarse for good mixing, the Sandwich glassworks were importing fine sand by packet boat from France and South America. James felt pride in being a member of his family.

The rays of the sunset resting on the finished pieces along the shelves, the sight of Master Jarvis busy after his men had gone home fascinated James. He stood still for a while, then stepped slowly through the doorway and closer to the blower. Still Master Jarvis did not notice him.

His ruddy cheeks swelled as he blew through the blow-pipe, the bubble of clear glass growing, thickening, becoming larger on the end of the pipe. From time to time he twisted it. Beside him lay his tools ready for instant use when the glass gather was right; the punty-rod for holding the hot gather, the tongs, shears, compasses for measuring, and the battledore for flattening the glass. It seemed that he must have some special piece in mind for he had no need of blowing his own glass now, with so many men and apprentices at hand during working hours. Larger, clearer the gather became. Master Jarvis turned as he transferred the glass from the long blow-pipe to the tongs. It was a gold-ruby bubble ready to shape into a goblet.

"James Lloyd," he exclaimed. "How is it that you are not at home doing the chores? This is not the hour for a boy of your age to be out sightseeing." It seemed almost as if Deming Jarvis felt himself caught off his guard, instead of young James.

"I like to see glass blowing, Gaffer Deming," the boy seated himself on a stool.

His eyes widened with excitement as Master Jarvis rolled the gather, blew it again lightly, set it gently upon the wet block, began tooling and trimming it into shape. Before the glass cooled he would engrave upon the plastic surface a delicately traced garland. He would put a threading made from the trimmings around the edge. The goblet he was making would be a rare beauty.

Master Jarvis felt called upon to explain. "The Mistress would have me, none other, make her a set of goblets. Each will have its own design engraved by hand; a garland, a horn of plenty, the great fringed thistle that grows in the marsh, the bellflower, and maybe a few birds."

"Those will be fine goblets!" James was sincere in his praise. "I have an ambition to be your apprentice, Gaffer Deming," he added boldly.

The glass-blower tipped his spectacles and looked at the lad. James was eager, standing straight in his hobnailed shoes and his homespun breeches, his tow head held high.

"The summer is upon us and I have learned my tables and can read the Bible from Genesis to Revelation," he boasted, although his voice trembled.

"I'll wager there's something about this work that the Bible doesn't mention," Master Jarvis said, "that glass has a soul and waits for the shaping of a master hand."

"I have been told somewhat of that at home," James agreed. "My father and Uncle Samuel say glass blowing is their life. They would choose none other."

"Spoken like a Lloyd!" the glass-blower said. "Come closer, James. You're a small lad. Do you mind that none of my apprentices is as young as you; that their first duty is to gather and split oak wood for firing the glory-hole, load and drive the bull-team, unload and stoke the furnace oven? My apprentices must go to school as well as work, either in the morning or afternoon? They have no chance to feel a blow-pipe between their lips for years maybe. All depends upon their skill and industry."

James hesitated a moment. The glory-hole, the great furnace oven where the glass mixture was melted in clay pots, vas a giant for eating up wood. That he had observed. Going to school half a day and splitting wood the other half did not sound hopeful. But he kept on with his appeal.

"I am told, Gaffer Deming, that you let a good apprentice work for himself after a time; and that when the bristles are worn from the glass-polishing brushes you give the backs to us for making little play carts."

Master Jarvis' eyes twinkled. He liked to be called Gaffer, because that indicated his skill in blowing. He noticed that James said *us*.

"That is true, in the case of good boys," he told James. "Also, I give my boys fifty cents for buying fireworks on the Fourth of July. You may report, if Thomas, your father, agrees, for work at seven o'clock tomorrow morning. Your father and Uncle Samuel will direct your work."

As he walked home the sunset over the marshes turned Sandwich to magic for James. In the afterglow that tinged the dunes James could see the colors of the glass that Master Jarvis was making; canary-yellow, purple, blue, amethyst, pale green, and the gold-ruby. The entire town held glass-blowing as its pride. Master Jarvis had built the eight-pot furnace with two chimneys in 1825 and the Cape Cod houses that lined the elm-arched streets. There was a Green with tall elms in front of the works and it was rumored that Deming Jarvis would soon build a horse railroad across the marsh to haul his glassware to Boston, and bring back sand and the oxides that, mixed with the melting batch, gave it those lovely colors.

There was comfort and a feeling for art in the little gray houses James passed. He looked in the bakeshop window, jingling some pennies in his breeches pocket. He went on. No foolish buying of sugar buns for a Sandwich apprentice, he decided. He looked in the shoe-shop, feeling the holes in his toes. That shop also he passed. The wages of an apprentice would hardly allow him one pair of shoes a year. But James was willing to go barefoot, holding in a dream the glass cologne bottle he would someday make for his mother. He might, also, make her a pomade jar. Glass-blowing, his father said, had brought in a new way of life. It had laid a fragile, and luminous touch upon the old homespun ways of the grandparents. Young ladies prinked in front of their dressing tables that were spread with glass scent bottles and pomade jars. They wore necklaces of bright glass beads. They dipped

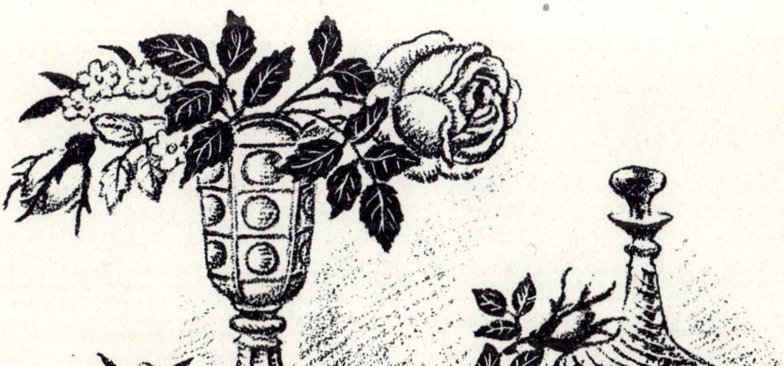

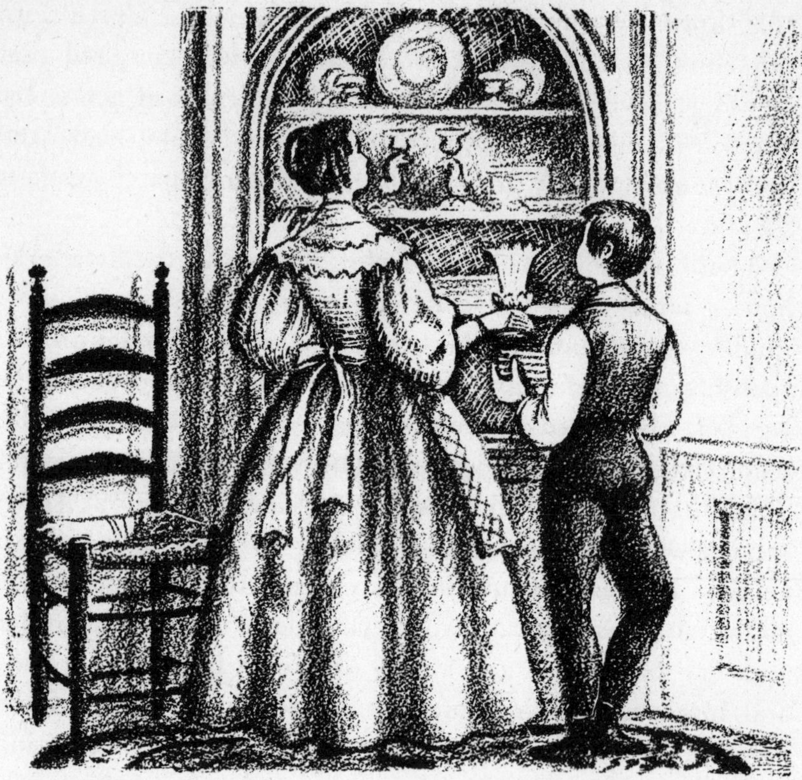

their finger tips daintily in the colored glass finger bowls that had come into fashion. James' mother could not have enough of the new colored glass dishes for filling her corner cupboards. Now he, a boy, was to have a part in making glassware. He ran. He would have to get the chores done early in order to be up and at work betimes in the morning.

That was a busy summer for the young apprentice. Oak wood is tough to split and heavy to load. A bull-team, even with the help of another boy, was a task to drive. Almost as soon as the glory-hole was stoked, and the pots of mixed batch set in for melting, more wood was needed. Some of the other apprentices had earned their right to attempt more lofty tasks. One was trusted to mix the sand, potash and lime, and the chemicals that gave the glass color. Another boy showed James with vast pride the trigger he had blown and shaped, a drinking glass that was made to test the skill of an apprentice. But eight-year-old James bent over his wood pile, stumbled along beside the team with an ox-goad, strained his back filling the glory-hole, and then began all over again.

The summer burned itself into autumn as Gaffer Deming's glassworks became more famous. He had the secret of making that brilliant gold-ruby glass for flowers and fruits used as decorations, and for goblets. He was making and sending all over the United States glass wig-stands, fancy bottles, flower vases, salts, and the sugar bowls that were needed since loaf had been superseded by spoon sugar. James' father and Uncle Samuel were too busy to heed him. So long as he did his work well no one asked whether his back and legs ached.

When Thanksgiving came, James sat down with the family to a loaded table that fairly glittered with the new glassware Gaffer Deming's men were allowed to buy at cost. The salts were all different in decoration, including the fashionable bee-hive and duck designs. The cup-plates, one at each place, were glass, both crystal and colored. They held the china tea cups as the Oolong tea was cooled and sipped delicately from the saucers. The vegetable and compote dishes had designs of fluted ribs and swirls, bellflowers, slender vine and leaf sprays, and the horn of plenty that symbolized our more prosperous land. The small glass sauce dishes that held cranberry jelly were engraved with rays, the star-and-fan, diamond and heart designs.

James ate until his head nodded over his second helping

of pumpkin pie. That night he dreamed that he had a blow-pipe in his mouth, puff, puffing, and twirling it as the bubble of the gather grew. He dreamed also that Gaffer Deming had invited him into his office and allowed him to read the secret formula for that gold-ruby coloring which was making Sandwich notable. But the day after Thanksgiving brought a cutting ice storm from the Cape. James' eyes were blinded with the snow-filled wind, it pierced his jacket and muffler as he shivered over to the works. His humdrum work began all over again.

Christmas brought a chance to make a gift to his mother and James selected a jade-green scent bottle and jar, to be paid for out of his wages. That green was a rare color, he thought, matching the late autumn sky when the nights were frosty, a greening apple, or the sea as one saw it down Boston way. The colors that came out of the melted batches thrilled James. Just a little of this or that copper, cobalt, lead, iron, saltpeter, borax, or chalk measured and stirred in the batch resulted in rainbow tints. That winter James was promoted to tending the clay pots. He helped skim the impurities off the melted batch before the blower dipped a pipe in it. It was pleasantly warm beside the furnace and James brought his school work over, staying after hours. He never made his play cart; he had a composition book in which he was secretly writing. He kept it locked, either at home or in a little chest at the factory. The other boys chaffed him:

"Poetry, maybe? You're getting ready for Valentine's Day?" But James refused to explain.

Sandwich glass was following the ways of a more care-free nation. It was the beginning of the happier nineteenth century and we were taking pride in a few luxuries. Sandwich-glass compote dishes, translucent blue, ruby, and amethyst goblets, apothecaries' jars in prismatic color, table pieces of life-size colored fruits with leaves and stems, and decorated glass lamps from Sandwich, all showed that Master Jarvis was an artist as well as a glass-blower. They were preferred to French and Venetian glass.

The seasons colored both Sandwich and James' work. The time came when he put on long jeans and was given a blow-pipe. Next he worked at a block with engraving tools. He learned the delicate task of packing glassware in sawdust for shipping. He rode to Boston on the new horse railway with boxes of luxury glass for the fine shops there. He also sifted and washed the sand upon the purity of which so much depended. He took note of the mixing of the batch as the precious powdered chemicals were measured on the brass scales, and added. He made sketches of the Sandwich bell-flowers, the birds and the garden posies that were favorite glassware designs. A day came when James could do gadrooning on bowls and pitchers; a separate gather that he blew and attached in fluting, swirls, and threading as ornamentation. As he learned, James' delight in his work grew. Glass, he discovered, held magic. He could spin it into threads, or mold it into a strong little figure of a dog or cat. It remained crystal-clear or the color of the rainbow, as he wished. He was a tall lad and a hard worker. He still spent evenings in the factory and secretly filled the pages of his composition book.

Working at Master Jarvis' desk one evening James thought that he was alone. The Gaffer was an important man and his Sandwich business took him frequently to Boston and

New York. Uncle Samuel was fussing near the glory-hole, gathering up bits of broken glass to be thrown outside on the cullet heap as waste. The boy was writing at the Gaffer's desk. He had been given that permission. The composition book was almost full and he had laid an alabaster-colored glass paper weight upon it to keep it open. The paper weight was as milk-white as a pearl and the rounded surface shone like satin in the lamplight. Uncle Samuel dropped in.

"Time to go home, Jamie lad," he warned. Then he lifted the ball of alabaster glass, holding it admiringly in the light. He examined it. "This is none of the Sandwich mixtures, lad! Where did you get it?" he exclaimed.

"I devised it," James explained. "From the washing of the sand to the melting of the batch, it is my own whimsey. The Gaffer has a secret for his gold-ruby color. So have I a secret recipe for this creamy color. Fancy it now, Uncle Samuel, as the base for a lamp or, engraved and gilded, to make a compote dish! It would be handsome."

"You have a discovery, Jamie!" Uncle Samuel set the opalescent ball on the top of the desk. "Wait until Master Jarvis sees it! I doubt not that he will add it to our glassware. By the way, he is to be gone a fortnight this trip and look as we may, we cannot find the formula for the mixture of the lead to go into the flint-green glass."

James turned the pages of his note-book and pointed to one. Uncle Samuel read excitedly. Then he turned other pages.

"So this is what you have been doing these late evenings; copying from memory the rules for the batches! Victoria-blue. Opal. Pearl-gray. Lilac. Rose. Turquoise. Iris. Lemon. Dove. Purple." He read the names of the colors aloud. "You have a master mind, Jamie. This book will be useful long after the Gaffer is finished with his glass-blowing. He carries his colors in his mind rather than on paper. We'll be at a loss when he goes."

"Written by the hand of my valued apprentice, James Lloyd," Deming Jarvis labeled the book of color formulas that was to be the guide for mixing the batches at the Sandwich glassworks for many years. James became the color expert of the glassworks. It always seemed that his pieces were brighter, more sparkling than any others. At last, though, his note-book was not needed. Machine-blown glass came in.

The seasons aged and the tides swept old Sandwich; they covered the glory-hole and the cullet heap at last. The factory had become a heap of bricks and all that remained of the glowing and beautifully designed glassware was the treasure in old cupboards and in museums. The buttons on an ancient gown within which shone little glass flowers and fruits, the glittering goblets, the glass doorknobs and curtain-ties, the cruets, decanters, and colored glass dishes that had made Sandwich the most famous of all American glassworks were scattered. The whimseys made in moments of leisure by apprentices and master blowers, little sets of dolls' dishes, glass

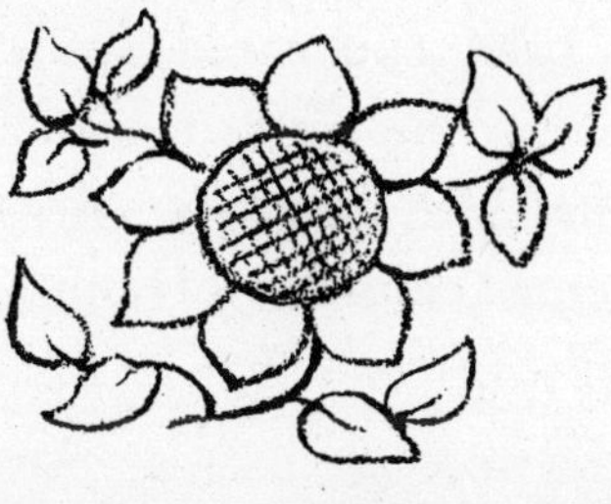

animals and birds, hats and canes, and bright little scent bottles that some seafaring father filled for his daughter with French perfume, hid themselves in attic chests.

The ruins of Sandwich covered their loneliness with greenery. Blueberry bushes and wild blackberry vines shielded the fallen walls and twined around the cullet heap. Sandwich glass-making was only a memory and the berry-pickers took possession of the ancient site. Blackberry vines can cut until the blood runs. A century after an eight-year-old apprentice had worked there at Sandwich, another boy, picking berries, jumped with the pain of a cut finger. It was a sharp jewel of ruby glass, not a berry vine, that had pricked him in the sand of the old cullet heap. A treasure had come to light, covered with ancient ashes and sand but glittering in the sunlight. He held it up, exclaimed, showed it to his companions. It was a broken bit of Deming Jarvis' gold-ruby glass, exquisite, scintillating.

Handmade jewelry had become the fashion and excavating at Sandwich began. There in the cullet-heap ruins bits of glass colored by Deming Jarvis' and the apprentice James Lloyd's formulas, were found. This glass was polished and cut, set in pendants, rings, and bracelets, and scattered its flashing color rays like sapphires, opals, rubies, amethysts, and jade. Today, Sandwich-glass jewelry is desired and rare. The shifting sands have washed away even the cullet heap. A few bits of discarded glass have been excavated from the creekside and among the sand dunes. The art of the ancient glass-blowers is lost to us but James Lloyd's story tells us of industry and faithfulness that helped color the precious jewels of Sandwich.

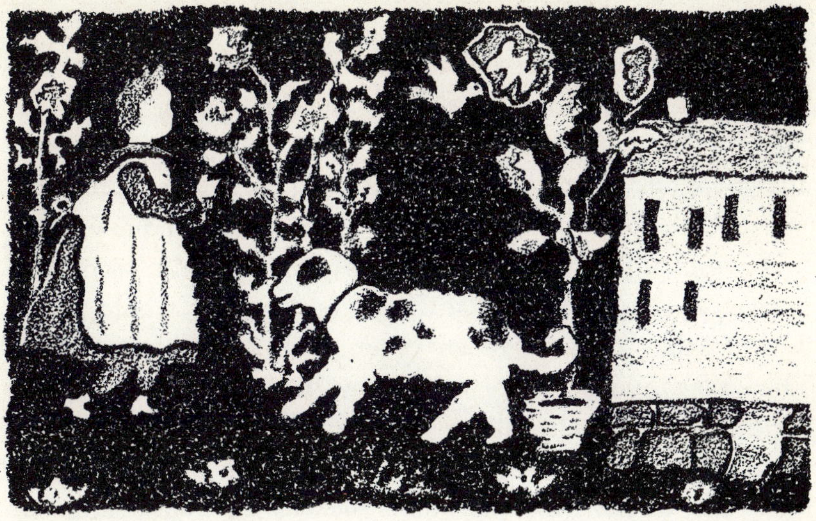

PICTURES IN HOMESPUN

IT SEEMED to Betsy Paine, standing at the entrance to the covered bridge and listening to the clop-clop of the stage horses on the wooden flooring, that the stage wheels were carrying happiness as well as Caroline away from her.

Caroline was Betsy's dear friend and she was going over to Boston to boarding school. She would be gone for the closed seasons, the Vermont autumn and winter. All spring, too, Caroline would be gone. She had promised to write but Betsy, remembering Caroline's glowing cheeks and sparkling eyes, her excited good-by— "Dear, it will be thrilling! I shall take up the pianoforte, needle-point, painting, and French—" felt that perhaps Caroline would forget her farm friend in Randolph.

Betsy knew that the Paine family was among the oldest in Randolph. Her father had driven there in his ox-cart. She loved the town; brown earth and blue sky so close where the hills lay in curves against the landscape, wooded valleys, the ancient white frame houses that the red barns clung to. Vermont was a folded state, all curves and color and hollows. But nothing changed in Randolph. September would be purple with grapes and crimson with apples. October would flame with scarlet maples, golden beech, and tawny oak leaves. Then all would be white with snow. Betsy would be unable for days to get to the village school except on her snow shoes. Each day would be like yesterday and a pattern of tomorrow. How she would miss Caroline! She turned as the rattling stage was lost to her sight at the other end of the bridge and started slowly home.

She passed the post-office where a hum of harvest talk drifted out. She walked past Caroline's new house, so beautiful in its Adam architecture, with a delicate white door that held the fanlight, white pilasters, and cornice. It was surrounded by great maple trees set out when the house was built. She stopped a moment to look across the rail fence that surrounded the Randolph Common, then followed a dirt road along which were houses like hers, their barns, woodsheds, and summer kitchens clinging to the house walls, their small panes of window glass looking out on hills and other valley farms. In the long winter evenings Betsy knew that the lights of those farms would make a pattern with the stars. She wrung her hands and tried to keep back the tears. She was twelve years old and she had never been to Boston.

Betsy found her mother outdoors, busily stirring a mixture of leaves, stalks, roots, and rags in the big brass dye kettle that was hung over a fire of pine boughs. With the first shut-in days, she would begin making hooked rugs. She hoped to finish by spring at least two rugs of good size. Two was the winter task of the Randolph women. Betsy was about to ignore the dye kettle with which she was too familiar but her mother beckoned.

"Now is the time to finish the dyes," she said. "Fetch another stick and help me stir, Betsy. I am experimenting with this cochineal the peddler brought over from Boston, but I like the natural colors best. I have an idea, too, that they will last longer."

Betsy found one of the smooth sticks that were used for stirring. She worked silently, looking in the earthen crocks of dyes that surrounded the kettle. Truly, she admitted, the colors were pretty. It was surprising what vivid tints and shades came from the gardens and woods. A yellow like gold was distilled from the stems, leaves, and flowers of wild St. John's-wurt. Other yellows were made from a suffusion of walnut, hickory, yellow oak, peach, sumach, and clematis leaves. Onion skin boiled down gave a rich dull yellow and saffron, a brighter yellow. Pokeberry root was good for making a red that had a rich purplish tinge. The precious package of cochineal that had traveled all the way from Spain to Vermont made a brighter red than did the cranberries and beets. Scrapings from old bricks boiled down to a delicate pink. When one wanted blue dye, there was the bag of indigo; also wax myrtle, garden purslane, and larkspur. Orange and brown could be had from a suffusion of the bark of butternut, hemlock, and maple trees. Tree moss, ash mint, smartweed, and unripe walnuts made a green dye.

Betsy's mother lifted a length of cloth from the dye kettle, rinsed it in cold water, and held it up to the sun. The red into which it was transformed rivaled the early-turned maple leaves in the door-yard.

"See, Betsy! It is rich looking!" But the girl did not look up.

"I can match almost any flower color," her mother went on. "Now this red could be our monthly rose or the fuchsias, the zinnia red or one of the turned maple leaves. Your grandfather's uniform up in the attic would make a pretty background for a rug with a pattern of flowers. This winter I have a mind to strip the uniform up into rags for hooking. That's work you could do, Betsy."

"Oh, Mother, I don't want to strip rags!" Betsy was close to tears. "I saw Caroline Stone off to school in Boston this morning. I'm going to hate the winter with Caroline gone. Every fall and winter is the same here in Randolph; housework, chores, stripping rags for hooking, making patchwork, nothing to see from the window but snow and bare trees. Caroline is going to learn French, painting, and the pianoforte. She has everything, Mother."

Betsy's mother pulled her spectacles down over her nose and looked at her rebellious daughter, not disapprovingly but with sympathy. She left the dye kettle and put an arm around Betsy's shoulders.

"There, there, don't cry! I know just how you feel. Randolph is a pretty spot when every garden is in blossom and the hills are green, when the brook is singing and there are berry-picking, picnics, and hay rides for you and Caroline. But I know how hard the shut-in days are, all alike and no pleasures unless we make them for ourselves. When I was a girl here in Randolph I had the same feelings as you, Betsy, that I couldn't stand it without a little excitement. That was when your grandmother taught me to make the stair-riser."

"Our stair-riser?" Betsy looked interested.

From the time when her short legs had hardly reached from one step to another, Betsy had studied and admired the stair-riser. The design showed a different picture hooked into the rug for each step of the staircase, and all so colored and mellowed that the pictures seemed like outdoors brought in. There were blue and gray doves first, then a step of apples, following that came a house, the Randolph Common with the rail fence, the farm horse, a bunch of garden flowers, dear old Tabby who had kept the barn mice down. All these pictures made climbing the stairs to bed, coming down to breakfast, a gay adventure for Betsy.

"Yes," her mother said. "Your grandmother taught me that the way to stand a long winter is to hook a rug to cover a bare floor with something as bright as outdoors. And there is enough brightness in our fields and gardens to last us in remembrance until the lilacs bloom again. Betsy, there is one thing that Caroline hasn't got. I know because I helped her mother settle their fine new house. It's got wall paintings and paintings of the family. There is a carpet in the parlor with cabbage roses but there isn't a single hooked rug. They scorned them. Now if you were to set your mind to it, you could make Caroline a pretty rug this winter that would make her think of Randolph."

"Would she like it? Wouldn't she turn up her nose at it?" Betsy wondered.

"You could try it anyway." The stick began swishing the dye around again, blending the colors. "I believe that right now Caroline wishes she were back in Randolph as much as you are wishing you could go to boarding school in Boston.

Help me get the housework done, Betsy, and this afternoon we will make our plans."

September flowers of garden and roadside seemed unable to give up that year. They bloomed late with vivid gold, purple, and red. The wild asters, the marigolds and zinnias, the dahlias and morning glories dazzled the eyes. But the first frost came in early October. Then, to make up for the faded gardens, every Vermont hill was covered with a rainbow of color. The maples turned first, each morning different in a massing of reds, yellows, and gold. The oaks showed their ruby and russet for a background. It was something to remember and Betsy, gathering a big bunch of garden flowers, bringing in colored leaves, saw it all with new light. She got out her box of crayons and copied the flowers and leaves on paper as patterns. She washed a burlap feed bag for the foundation of her rug. She stripped rags and dyed them to match her patterns as well as she could. Her father made her the wooden frame on which the burlap would be stretched and they made a trip with the horse and buggy down the road, through the mysterious twilight of the old covered bridge, as far as Montpelier to buy Betsy a hand-wrought hook from the blacksmith who made them skillfully from nails.

"I feel excited," she told her father as they returned. "I don't mind the leaves dying this year."

"Leaves don't die," he explained. "They just ripen along with the corn and apples."

With the first dull days of November, when the countryside was wrapped in gray and the dusky kitchen needed a great fire for light and comfort, the rug-hooking began.

Betsy's mother had decided upon a butternut-brown background within which she would hook bright autumn leaves copied from those that Betsy had painted. The border of her rug would be a New England twist, like a skein of yarn, in lighter brown. That would make a gay patch of color for the upstairs guest room where the cherry-wood four-poster desk, and the yellow wooden rocking chair were. Her second rug might show the Randolph meeting house.

Betsy was to use the soft blue-gray strips of the old army uniform as a background for her rug. The center was to be a great bouquet of garden flowers, one big pink rose, with blue morning glories, delphinium, and shades of leaves from jade green to moss green. The border was going to be a floral band of rosebuds and leaves. The burlap was stretched tightly on Betsy's frame. She drew the pattern on it with a stick of charcoal. Ranged about the kitchen were the dye jars and a line stretched across one end of the room held the strips of drying colored cloth ready for threading on the hook and drawing up and down through the coarse mesh of the burlap. There was a pile of motley colored strips in one corner into which she would dip. In addition to the dyed strips and the lengths of the old uniform there were some silk bonnet ribbons; those would add softness to the flowers. She quickly learned to hook; to draw a narrow loop of cloth up through with the hook making the outline of the pattern first, then filling in.

Presently the snowdrifts reached the tops of the kitchen windows. The wind sounded like a pack of howling wolves. A weak sun made no impression on the cold. Her father, bringing in a great pile of firewood, brought also the prophecy of worse weather.

"The vane is pointing north-east," he said, stamping his boots. "It's a good thing I built the covered passage to the barn and the stock."

But Betsy hardly heard. No longer was she lonely nor did she long to escape from the humdrum days of a Vermont winter. With the threading of her hook, as she saw the pattern of the rug beginning to take form and color, she brought summer into the house. Carefully drawing loops of colored cloth, worsted homespun, hand-woven linen, linsey-woolsey, and the silk ribbons up through the mesh of the background, she hooked the bouquet that gave life to the rug. It would take weeks to fill in the flowers, and hooking in the background and the border would continue until spring. Betsy's mother hooked fast. Her hook was worn smooth from years of use. As she placed the shower of bright leaves on her length of background burlap, she talked.

"Someday, maybe in your time, Betsy, these hooked rugs will tell stories. All up and down the coast of New England women have hooked pictures into their rugs. There's the Boston Sidewalk pattern made of little colored blocks fitted together by the Boston ladies; and in Salem they hook the Wentworth Brick pattern in gray and rose like one in Governor Wentworth's parlor. I'm told that the Nantucket Scroll is fashioned like the swirls of seaweed, the waves, and the sands, hooked in green and gray. The Maine Scroll is designed from sea shells that are pretty in color. The ladies whose husbands sail the seas put the colors of Paisley shawls, of Dresden china, and imported India prints in their rugs. There are a hundred patterns to choose from; the cornucopia with colored fruits spilling out of it; that makes a rich center. The mountain and hill folk like to hook into their rugs

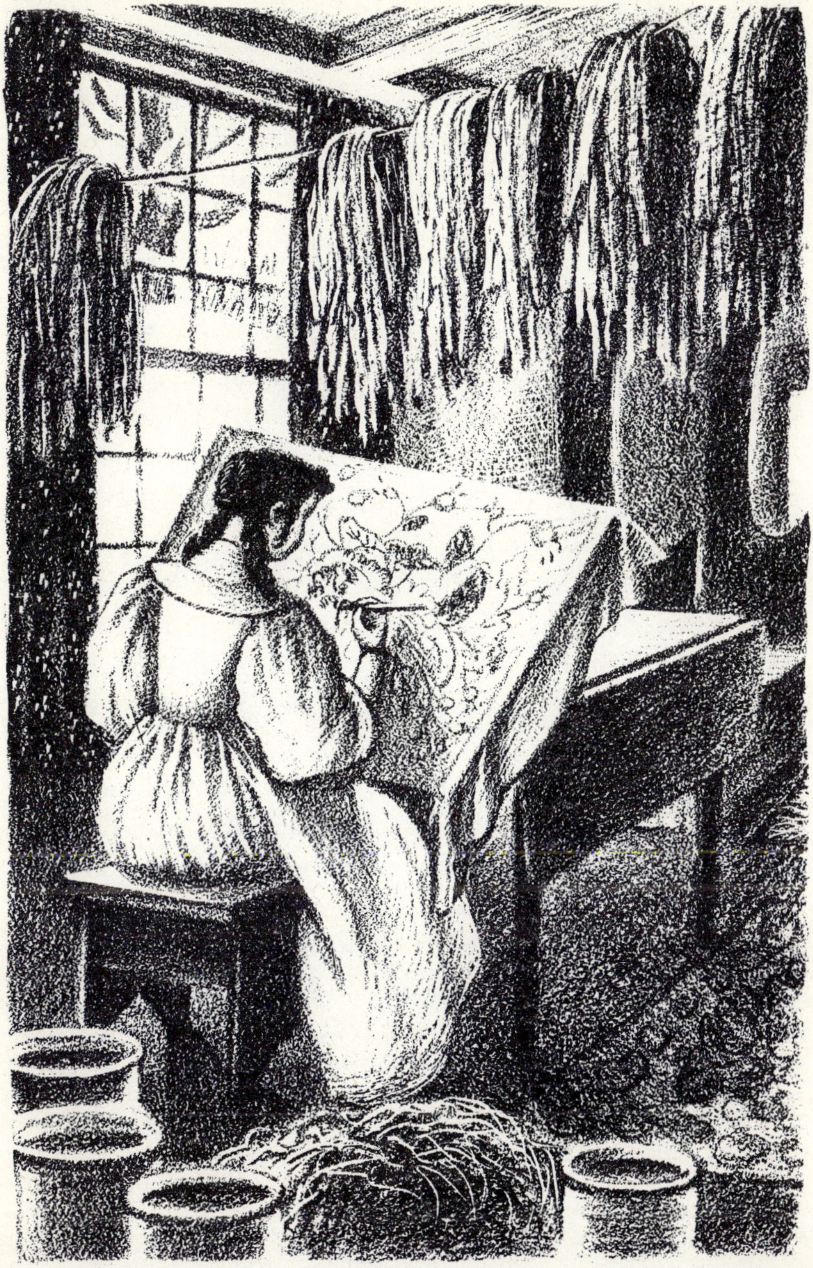

pictures of dogs and cats, their farmhouses, the village church, or the town hall."

"I hope Caroline will like her rug." Betsy was so intent on her work that she hardly heard her mother. "I made the flowers crooked at first but now you may almost smell them."

Caroline came home for the summer vacation. Her Boston bonnet and hooped skirt, her portfolio of water-color scenes, her fringed green silk cape were impressive. The winter was over, syringa and tea roses scented all the gardens and Betsy met Caroline at the bridge.

"Come home with me for tea, Betsy," Caroline urged. "I want to tell you all about how the girls dress in Boston and there's a present for you in my carpet bag."

Betsy's feet dragged as they crossed the threshold of Caroline's house. This was a different Caroline from her friend of last autumn, so stylish and wearing a glow of Boston airs and graces. She followed Caroline up to her own room slowly, stopped in the doorway.

It was a pretty room, the four-poster draped with a dotted-swiss tester and valance, the windows curtained with the same and tied back with blue ribbons. The wall paper was blue, in the new striped pattern that had recently become the fashion. The floor boards were painted gray. Lying like a bit of blue sky dropped down to frame an old-fashioned bouquet, lay the hooked rug that Betsy had made. The flowers looked as fresh as if they had been picked that morning. The buds of the border seemed ready to open. The dye that held the essence of nature's own colors reflected the garden from which the rug took its design. And the hooking was well done. Betsy had spent all winter making her work perfect.

Caroline was silent, at first with surprise, and then delight. She threw her arms about Betsy's neck, her Boston bonnet and hooped frock crushed in a great hug.

"It is beautiful. And you made it yourself, all for me? I do thank you, Betsy! Now I will tell you a secret. I was homesick in Boston. I wanted to leave school and come back to Randolph. If my parents will give their permission, I shall go to our village school with you next term. I have brought you a piece of poorly worked needlepoint to make up into a hand bag." She stopped to open her carpet bag and take out the needlework. "But, Betsy, dear, it is not half as fine a gift as your hooked rug. The pattern was drawn by my teacher and she helped me with the stitches."

"I love it!" Betsy told her. "I wanted a hand bag for Sundays. But the nicest gift is you, Caroline, I thought you would come back from Boston stuck up. Mother said to make you a hooked rug, but I was sure you would turn your nose up at it."

"Well, I didn't." Caroline knelt down and traced the flowers of the rug with her fingers. "Is it very hard to do, Betsy? I brought back a box of water colors and we might make our own designs for next winter's rugs this summer. I'm almost sure that I shall be here to join you in the hooking when autumn comes."

"Oh, Caroline, we will!" Betsy's eyes shone.

The hooked rug with its background of old uniform blue-gray and the New England bouquet in the center held generations of footsteps, glowed with color and at last softened and mellowed to the tints of a Persian carpet. It wore well, for the fabric of the backing and the cloth of which it was hooked were hand-spun and woven. The colors distilled fron roots and leaves were more permanent than any of the chemical dyes that supplanted them. And Betsy Paine of Randolph, Vermont, born in the year 1825, became one of our most notable designers of the hooked rug. As their value increased to hundreds of dollars for the best preserved and most colorful rugs, when museums showed them as examples of the inner beauty that our ancestors felt, lonely and shut in for many months of each year, Betsy's rugs became sought after.

There were other precious hooked rugs, many of them wrought by unknown workers. A primitive farm rug had a design of a fence, the orchard, duck-pond, house and barn, and a border of flowers, crude and out of proportion but inspired by the worker's love of home. Stair-risers that took several years to finish were panoramas in homespun and color of the scenes that winter shut away from the farm people. The austere lines of mountains and hills, lonely roads and the plain architecture of the New England scene, were hooked into rugs in geometric patterns of angles, triangles, diamonds, and squares. Because the solitude of long winters brought the farm animals close to humans in their need for care and their offer of friendliness, the barn cat, the old sheep dog, a turkey, goat, hen, and chicks, sometimes the pony, a cow, or a deer were used in the center of the rug, the drawing untaught but spirited and bright.

At last, as bare wood floors from Maine to New Jersey and down along the bleak Atlantic Coast began to glow with these hand-dyed, hand-hooked rugs, they painted their own canvases, a story as well of a good way of life. The Heroic Rose, the Maine Scroll, the New England Twist, the Wentworth Brick, the Nantucket Scroll, the Dresden China, the

Wedgwood Plate, the Boston Sidewalk, the Banded Floral, the Star, the Single and Double Cornucopia, the Floral All-Over, the Great Dane, Fall Leaves, and a hundred other designs grew from the gardens, fields, farms, and foothills of our ancestors:

Hooking a rug was a slow piece of work. The gathering of dye materials, stripping and coloring the rags were also painstaking. Spinning, weaving, and doing farm chores came first; making a rug was a pastime. So, today, Betsy's rugs are rare indeed. Also prized are those of the other rug designers, unknown and celebrated. Machine-hooked rugs made of chemically dyed fabrics try to take the place of the beautiful old ones. The recipes for extracting dyes from vegetables, flowers, roots, and leaves are lost, for only in rare instances were they written down. They were preserved in the minds of the farm people, handed about from one farm, one village, to another. Our machine-made hooked rugs lack also the marks of the old ones; the initials of the maker in one corner, the irregularities that only increase their charm, the name of the farm dog perhaps misspelled and hooked in beneath his portrait. The Revolutionary uniform, the best-bonnet ribbons, the scraps of a wedding or party dress, the calico that came from the Indies by clipper ship. These can never be discovered in a rug made today.

The story the old hooked rugs tell is the same, no matter how widely the designs and colors differ. From bleak fishing villages, Colonial towns, New England hill-towns, and hollows, each rug speaks of our forefathers' search for beauty in hardship, monotony, and loneliness, and the reward of that search.

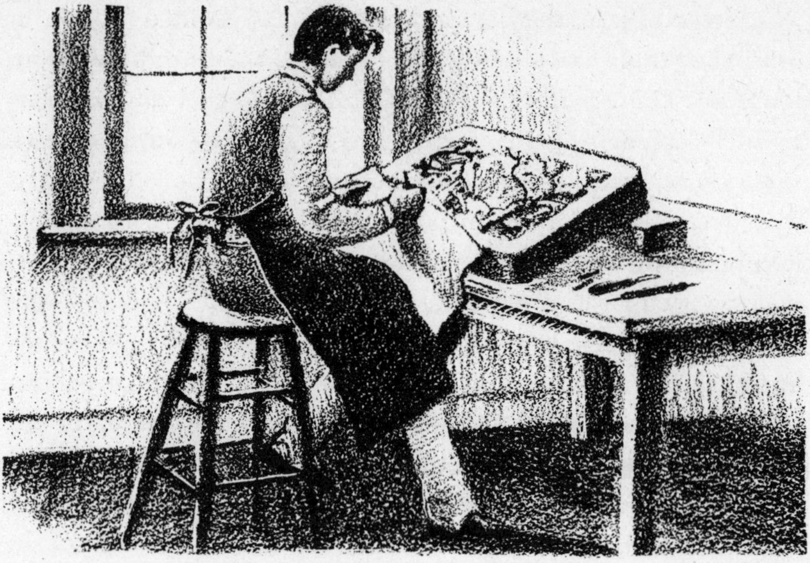

HOME TO THANKSGIVING

THE November wind swooshing and shrilling around Boston Common fairly took Nathaniel Currier off his feet. He shivered, for his jacket was none too thick. He knotted his wool tippet closer and pulled down the earlaps of his cap. He was waiting for the stage that would take him home to Roxbury for Thanksgiving. It had been months since he had been allowed to leave his work at Mr. Pendleton's lithographing firm in Boston. Mr. Pendleton's was the first firm to turn out printed pictures successfully in our country and Nathaniel, fifteen years old, was proud to be one of his apprentices. Still, that had not kept him from being hungry for his grandmother's ginger cookies, his mother's apple pies. And the long hours in the shop when, some days, all he did was grind the sanded stones to velvet smoothness for the lithographing tools, were wearisome.

Home for Thanksgiving! Nathaniel squared his shoulders, whistled above the gale and saw the home farm in imagination precisely as it would look.

Massachusetts country was bitter in November but the snow would be piled in fluffy drifts around the home fences and barn. The air would be icy clear and as an open sleigh drawn by a spirited horse brought his aunt and uncle to the door, the sleigh bells would ring a lovely tinkling tune. On the porch his grandmother and grandfather would welcome the company. Just behind them, in the doorway, his mother in her cooking apron, a shawl pulled on hastily and the little ones clinging to her, would smile a greeting too. Good old dog Rover, a bit lame but still the guardian of the sheep, would bark and wag his tail. He, Nathaniel, would be doing the chores, easy now in comparison with his Boston job. Smoke would trail from the chimney and from the opened door would flow the scents of Thanksgiving, spicy cake, rich mincemeat, fruit pies, and the roasting turkey. They would all sit down to the feast and his grandfather, at the head of the table, would ask the blessing, giving thanks especially that Nathaniel was doing his best at Mr. Pendleton's in Boston. Well, he was learning the business fast; that Nathaniel knew. He was just about to lift in fancy a turkey drumstick to his mouth when a news sheet, blown from a boy's passing wheelbarrow, flew straight into Nathaniel's face, blinding him for the instant.

He grabbed it, ran shouting, "Hey, here's one of your News Letters! Hey there!"

But the boy did not hear him. News sheets were prized

and important at that time, the year 1828. Our country was progressing.

The stage was late. Nathaniel braced himself against a lamp post and read the news. It always thrilled him. As he ground the stones or mixed ink at Mr. Pendleton's he wished that he might have a share in getting and distributing the news. Lithography, Mr. Pendleton said, was going to do great things for the news sheets. Pictures in newspapers were a possibility of tomorrow. Nathaniel, reading on, agreed with him, but he had an idea of his own, secretly cherished, on the subject. Now, if he were the printers of the Boston News Letter he would—. He whistled louder at the magnificence of the idea. For a moment, the white drifts of snow, the blue sky, the red barn, and the painted sleigh were lost in the boy's mind. He was startled by the heavy hand on his shoulder. One of Mr. Pendleton's other apprentices, out of breath, grabbed his arm.

"I feared you'd caught the stage, Nat. We've just had a big order for prints and Mr. Pendleton says he'll need your help. We're to keep the shop open on Thanksgiving Day. Come along, lad. It's tough losing your holiday, but Mistress Pendleton promises us extra rations for the day."

Nathaniel stuffed the news sheet in his pocket and followed the other lad, his shoulders bent against the wind. The mixing of the ink, he knew, would be his share of that overtime job.

"Everything you do, Nathaniel Currier, is accomplished with speed and skill," Mr. Pendleton had told him. "Your inks are more smoothly blended than those of any of the other boys."

Nathaniel reviewed in his mind the recipe for lithographing

ink that Mr. Pendleton had brought with him from England. The items punctuated his footsteps:

Beef suet	¾ of a pound
Goose grease	8 ounces
White wax	11 ounces
Castile soap	24 ounces
Gum mastic	2¼ ounces
Shellac	10 ounces
Gas black	4 ounces

A mess! But Nathaniel knew how to blend the stuff fast and smoothly. There was the door of the shop. Thanksgiving was lost for a year, but as he went in, took off his jacket and put on his ink-daubed apron, Nathaniel Currier repeated to himself, "Now if I could scatter the news, I would—" His thought was almost too mighty to even whisper.

Melting snow, a green Common, hot sun on the bricks of Beacon Hill, so the seasons went, as Nathaniel worked diligently. The business of reproducing pictures on stone was arduous but gave good results. Nathaniel became a skilled grinder; his stones took drawings well. The stones were rectangular, yellowish-gray, eight inches by about a foot thick. When one was ground, Nathaniel would sometimes grasp a sharpened black crayon and sketch a picture. The world went by outside the shop, along the narrow Boston lane, but the boy's eyes carried him farther. Sometimes he sketched one of the new locomotives then being built in the West Point shops. More often he drew the outlines of a country road and an old farmhouse and barn at the end.

When the sketch was drawn in boldly black lines Nathaniel washed the stone in gum and acid that bit out the surrounding parts not covered by the crayon. Then he bathed the stone in water and applied ink from a roller. Last, a sheet of paper was placed on the inked stone and stone and paper were put in the press. When the paper was pulled from the press, there was a black-and-white lithographed picture. Nathaniel worked fast as well as deftly.

The year after he went to work in Boston, 1829, the first locomotive pulled some wooden cars on wooden rails from the new station in Carbondale in Pennsylvania. That puffing, belching locomotive with its great grimy smoke stack came from England but in two years we made our own steam engine and named it *The Best Friend*. Sometimes Nathaniel went over to the waterfront to see the arrival of the new steamboats that made the long trip from Boston and New York to Liverpool. Once he saw a great two-wheeled invention unloaded, called a gentleman's cycle. They were making cycles in England and racing them was soon to become a popular American sport. The old sailboats were replaced by the new racing yachts and all up and down our riverways smaller steamboats plied.

Once Nathaniel met an oddly dressed youth there on the dock, waiting for the steamer to New York. He wore padded blue trousers, a white shirt, and a round straw hat with a ribbon band, of which he was very tender.

"You going to be in a show, Bub?" Nathaniel asked him.

"Not on your life," the boy swelled with pride. "I'm going to play in a match of baseball on the new diamond they've laid out down at Cooperstown, New York. Hope the wind doesn't blow away my hat. The gentlemen baseball players wear tall hats but the young men sport these straw boaters."

New York! That was already a magic-sounding name.

There must be more news pictures waiting to be drawn there than in Boston.

From season to season Nathaniel had cherished his idea, trying to see it in reality, decorating it. At last he bundled together a few stones, crayons, his formulas for acid and ink, and his clothes. He took passage south. He worked at lithography a while in Philadelphia, then in New York, still turning his idea over in his mind, shaping, and coloring it. Also he saved his wages.

There he was at last, a young young-man of twenty, tall, blond, with sharp blue eyes. He stood on a ruined New York street, thrilled, not discouraged, at the great fire of 1835. It had been the most disastrous fire New York had ever known, raging fiercely for two days. Six hundred warehouses were gone and the city had lost twenty million dollars' worth of property. Nathaniel had seen it, the flames, the scarlet of the firemen's great hats, the painted engines, and the blue-gray curtain of smoke, the jagged lines of ruin, the smoldering flames. The devastation of the New York waterfront appealed to him. The smoking ruins that still blazed against the green water and the blue of the horizon would make a thrilling picture, Nathaniel thought. Also, that might be a good time to pick up a small piece of property cheaply and locate a discarded press that he could repair and use. He ate scarcely anything at that time, his dreams being sufficient food. He hoped that his hoarded wages would stretch to cover his plan. That plan was definite at last and, he believed, practical.

The United States had a new word, news. There were several newspapers but printed in small type with no pictures. All the world loved a colored picture; Nathaniel knew that. He was going to try and get out colored pictures of the news fast, almost as soon as something important happened. He was going to peddle his colored lithographs on the streets of New York, damp and limp if necessary from the presses, but newsy. His brain whirled with their subjects. Racing yachts on blue waters, puffing locomotives, trotting race horses with gaily dressed jockeys astride. Pioneers going out West in their leather and red flannel shirts. The green grass of the baseball diamonds. Fashionable ladies in brilliant silks, little girls in the new striped stockings and tasseled boots, small boys in their first long trousers. Inventions. Adventure. Sports. Fashion.

Also, Nathaniel was homesick with his memories; the flaming forge of the village blacksmith back home in Roxbury where he had loved to watch the farm horses being shod; his grandfather's preparation for market day in Roxbury as he loaded the farm cart with vegetables and fruit, and the turkeys and cocks whose gay feathers added to the color; a farm harvest golden with shocks of grain and bright with the blue smocks of the harvesters. Colored news pictures from the Currier shop, he believed, would become as sought after as the newspapers. In three or four days after an accident, a sports event, a record locomotive-run, a picture of it would be on the streets of New York, peddled for fifteen to twenty-five cents. That would be his business, making news pictures. But Nathaniel's heart followed the seasons along a New England countryside.

Early one morning a boy about the age of Nathaniel Currier when he began his apprenticeship wheeled a pushcart up to the front of a shop on Nassau Street in lower New York.

It was a cluttered place. Colored prints hung in the windows, on the walls, and were piled on long sidewalk tables.

A tall man with keen blue eyes stood in the doorway. "Good morning, sonny. They're almost dried. Come in and wait a few minutes. Come in and look around."

That was what the boy wanted. He never tired of poking about the floors of piled lithograph stones, looking at the jumble of pictures that, framed and unframed, covered the walls. He climbed up dusty stairs to the fourth floor that was reserved for the artists who drew the scenes and the lettering on the lithographing stones. Mr. Currier had taken in a partner, a youth whose father was superintendent of Bellevue Hospital and whom Nathaniel had seen in the Bellevue gate cottage, drawing in a vivid self-taught way. James Ives could usually be found on the artists' floor of the shop. There were a number of noted draughtsmen there, Louis Maurer, Thomas Worth, Arthur Tait and, best of all in a newsboy's eyes, Fanny Palmer. Fanny had been working for Currier and Ives ever since she wore her curls down her back. She looked up from her crayon as the boy leaned over her shoulder.

"A great day for Mr. Currier and Mr. Ives," she said, jumping up. Fanny was as lively as her pictures. "Come with me up to the coloring room and see for yourself what we have finished."

Together they climbed to the top floor where a long table was circled by colorists who worked like machines. Their color washes were put on with rare Austrian colors, one at a time. A scene from a skating carnival in Central Park was being painted as the boy and Fanny Palmer entered the room. It was a black and white print as the first girl took it and deftly laid on a blue sky. A second colorist washed in the lake.

So the color flowed from one brush and another until the print showed bright splashes of blue, rose, crimson and green of the dresses of girls and ladies beneath their furred coats, the colored coats of men, the gay tippets of boys, the red and yellow sleds, and the silvery skates. The boy lingered to watch the painting. He had never been so far uptown as Central Park, nor did he own skates. The pictures of winter fun, growing from hand to hand, thrilled him. But Fanny Palmer pulled him away to another table where a mass of drying prints dominated the entire room.

"There it is, our masterpiece!" she exclaimed. "Did you ever see such red flames, such brilliant firemen's hats, such detail in depicting a New York fire engine? It is our new set of prints that you are to begin peddling today, *The Life of a Fireman*."

"You speak the truth, Fanny," the newsboy agreed.

He followed the sequence of the pageant in scene and brilliant paint. *The Night Alarm* came first. A yellow flame from the gas lamp in front of the engine house pointed to midnight on the clock face of its tower. A dozen men in red dragged out the engine. The background was blue-gray with smoke. Next was *The Race*. A glowing mass of flames colored the background. Trumpets were being played. The engines passed the green of City Hall Park and the City Hall. Speed was drawn in every line. Third came *The Fire* with hose playing on a red glare of flame that poured from the windows of one of the new tall three-story houses. A fireman was rescuing a child from a window. *The Ruins* was the last picture in the series. The firemen were starting for home. Smoking ruins were colored gray as a background for the bright hats and the painted fire engine.

What a set of prints! Scarcely waiting to thank Fanny, who gathered up the pictures and followed him, the boy ran, two steps at a time, down stairs.

On the main floor wooden bins built against the walls held the prints, the subjects separated by sheets of heavy paper. Mr. Currier made his selections for filling the pushcart. Prints of the recent horse races up at Saratoga Springs, the jockeys clinging to the horses' necks and making bright color splashes in their blue, red, and green jackets. *Across the Continent,* a picture of pioneering in which a cross-country locomotive spouted black smoke, some blanketed Indians watched from the plain, a crowd in leather and gay bonnets and shawls waited at the tiny log settlement for the train to draw in, and in the distance were green woods and blue mountains. These were popular prints, sure to sell, but on the top of the cart Mr. Currier laid the sets of prints that illustrated *The Life of a Fireman*, fresh and exciting.

"Well, I'm off, sir." The boy lifted the handles of the pushcart, but Mr. Currier stopped him.

"Not so fast, sonny."

He took from one of the bins his favorite picture and once more looked lovingly at the details, the soft and mellow colors. A farmhouse and barn, a sleigh with gaily dressed guests drawn up in front of the porch. Grandfather and Grandmother waiting to welcome them.

Mr. Currier had a sharp nose for news. Among his pictures popular in New York, peddled throughout the United States and even going by steamboat to Europe, were Niagara Falls in natural color, the Mississippi River showboats, baseball matches on bright emerald diamonds with color touches on the boys' hat bands, George Washington's birthplace on the

Potomac set within an old-fashioned garden, and even a *Rocky Mountain Scene,* the blue peaks touched to rose, a long sunny road, and the blue wagons, brown oxen, and red shirts of the drivers on the foreground. But Mr. Currier's favorite print was *Home to Thanksgiving.* He tacked it to the front of the pushcart as he had several times before.

"Now you're ready," he told the boy.

The newsboy turned away that Mr. Currier need not see his grin. *The Life of a Fireman* and all those other pictures would sell like hot cakes. But *Home to Thanksgiving!* Nobody in New York wanted to be reminded of going back to the farm. The ambition of country folk was to get to New York. Had he not tried to sell that picture that Mr. Currier and even Mr. Ives, too, seemed to be so fond of? The sample was getting a bit worn although the colors exposed to sun and air had blended and softened to mellow tints. He carefully tacked some news pictures to the sides of the cart, spread out the fire pictures on the top and rattled off, calling shrilly, "*The Life of a Fireman* in four scenes. Big and bright. Twenty-five cents a piece or seventy-five cents for the four. *The Life of a Fireman,* a Currier and Ives bargain. Here you are, fresh from the press, while they last!"

Pushing slowly home for noon dinner, the newsboy watched the breeze flapping *Home to Thanksgiving* that still hung like a banner on the front of the cart. All the other pictures had sold. He took courage to speak to Mr. Currier as the lithographer counted out the coins of his selling commission.

"You'll excuse me, Mr. Currier, but this country picture? Nobody seems to want it. Nobody wants to go back to the farm; they all want a chance to come to the city."

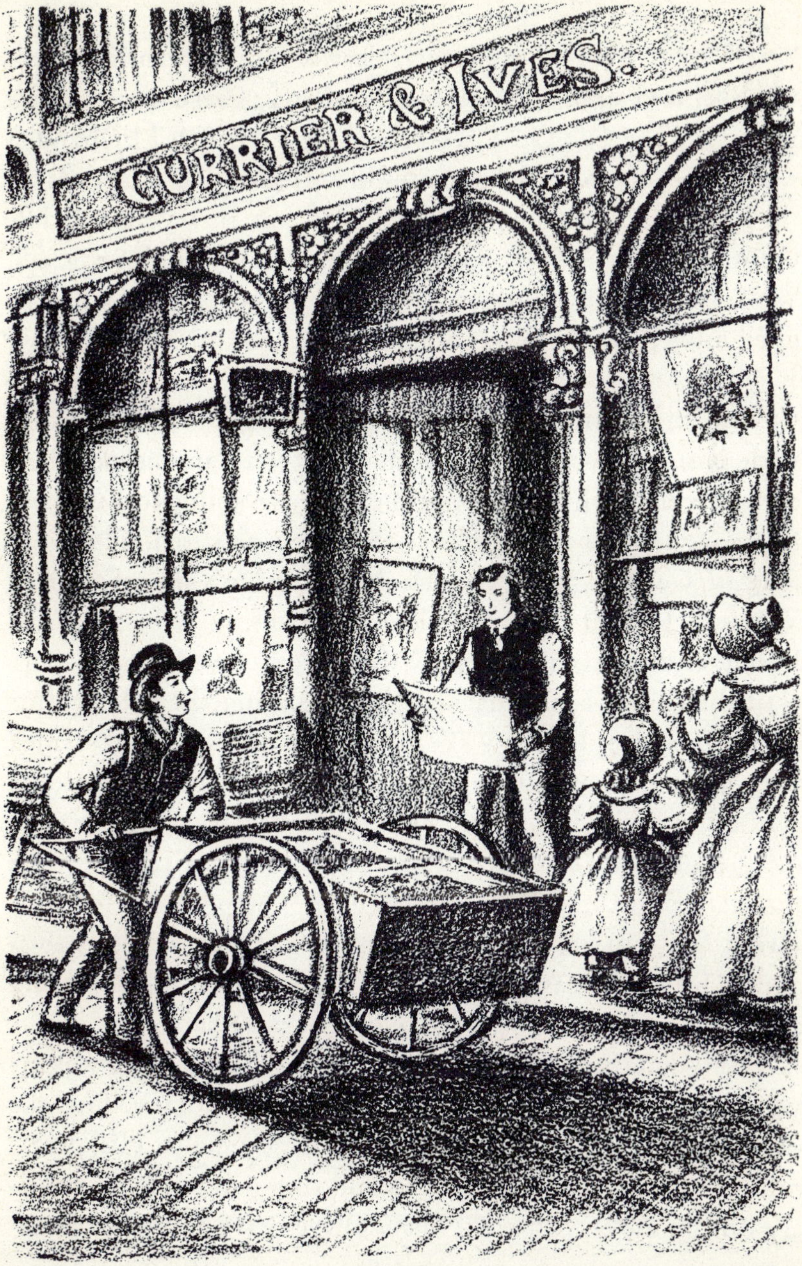
CURRIER & IVES.

Mr. Currier put the unsold picture in its old place in the bin. With it were other pictures dear to him, carefully drawn, well printed and colored from nature. There were *Maple Sugaring, The Old Grist Mill, Husking,* all painted by hand as were the other country pictures in soft glowing washes from the Austrian paint boxes. He decided not to try and peddle them for a while. Perhaps, he thought, they would never sell. Well, his growing business allowed him to picture what he liked as well as the news pictures.

Mr. Currier and Mr. Ives continued to get out lithographs with great speed, have them on the streets, in the peddlers' carts, on the trains, and even on steamers going to Europe a few days after the happenings that they pictured. The wedding of General Tom Thumb, Mr. Barnum's dwarf. Queen Victoria. United States Presidents; Madison, Jefferson, Van Buren, and Lincoln. George Washington copied from a portrait. Benjamin Franklin. These were among the color prints of notable people. New York pageantry, the streets filled with horse-drawn cabs and victorias, brilliant parasols, feathered bonnets, and dolmans, and gentlemen wearing the new colored gloves. *The Chicago Fire,* a magnificent picture with the waterfront in crimson and yellow. The public often preferred Mr. Currier's and Mr. Ives' news pictures to a newspaper. From the east to the west, north to south, they hung on parlor walls or lay in portfolios on center tables.

Then something unexpected happened. The camera was invented. The boy Nathaniel Currier's dream of speeding the news in pictures had been realized handsomely. His prints numbered about seven thousand and they pictured our country on the move. But sooty locomotives gave way to streamlined trains. Ancient victorias were replaced by automobiles. The covered wagons were pushed off the roads by motor busses. The cameras were speedier than the old lithographing stones; they even took to the air. Newspapers and magazines with colored illustrations were delivered from door to door, town to town, faster than Mr. Currier and Mr. Ives could peddle their lithographs. The bins in their shop gathered cobwebs and mice. That was a pity for the old bright prints had represented a miracle of speed. They pictured just what the growing United States had wanted in the nineteenth century.

With the years we changed again. Our nation was moving a little too fast and we slowed the automobiles and busses. We found the cities to be too crowded, and we returned to the country. It was still there, with brooks and pine woods, big barns with haymows, fields yellow with the harvest, and the doors of farmhouses open when Thanksgiving came. The colored prints of Mr. Currier and Ives were collected from bins and attics. Newspapers advertised for them. The first ones that had been colored with the old washes were sought after. The subjects, too, were given preference by collectors and a strange thing happened. *The Life of a Fireman, The Lightning Express, Clipper Ship, Westward the Course of Empire Takes Its Way,* were in demand and high prices were paid for them. But the country pictures into which the skill of Mr. Currier and his artists had put love as well as color were snatched from obscurity. They were hung in great collections, and decorated country houses in their ancient and mellowed tints. They showed a way of life that had made a great nation. The best-loved one of all, the scene that a lonely boy had seen from a bleak Boston street corner, became a legend as fourten hundred and fifty dollars was paid for the first edition of *Home to Thanksgiving.*

A Record of Prices Paid by Collectors for Early Currier and Ives Prints but Their Values Are Increasing

Home to Thanksgiving	$1,450
Other prints of the same	$975
	$900
	$825
	$800
The American National Game of Baseball	$1,500
Rail Shooting on the Delaware	$4,000
First of our sporting prints, Set of Six	
Emigrants Crossing the Plains	$875
Express Train	$850
Night Scene at an American Railroad Junction	$300
The White Mountains	$310
Maine Lighthouse	$550
The Trout Stream	$450
The Happy Family	$900
Winter in the Country	$500
The Old Grist Mill	$450
The Old Homestead in Winter	$425
The Life of a Fireman, single print	$320
Central Park. Skating Pond	$425

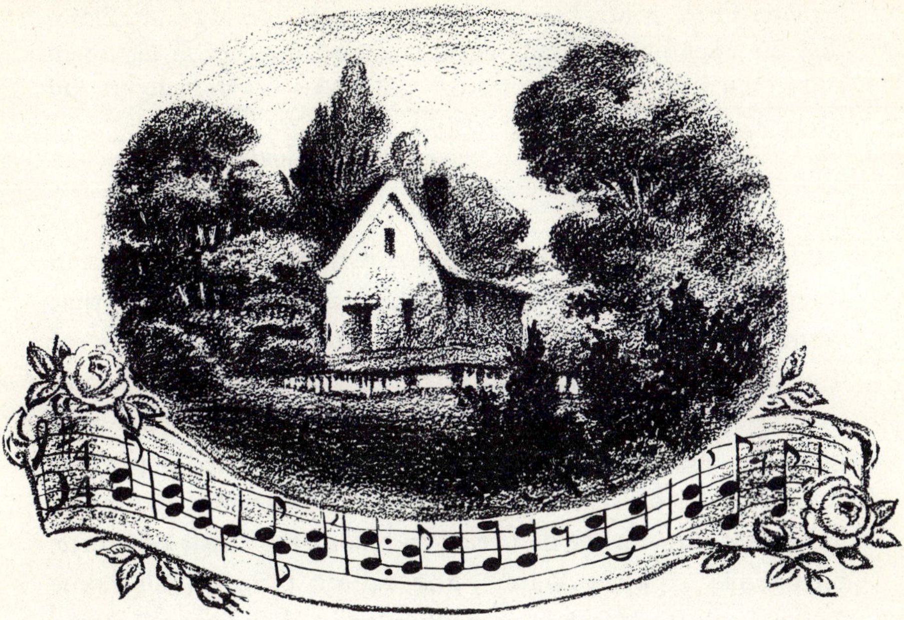

HE SET AMERICA TO MUSIC

STEPHEN's fingers ached but he wrote on:

Dear Mother:

It was jolly driving over here with brother William. Three hundred miles from home in an open sleigh, with bells on both horses and friends to visit all the way. William is now keeping store at Towanda and I am alone here at Athens, boarding at Mr. Herrick's and going to the Academy.

You and Father were right in sending me here. I played my flute and the piano instead of studying, but this is a lonely place. I walked out to Tioga Point one day after school. When the ice melts it will be pretty there, the Susquehanna River singing as it flows into the Chemung. I am taking philosophy, grammar, and arithmetic at school.

Well, I must tell you that I have no place to study as the

little ones here at Mr. Herrick's keep up such a crying and talking that it's impossible to read. There is a good fireplace in my room and if you will just say the word I will have a fire in it nights and learn something. I must stop writing as I am very cold.

Your loving son,
Stephen Foster.

He stamped on the bare floor and flung his arms to keep warm, a tall boy for thirteen, with black hair, dark eyes that wandered from everyday matters into his special land of dreams, and a sensitive mouth that drooped now with homesickness. He opened the carpet bag that had been his only luggage, to get out a stick of sealing wax. A folded paper was tucked under his shirts. He opened it and hummed the music he had set down as he had tried to record the rustle of leaves, bird songs, rippling waters, and falling twigs in his home woods back in Allegheny. Stephen twisted the music into a lighter for the fire he needed.

It was right that he should have been sent away from home to learn something useful. The Fosters were a large family and times were hard. He remembered his mother, loving music and able to write verse but now turning old clothes into new, getting the children off to school with full lunch boxes, marketing, keeping the old white house as neat as a pin, reading to him, Henriette, and Dunning beside the coal grate after supper. No matter how many tunes ran through her head, she never took time to sit down at the piano and improvise. He was always doing that, when they were skimping to pay for his schooling back in Allegheny.

Stephen lighted his candle and melted a drop of the sealing wax to fasten his letter. Downstairs, the Herrick children were still brawling in deafening discord. He put his flute to his stiff lips and blew a few notes. They jigged themselves into a plantation tune that the crews of the flat boats coming up from New Orleans sang. When Stephen went over to the Allegheny wharf to meet his father, home from a trading trip down South with sugar, coffee, and calico prints, he caught every note of those roustabout tunes. As he played his flute the noise downstairs quieted. He changed to the minor of a Negro spiritual that he had remembered on the Sundays when Olivia, who chored for the Fosters, took him to her church.

He had been nine then and he ran a theater in their old carriage house. The Foster boys and girls, Susan Pentland, their neighbor across the picket gate, and occasionally the old Negroes, Cuff and Ginger, who carried trunks up from the wharf, sang minstrel songs for an audience who paid in copper pennies. They sang very well, too, accompanied by Stephen's guitar; "Zip Coon," "Long-tailed Blue," and "Jim Crow." They all shared alike in the profits but Stephen was manager. That was the year 1835 and minstrelsy was the fashion. With blackened faces the minstrel shows had made Negro songs popular but they sang without taste or feeling. Young Stephen's amateurs had composed a bit under his direction; they had harmonized one song already that they liked. They called it "Away Down South Where the Corn Grows."

Indeed, he thought, home had been worth higher marks in school. Their house back in Allegheny faced the Common. The river was near and the growing town of Pittsburgh lay on the opposite bank. Kentucky was not far away and Stephen visited there at an old mansion with wide green lawns, shade trees and a grove in Bardsville. With his older sister Charlotte he had rare good times there. Jane McDowell back home had been a fine playmate too. Stephen used to make her bouquets daintily wrapped in lace paper and, being too shy to present them, old Black Joe who worked for the McDowells did it for him. He wished that he might hear even the gruff barking of the McDowells' dog Tray. All these memories had become precious.

They used to sing at the Kentucky home in Bardsville, gathered by candle light around the piano, Charlotte playing the accompaniments. The McDowells' Joe in Allegheny whistled jig tunes as he polished the silverware or tended the flower gardens in Jane's home. Echoes of home music thrilled Stephen, but America sang to him too as he fingered his flute in the chilly boarding-house room. From the Allegheny Common he heard in his homesickness a fife and drum corps marching to the rousing measures of "Hail Columbia." He piped that also on his fife, tramping up and down the room to fight the cold.

If he could only see the folks at home, just for a short visit! The old folks at home, Stephen called them to himself lovingly. His sweet-faced mother in her lace cap and shoulder shawl. His father, rugged in a great ulster and fur cap, as he bargained with the river boatmen. His brothers and sisters all older than he; Charlotte, Ann, Henry, Dunning, Henriette, and Morrison. Olivia, smiling as she served them with great platters of chicken and yams, waffles and hominy, was a person to miss also. Stephen laid aside the flute, blew on his fingers and sat down to work out tomorrow's sums.

A rap at the door interrupted him. Coals perhaps through the generosity of his landlord! But no. As Stephen opened the door a red-cheeked country boy in a sheepskin coat and cap with earlaps came in. His skates hung over his shoulder.

"I'm Willie Blake," he explained. "You're the new boy at the Academy, I take it. Whew, it's cold here! The way to get warm is to exercise. There's good skating out at the Point and some of us boys have a sleigh outside. Come along!"

"All right, I'll do that." Stephen closed his arithmetic without a regret.

The sleigh bells rang out a jingling call. He could leave the letter at the post-office. He threw on his ulster, tied his muffler tightly, and found his skates. As he started off with Willie he whistled a few bars that had been running through his mind, unwritten but haunting:

Way down upon the Suwanee River.
(Suwanee had just the right number
of syllables. Much better than
Allegheny.)
Far, far away.
That's where my heart is turning ever,
That's where the old folks stay.

It eased Stephen's loneliness to improvise, set his loneliness to music.

A letter from home brought an order for a basket of coals every evening and Stephen's fireplace glowed and crackled for his home work. He invited Willie Blake in to parse and figure but Willie was no scholar. They sat on the floor and cracked nuts and roasted apples.

"Listen, Willie, that log is singing!" Stephen said.

"Shucks, Stevie, you're off again. It's only green wood sizzling."

"When Jeannie McDowell and I used to roast apples back home, their old Black Joe put on a big back log for us."

"You like girls, Stevie?" Willie asked curiously. "Me, I don't care for them so much. Frances Welles, though, over at the Academy, is as good as a boy outdoors, knows the Indian trails, can build a fire with flint and tinder. Well, let's get on with this home work."

But Stephen was fingering his flute. Downstairs, again, the young Herricks became quiet and an older one timidly picked out a piano accompaniment with one finger as the boy piped,

> Way down upon the Suwanee River,
> Far, far away—

Willie Blake listened open-mouthed.

"That's a pretty piece, Stevie," he commented. "I'd like to learn how to play it."

"All right," Stephen held out the flute. "You do my home work and I'll teach you to play 'Hail Columbia.' "

"It's a bargain," Willie said solemnly. It was a poor bargain for both boys. Willie never learned fingering and Stephen's school work suffered, but he grew more at home in Athens.

Winter melted into spring. Athens, where old Indian roads came together at Tioga Point, the meadows and banks were lushly green and the willows along the Susquehanna tossed their branches in the soft wind, was pleasant. The yellow blooms of the chestnut trees danced. Little tributary streams sang as they bubbled over their stones. Stephen and Willie, truants often from the Academy, heard the notes of red-winged blackbirds, bluebirds, and larks. In the little town new life broke out in sounds. One Saturday a dancing bear wearing a string of bells lumbered along the main street. All the mules wore bells too. Thatchers with bundles of straw on their backs, glass-blowers, and turkey-drovers traveled along old paths from Tioga Point to town, singing and whistling for pleasure in the spring. The herb and perfume sellers called their wares in a musical sing-song. The brass band blared marching tunes, practising for the Fourth of July which was not so many weeks away.

Willie and Stephen, stretched out on a bank above the river one school day in June, were thoroughly enjoying themselves. Willie had picked a bunch of bluebells and was thoughtfully arranging and tying them with grass. Stephen was filling music paper with pencilled notes.

"I shall call this 'The Tioga Waltz,' Willie." He spoke more to himself than to his unfeeling but loved friend.

Willie would never be a musician but he had fought for Stephen in the Academy yard until Stephen had learned to use his fists.

"I don't know how long we can keep this up, Stevie." Willie looked anxiously in the direction of town. "I am getting behind in my own arithmetic to say nothing of yours."

"I am composing a waltz because everything seems to dance in the spring," Stephen explained. "If you look carefully at those branches you will see that the winds turn them in circles. The whippoor-will has a three-quarter note song—"

"I give you up, Stevie," Willie groaned. He put his bouquet in a spring of water and opened his lunch pail. "There's enough for two." He offered cheese and doughnuts. "Let's eat and then sleep."

He stretched out on the grass and closed his eyes. Stephen was so occupied with his composition that he did not hear the girl's footsteps until she was there, right upon them, their schoolmate at the Academy, Frances Welles. A good play-

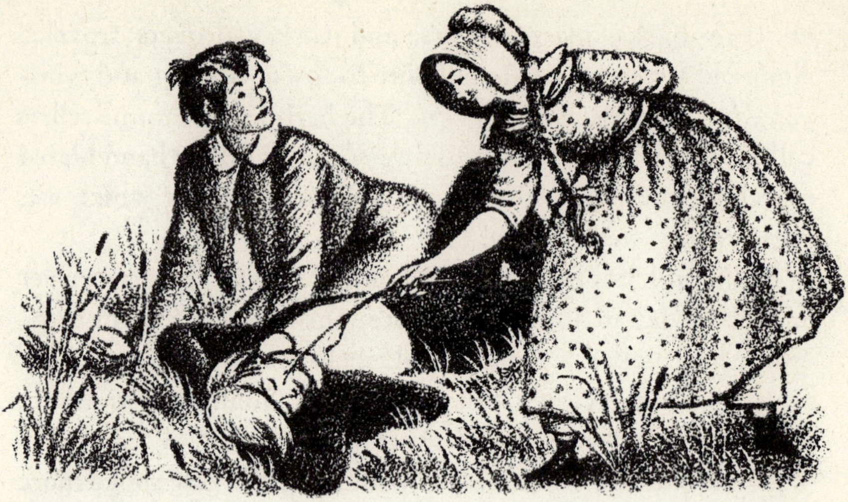

mate, too. She stood in front of them, starched and proper in her pink polka-dotted frock and sunbonnet, pulling at one flaxen braid. Stephen jumped up but Willie kept on snoring. Frances put her finger to her lips as Stephen started to speak. She pulled up a long grass blade and tickled Willie's nose. He sneezed, woke with a start, and looked ashamed.

"So here you are, two lazy truants!" she said. "Don't you know all the bad marks chalked up against you, and the term ending on the Fourth of July!"

"That is my birthday!" Stephen commented.

"And all the more shame to you, Stephen Foster," she scolded. "Suppose you are sent home in disgrace on your birthday!"

Stephen had thought of that himself. Willie bounded over to the spring for his bouquet of bluebells.

"I picked them for you." He offered them to Frances.

"Look, Frances," Stephen found words now. "I am writing a waltz, 'The Tioga Waltz.' I shall dedicate it to you." He wrote at the top of the music with a flourish,

To Frances Welles

"What do you think we ought to do, Frances?" Willie's round face lengthened with anxiety.

"Run!" Frances gripped a boy with each hand. "If we hurry," she gasped, "you won't be late for the afternoon session. I shall tell the master that you, Willie, had a stomachache that detained you. But Stephen was better engaged for he is a great composer of music!"

The Fourth of July came in with a parade of the Athens militia and the brass band tootling at the head. Willie and Stephen with C's on their report cards were passed on their promises to do better another term and sat in the front seats of the Presbyterian church at the finals of the Academy. Frances, as ruffled as a daisy in her white frock, looked anxiously but with pride at her two friends in need; Willie flushed and sweating in his tight collar and new shoes, Stephen pale but happy with a secret close to his heart. He wished that his mother were there for his birthday. She had sent him a new jacket with a velvet collar and a flowing black necktie cut from the polonaise of her best silk dress. Brother William had closed store and come over for the exercises. From cottages, farms, and town houses the Athens folk had come in their crinolines and stovepipe hats to sit expectant in the hard bull-pine pews, look expectantly up at the old pulpit painted ox-cart blue, where the Academy master stood to call out the marks. There were prayers, and an address then—

Abby Baxter—Average A
Alonzo Cutter—Average B +
Ebenezer Drew—Average A —

One by one the students went up to the platform to receive their report cards.

Stephen Foster—Average C
William Blake—Average C
Frances Welles—Average A

Sighs from the audience, and then applause as the C's were forgotten in Frances' A, were silenced when the schoolmaster made an announcement.

"The skill in musical improvisation by one of the Academy pupils, Stephen Foster, has compensated for his poor record. 'The Tioga Waltz,' written for three flutes by Stephen, will now be given its first public performance."

They went up front, Willie's shoes squeaking all the way. Frances stood in the middle, with a boy on each side. Willie got off to a bad start but Stephen's sure clear fluting set him right. One, two, three! The parents began tapping in time to the bright melody. Stephen's tune danced with flowing brooks, sang with merry bird calls, and rustled with forest leaves in summer zephyrs. Light, gay, with Willie's accompaniment and Frances' noble help, "The Tioga Waltz" thrilled, rippled, floated to its end. They were confused by the applause that began, continued, did not stop.

Willie whispered, "Play that other tune, Stevie, the one you made up when you were homesick."

Stephen's fingers found the notes. His eyes saw beyond the listeners, way back home, as the flute cried with wordless longing.

Way down upon the Suwanee River,
Far, far away.
That's where my heart is turning ever,
That's where the old folks stay.

Stephen's marks were better his next year at the Athens Academy, but he went home to stay at the end of the spring term. The entire family, his mother most of all, wanted him. She had decided that Stephen should have piano lessons and so enter the great music world of Mozart, Beethoven, and Weber. His father wanted to take him to call on a visiting Englishman, Mr. Charles Dickens, then in town. His home had never before seemed so precious to Stephen. He learned the principles of harmony, but simple improvisation pleased him better. When he was sixteen a local music publisher printed his song, "Open Thy Lattice, Love." The inspiration was his secret but the white latticed gate that opened into Susan Pentland's garden had made him compose that melody. The sales provided him with all the music paper he needed.

With the years Stephen Foster's songs echoed from north to south, east to west. They set all America singing of home and country, friends and the everyday doings of our growing nation. They recorded the unwritten folk music of the Negroes. They were beloved because the composer had harmonized precious memories. They were published by the thousands in sheet music form with pictures on the covers. They took places of honor on home pianos, were sung by white and colored people alike. They thrilled with hope and dreams, patriotism and faith.

Loved most of all was "The Old Folks at Home," the song of homesickness that the boy Stephen had improvised out of his own loneliness in a chilly boarding house and later given words. "The Tioga Waltz" had its day, but the songs were whistled, orchestrated, chorused, hummed, programmed everywhere. "The Old Folks at Home," today the most widely printed song in collections, was learned and rendered by Christine Nilsson, the Swedish prima donna, when she first gave a concert in New York in 1872. Echoing the boy Stephen's lonely days were "Happy Hours at Home" with a picture on the cover of a lady playing the piano; "My Old Kentucky Home" in memory of playdays with the children at the white-pillared mansion in Bardsville; "Old Black Joe"; "There's a Good Time Coming"; "Old Dog Tray"; and "Jeannie with the Light Brown Hair," that song of Stephen's best-of-all girl. "Oh, Susannah," and "We Are Coming, Father Abraham," were grand fife and drum tunes for Lincoln's soldiers. "Down Among the Cane Brakes," "Nelly Was a Lady," "Sitting in My Own Cabin Door," were songs whose phrases had drifted up the Mississippi and Ohio to a boy who watched the river boats with his father. These and almost two hundred other popular songs Stephen Foster wrote.

Voices of minstrels, old banjos, and fiddles were stilled at last. The tinkling keys of square pianos yellowed and their strings rusted. Blue and gray of the War Between the States faded and were replaced by khaki. Blues and swing crowded out the waltz. Stephen Foster found himself at last in another homesick place, a New York lodging house, alone, ill, but still hearing his country's voices. He always had poor marks so far as worldly success goes, but turn on the radio! Encore a concert star! Open that new collection of songs everybody loves!

"Way Down Upon the Swanee River."
"Jeannie With the Light Brown Hair."
"My Old Kentucky Home."
America set to music by Stephen Foster!

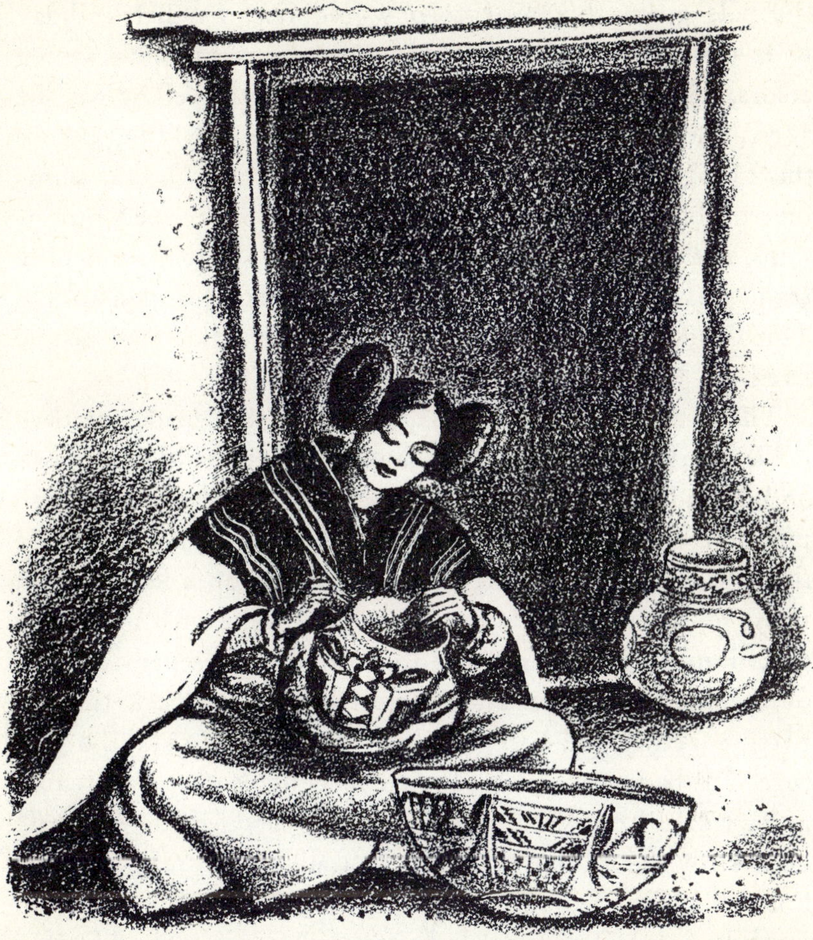

THE YELLOW BOWL

FROM where she stood, at the top of the sky-ladder, Nampeyo could see all of the First Mesa, her home. Terrace upon terrace of stone houses. The pink of peach bloom that covered the sand dunes. Freshly plowed fields where soon the pale green shoots of corn would rise. Farther still lay wide plains touched with the colors of bright sand; sacred colors, white for the East, blue for the South, yellow for the West, and black for the North. Her whole world lay before this Hopi girl; the Painted Desert of Arizona, the far glimmer of blue rivers, the distant line of snow-topped mountains. A thin spiral of smoke told Nampeyo that the morning train was pulling in. Yesterday and today blended in the Third Mesa, but it was yesterday in which the Hopi people lived.

There, at the top of the natural steps that made the sky-ladder in the rocks, Nampeyo saw the Medicine Man at work on his sand painting. He bent before the Hopi shrine, a high pile of rocks out of which grew flowering shrubs and wild flowers. He was designing a sacred picture on a flat space in front of the shrine, sifting the colored sand with incredible precision through thumb and fore-finger. The separate colors of the sand filled small containers of juniper bark that he fitted together and laid on mosaic-fashion to make the picture. He had outlined a plumed serpent in the center and, as he worked outward, the figure was blocked in with half circles for the rainbow, circles for the clouds, and geometric lines that outlined rain and lightning. The Medicine Man looked up as he heard the light tap of Nampeyo's red leather boots. A smile broke the mass of wrinkles that made his face a map of Hopi character.

"So our Nampeyo is now a woman," he commented. "Last week you were a little girl, running races and playing with your Katchina. Your black braids flew with the breezes and your feet were as swift as the wind. Today your hair is worn in butterfly coils behind your ears. You have silver and turquoise jewelry at your throat and on your arms. Your long dress is cut from the White Man's cotton."

"I shall not go to school any longer," Nampeyo told him. "I am thirteen years old. When I grind the corn meal for my mother I shall save a few grains to feed the butterflies, for they know how to make themselves beautiful and will teach me."

The Medicine Man frowned. "A Hopi girl does not need to think of her face but her soul." He added soberly, "You have a straight back and dark, far-seeing eyes. Your mouth is a scarlet bow and your voice is as clear as that of a bird. Take no pains save to be a good member of the Mesa."

She laughed, "My boy friend says that the Hopi girl who wants to sing should cherish the mocking bird, who is never the same but always repeats in his tune the opinions of others. Old man, do you know that my boy friend has already begun weaving a wedding shawl? It will be of the finest white wool with a border that shows raindrops, butterflies, birds, and clouds."

"Do you know the meaning of the wedding shawl?" he asked. "It is a garment of brightness in which the bride may walk fittingly where birds sing and the grass is green."

Nampeyo hummed a few bars of a chant. The sun made the Medicine Man's sand painting glitter as if each grain were a tiny jewel. Spring caressed her cheek. No dull lessons in school for a girl old enough to wear her hair in those great black coils that gave her face dusky wings! She couldn't be serious, but the Medicine Man held up one wrinkled hand.

"Do you know what you are singing? That is the Hopi chant of beauty. Repeat the words after me."

" 'As it used to be long ago, may I walk.' "

Nampeyo echoed the words:

As it used to be long ago, may I walk.
May it be beautiful before me.
May it be beautiful below me.
May it be beautiful above me.
May it be beautiful around me.
In beauty is it finished.

Nampeyo ended the chant, " 'In beauty is it finished.' "

A shrill whistle split the air. The Medicine Man gathered together his containers of colored sand, rose and started down the steps in the rocky terrace.

"The train is in. I must meet it with the curios the tourists want; my hurried weaving with factory-spun wools and cheap dyes for the blankets, silver ornaments hammered to suit the tourists' price, and the pottery." He sighed. "Nampeyo," he warned as the girl joined him and they descended to the Hopi village, "the fine yellow bowls of our fathers are gone. Only fragments remain in the ruins of old Hopi towns. They were beautiful, molded generously with room to breathe from the design of birds' nests, fired with the strong life colors of our race. White was laid on the yellow to signify the light of morning, red, for the glow of evening, and the border was bright with the colors of the rainbow. Our earth still holds the same colored clays but the art of using them is gone."

"Good-by, Medicine Man."

Nampeyo gave a little dance step as they came down to the terrace where she lived and he continued on his way to the railroad station. She liked the old man. He had given her the Katchina which she now took out of the deep pocket in her skirt. But the Medicine Man was old-fashioned, the boys and girls thought. They respected but did not heed him.

She held the small figure of the Katchina up to the sunlight. That was no ordinary doll. It was carved of soft cottonwood, the sacred wood of her people. It was painted in patterns of the tribe's beliefs; the feathered head-dress, flat painted feet, embroidered skirt, and masklike face were in imitation of the Rain Dancer's costume. When she was a child the Medicine Man had led the Rain Dancers and given the Katchina to Nampeyo. All the little ones of the village were given these dolls made in the Kiva by the dancers and held in reverence by the boys and girls who received them.

Now Nampeyo, being thirteen, must give up dolls. She was sorry about that. She had met a girl from the East once at the railroad station who had told her of the fluffy-skirted, blue-eyed dancing doll, a boudoir doll she had called it, that sat upon her bed at home. That girl had laughed at the stiff Katchina Nampeyo carried with so much pride.

"Does the boudoir doll speak to you?" Nampeyo had asked.

"Speak!" the girl had ridiculed Nampeyo. "You are an odd girl to believe a doll can talk."

Remembering this, Nampeyo came home. In the one large room of their house her mother was grinding the last of the winter's corn on the great stone in the center. It was a pleasant room hung with gay blankets, the family's clothing, and the ceremonial masks. Low couches covered with more soft blankets lined the walls. Nampeyo had enjoyed a free childhood; coming and going as she pleased, never scolded unless she touched a dancing costume or a painted mask, never frightened except when she was warned against fire or falling off a cliff. Now she would be a young woman in that room. She started to hang the Katchina on a hook in the adobe wall beside her mother's old doll. There it would remain, a relic, to be revered but not touched.

But an impulse stopped Nampeyo. She seated the Katchina, stiff and staring, on the white wool of her bed blanket. A boudoir doll? Why not?

Her mother smiled assent. "Wait a while before you put it away. Your grandmother used to tell me that the Katchinas were the spirits of living Indians who had their homes in the mountains. In the summer they descended secretly to the valleys, bringing us gifts of sweet melons and corn from their immortal farms. And your grandmother told me, also, that a Katchina doll has a message for those who can hear. Let it remain there on your bed, daughter. I fancy it humiliates a Katchina to hang from a hook."

Nampeyo had a busy day. She watched the sales the Medicine Man made to the tourists. She helped with the corn grinding at home, swept the floor, kneaded bread and weeded the new garden. After supper, she sat a moment on the edge of her bed beside the Katchina. It was fast growing dark. Shadows of long garments and masks were thrown from the wall upon the clay floor and Nampeyo could imagine them alive. The Katchina's eyes were bright. Nampeyo was alone. Her father and brothers were working down in the valley where the men lived in a camp until the fields were plowed and planted. Her mother had gone to teach a weaving design to a neighbor. The inanimate objects of the room seemed alive to the girl. The eyes of the Katchina seemed to move, then rest on a dark corner. Echoing among the cliffs came the notes of a drum. Their deep tones beat through the night,

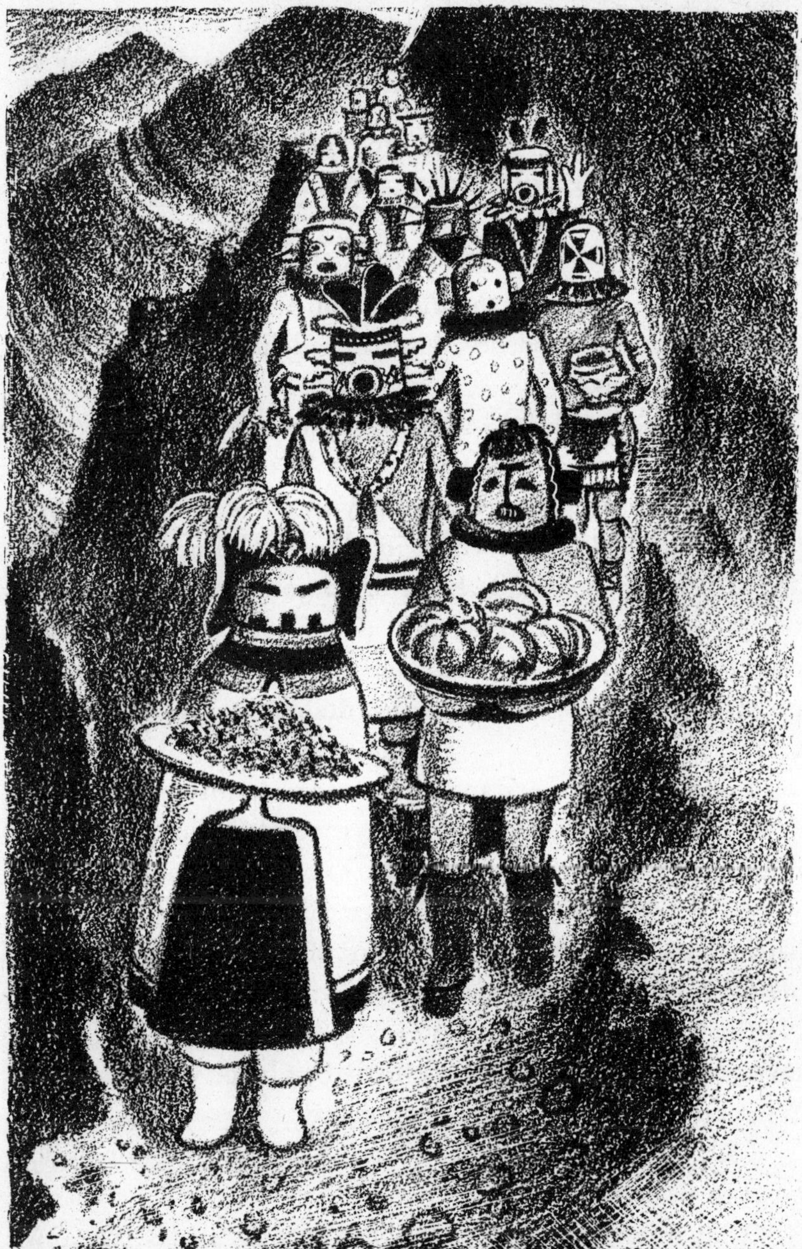

closer and closer. Nampeyo ran out of the house trembling, almost fell upon the Medicine Man who was drumming his footsteps home.

"The Katchina is alive!" Nampeyo gasped. "It is looking toward something in the room that I cannot see." She clung to the old man's hand.

"Foolish little girl!" He smoothed her hair. "Show me." Together they entered the dim room.

"There, in that corner. She turned her eyes that way," Nampeyo gasped.

"Then the Katchina wanted us to follow her eyes. Come, let us see what these dusty things are."

The Medicine Man led Nampeyo to a discarded heap of pottery tools. He lifted them in turn, blowing off the dust. There were spoons made from dried gourds, colored pebbles for polishing, paint brushes made of soap weed, some old round molds, the stones left from an ancient firing kiln, and pointed stone tools for drawing designs on the surface of soft clay.

"Your grandparents and their ancestors of ancient times made good pottery," he said. "They molded and decorated it slowly, in peace and well-being. They did not mold cheap ware for the tourist trade. Your family has kept these tools because they were precious. Even these gourd spoons were blessed by the Hopi priests. Look at your long nimble fingers, Nampeyo. When you were a very small child you used to dig up our colored clays and shape little bowls for your Katchina. Who knows what a doll remembers?"

"I like the feeling of clay. Perhaps I could mold a yellow bowl in beauty now?"

"That might come to pass," the old man said softly. "We

still have clay in the same colors as when the Katchinas came down from the mountains bringing seed in pottery bowls to the Hopi farmers. They copied the bowl of the sky in shaping it. They drew pictures of the rain, the crescent moon, the hills, and the feathers of birds on their ware. The old Hopi potters thought they were making up their designs as they worked but, no, the Katchinas were guiding their hands."

Nampeyo's eyes shone. "Could I make a bowl, a yellow bowl, all myself?" she begged. "I can't play with my doll any longer, but I should like to keep the Katchina as a companion."

The old man nodded his head. "So it shall be," he agreed. "When you have finished your home duties, bring the Katchina up the rock steps to the shrine. There we will collect and sift our colored clay, yellow, red, and white. We will build a kiln and look about us at the sky, the earth and the birds and beasts for our designs. You shall be a potter, Nampeyo. Would you like that, my girl?"

"Oh, so much!"

She held his gnarled hand in thanks and watched him as he started to climb up, up, to his house, the dark trembling with the first stars and his drum beats thrilling back, bringing old, better Hopi days to life. Then she went inside and lay down beside the Katchina holding the doll close, and was soon fast asleep.

All spring, all summer, Nampeyo spent her free time with the Medicine Man. The other young people wondered at her interest in the old priest and his strange fancies. Sand painting had gone out of fashion in the First Mesa, and the pottery on sale at the railroad station was quickly turned on a wheel and painted with stencilled colors in patterns that meant nothing. But Nampeyo and her ancient friend were keeping a secret. It took months to work out.

The clay that they dug out of near-by pits had to be finely winnowed through a basket, then the fine pure earth that was left was again sifted through a blanket. They built a stone kiln near the shrine and gathered cornstalks when harvest time came, for drying and feeding the fire. The paints had to be mixed; black was distilled from the bee-plant and stored in earthen jars. Laying black on the colored clay was an old Hopi painting art. An orange-red paint was made from iron deposits in the earth. Their kiln had a grate that the Medicine Man found in some ruins on which the pottery rested as it was slowly fired. As it hardened the pottery would turn yellow, orange, or brown, according to the skill of the potter. While they made ready for modeling a bowl that would be the most beautiful Nampeyo had ever seen, the Medicine Man talked to her, explained what each step of the art meant to the Hopi people.

"Roll the clay into smooth long coils," he told her. "The overlapping of these coils will build the bowl high and smooth for the painting. Shape it from the inside out and then smooth it with your tool. That sharp stone is for drawing the design. Choose an old picture; straight lines and curves may be combined to show the rain filling the earth with running water; a cross will be a star; a half circle draws the crescent moon. Fill in your lines with paint, earth black or red. We shall dry the bowl in the sun a little and then fire it. Ah, my child, you take to the art as if the Katchinas themselves had taught you."

The Katchina watched through the months Nampeyo

spent learning. It stood on a step of the rock stairway or peered with its sharp little eyes out of Nampeyo's pocket. As Nampeyo mixed clay with powdered rock and water for hardening the clay, rolled the long coils and wound them into deep bowls that would fit the molds the Medicine Man carved, drew and painted the designs in black or deep red on yellow, tended the firing, she grew in artistic skill.

"Will anyone like our work?" she asked her old friend as another spring came to the Third Mesa.

Again the plowing and planting began; the bleating of new lambs was heard, and the whistle of the trains came up to them from the valley.

"Wait and see," he told her. "Today we shall take our work down to the station. Your pottery will be different from the cheap ware the tourists expect to buy as souvenirs of Hopi art. Never, in my long life, have such beautiful bowls as yours been displayed."

One spring day a train emptied itself of curious travelers at the railroad station of the First Mesa. They swarmed the sunny platform and crowded about an old man who wore the ancient blanket and head-dress of his ancestors. Beside him was Nampeyo, her eyes shining with pride. About the two were set the pieces of pottery for which their people in the beginning, for centuries back, had been famed. The smoothly shaped bowls gleamed in polished surfaces from the firing. The designs were the life patterns of the Hopis; precious clouds dripping rain for the crops, the heavens at night full of stars, the feathers that covered their friend the eagle, the glowing colors of the earth at harvest.

Nampeyo's friend, the girl from the East, was one of the first off the train. "Here you are again, Nampeyo!" she laughed. "And your hair is up in the butterfly coils. What a lovely turquoise bracelet! But, oh, my dear, there is that funny old doll sticking its head out of your pocket. For shame, when you must be at least fourteen years old!"

Nampeyo's rosy cheeks deepened in color. But before she could think of anything to retort, a man separated himself from the others, lifted a yellow bowl of Nampeyo's making, and exclaimed as he held it with tender grasp to the light. "Who made this?" he asked the Medicine Man. "It must return with me to the Museum. It is a perfect example of the lost art of Hopi pottery design."

"Who but our Nampeyo, inspired by the tradition of the Katchinas, Professor," he replied. "She is now a young woman and she plans to give her life to the art of her ancestors."

"But the Medicine Man taught me," Nampeyo hastened to break in.

"Look, daughter," the professor said, turning to Nampeyo's friend. "Never has our Museum had so beautiful an offering. Ask this girl to explain it to you."

The Katchina listened, forgotten in Nampeyo's pocket as the two girls talked, fair curls flying close to the dusky ear-coils, blue eyes and brown shining as Nampeyo told of the joy of making the yellow bowl. The weaving, the jewelry designing of the First Mesa there in Hopi land were forgotten in this surprising revival of a forgotten art. Nampeyo was the star, the Medicine Man the hero of the occasion.

Spring faded into summer. The sun ripened the corn and melons, winter came with long days for kneading more clay, modeling and painting more colored bowls in Nampeyo's home. Another year came, and she was there at the station with even more beautiful examples of her work; bold black designs of birds, tadpoles, the dragon-fly, leaves and flowers on pale cream slip; the humming-bird, conventionalized ears of corn and butterflies on orange, yellow and cream pottery.

As long as he could the Medicine Man taught her and explained the meaning of her work to visitors to the First Mesa. She wore the wedding shawl, and ground her own corn. Then Nampeyo was alone with her art. At last she was blind, but her fingers had wrought the art so long that she did not need her eyes. She sat on a sheepskin, surrounded by her work, still offered ancient Hopi pottery to those who cared to learn from it.

Not a story girl, but a real person in our art life was Nampeyo. Her long life was given over to the revival of Hopi pottery making. Because of her work preserved in museums and carried on by her pupils, we may learn the meaning of art in the lives of a primitive people in our land. The people of the First Mesa followed her lead. As we study the design of curves, lines, steps, triangles, and crescents in rich colors on her bowls, as we translate them into the symbols of Hopi life, we find that useful things may be beautiful, that beauty may last longer than men and machines.

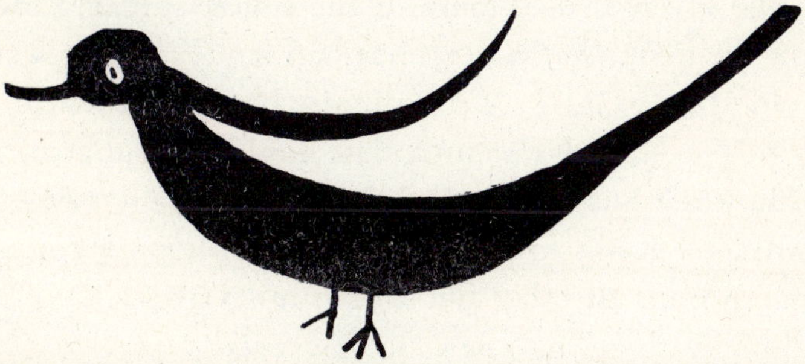

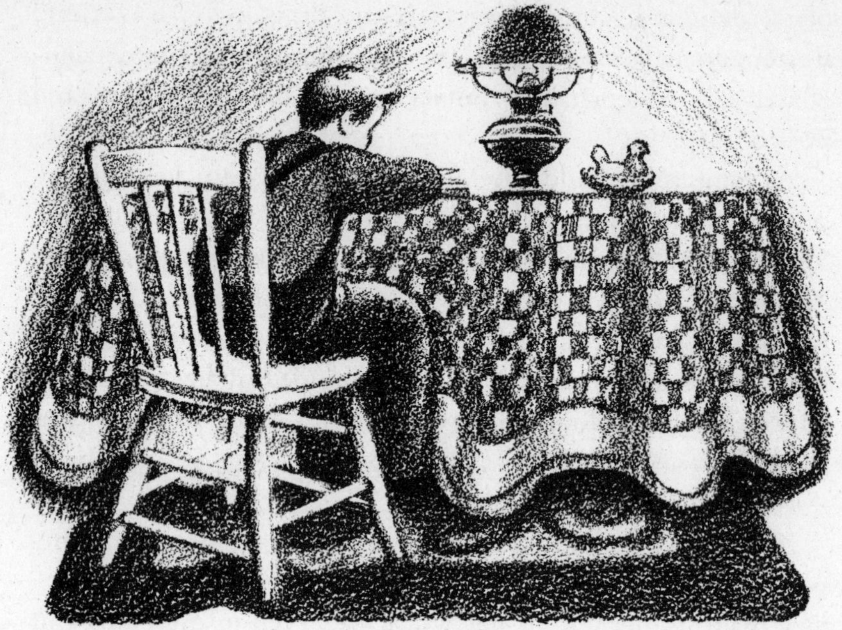

AMERICAN GOTHIC

IT WAS the pleasantest time of the day there on the Iowa farm, after-supper time. Grant Wood sat at the kitchen table, cleared and covered with the red-and-white checked cloth. The green-shaded lamp in the center spread a mellow light on the book that a neighbor had lent him. He was ten years old that year, 1902; a plump boy, short, with blue eyes, a pug nose and a mouth that could be stubborn if he liked. He was a busy boy, helping his father raise sweet corn and tomatoes, going to the district school, hoping for a trip to Cedar Rapids that lay but thirty miles away. One could visit a library there, he knew, see pictures.

But what was the need of traveling, Grant thought? Here, spread open upon the table, lay a dream world ready for him to enter. It was a copy of *Grimm's Fairy Tales* that a neighbor had lent him, fascinating with its colored pictures.

His eyes had always seen farther, found richer scenes, than the other children at school. The green of the cornfields changed through his vision to brilliant blues. The earth touched by sunrise and sunset, mists and high noon became rose-pink and purple. The faded blue of the threshers' overalls, the crimson, purple, and gold of his mother's jellies in their Mason jars enchanted Grant. He settled down to enjoy the pictures in *Grimm's Fairy Tales,* longing to paint one himself.

There was one most enchanting picture of barnyard hens like his own Leghorns and Plymouth Rocks, massing their bright plumage around a gaudy strutting cock. As he scattered corn for their fowls, Grant had noticed each curve and line, tint and shade of the flock. Now, with that picture before him, he felt like a painter. But a shadow crossed the threshold. He felt a kindly touch on his shoulder. A firm earth-stained hand closed the book.

"You must return this book." Grant Wood's father told him. "It is a volume of fancy. We Quakers read only the truth."

Grant's face tightened into lines of stubbornness, wrinkled as he was close to tears. Then he smiled. It was a proud heritage, his father had told him, to be born a Quaker, especially to be born of pioneering Quakers. After all, he did not need *Grimm's Fairy Tales* to show him pictures. They spread out before him from cornfields to the sky. He put the book under his arm and started over the fields to return it.

As he trudged along, he turned the pages of the picture book that was growing in his mind. Everyday pages, but all the better for their homeliness.

Some of those everyday pictures had come to him in the late afternoon of the home barnyard as he fed the fowls. Arbor Day at school painted another one. Back of the school lay a checkerboard of plowed fields with new corn sprouting in green blades. The little school itself was a white spot outside of which Grant and a few barefooted boys and girls in blue jeans and gingham, with the school-ma'am, were gathered about the slender young tree they had planted beyond the school door. That was one picture to keep, and it had highlights, for his father had passed by in their farm wagon and waved to the Arbor Day party. No refreshments, no musical program, no speeches, just starting a new tree, but that had made it an occasion.

He saw their evenings at home popping corn. His father, seated in a wooden chair, held a yellow bowl in his lap into which Grant and his brothers piled the white balls of bursting corn, each kernel a different shape, golden with the melted butter they poured on. He remembered the time of the threshing when farmhouse and barnyard had been a picture cut through the center into scenes. In one, his mother and the other women bent over the stove cooking and carrying big platters of food; another scene was painted in the boy's memory by the long table at which the threshers sat in their farm clothes, all alike, blue overalls and checkered shirts; the far scene was the yard where his father was washing at the water trough, a horse waited and the hens were crowding toward the threshold.

Good pictures, these! Grant thanked their neighbor for the

book; explained with a lift of his head. "It is ever so nice, but we Quakers read only true things."

He thought as he came home, "True things make the best pictures too!" He had a scant half hour before dark and he went into the house. He had a studio and he was going to work in it until bedtime.

Grant Wood's studio was under the table. The checkered red-and-white table cloth draped itself over the edges tent-fashion and was lifted at one side to let in the light. Grant had some sheets of the cheap cardboard that came as partitions in the boxes of soda crackers they bought in Cedar Rapids. He had a red crayon and he was drawing on a cardboard his pet Plymouth Rock hen, each feather etched and counted. It was as satisfying as the farmyard of the Brothers Grimm.

When Grant Wood's father died, the boy gave up his kitchen studio. That was because he had become the man of the house. The family moved to Cedar Rapids where his mother bought a home with garden space. That was a bold move, with the father gone, and Grant raised vegetables to sell, milked the doctor's cow and sold water from the artesian well to help support them all. They had been a prosperous family until the father went. Now, instead of drawing after supper, Grant Wood watched the kitchen door anxiously. He had heard what the neighbors were saying about the Wood family; that he, a boy, was helping keep the wolf from the door. No one had ever seen or heard a wolf there in town but that only increased the boy's concern. He must work harder. Drawing had to be a luxury, chores and gardening came first.

He was graduated from high school. Later an Iowa school

had a new teacher one day. It was a class of tough boys and the last teacher had given up, for they preferred outdoors to the schoolroom, sticks and stones to arithmetic. The new teacher was a thickset, blue-eyed young man with a cheerfully tilted pug nose and light russet hair. He wore overalls. He must keep his school job and earn a suit. But he liked the job and the tough boys. When a number of them stayed out in the school yard, tardy in returning after recess, the new teacher invited the rest of the class to join them and they chose objects and scenes in the surrounding fields and town that they would like to paint or model in clay or even build with wood and cement, if they played fair with the three R's. As Grant Wood, the teacher, stood in the school yard, watched the barefooted boys in overalls and suspenders, he saw again his own schooldays, the picture of Arbor Day that he had painted in dreams when he was ten years old.

Teaching school and later working in a jeweler's shop to pay for his tuition at the Art Institute of Chicago filled the years from Grant's boyhood to his young manhood. The wolf that had threatened their home doorstep became only a nightmare. It was a time of nightmares. Our country was close to the First World War. People as well as nations were in disruption. Grant Wood felt that the home folks might need him. He went home and found this to be true. The Cedar Rapids home had been lost and his mother and sisters were living with an aunt. The wolf had found their doorway.

The way to kill a wolf is to fight it. Grant bought a lot for fifty dollars in the wooded hills of Kenwood near by, paying one dollar down and promising one more dollar each month. The house that he built on it was little more than a one-story shack but berries, mushrooms, and rabbits were

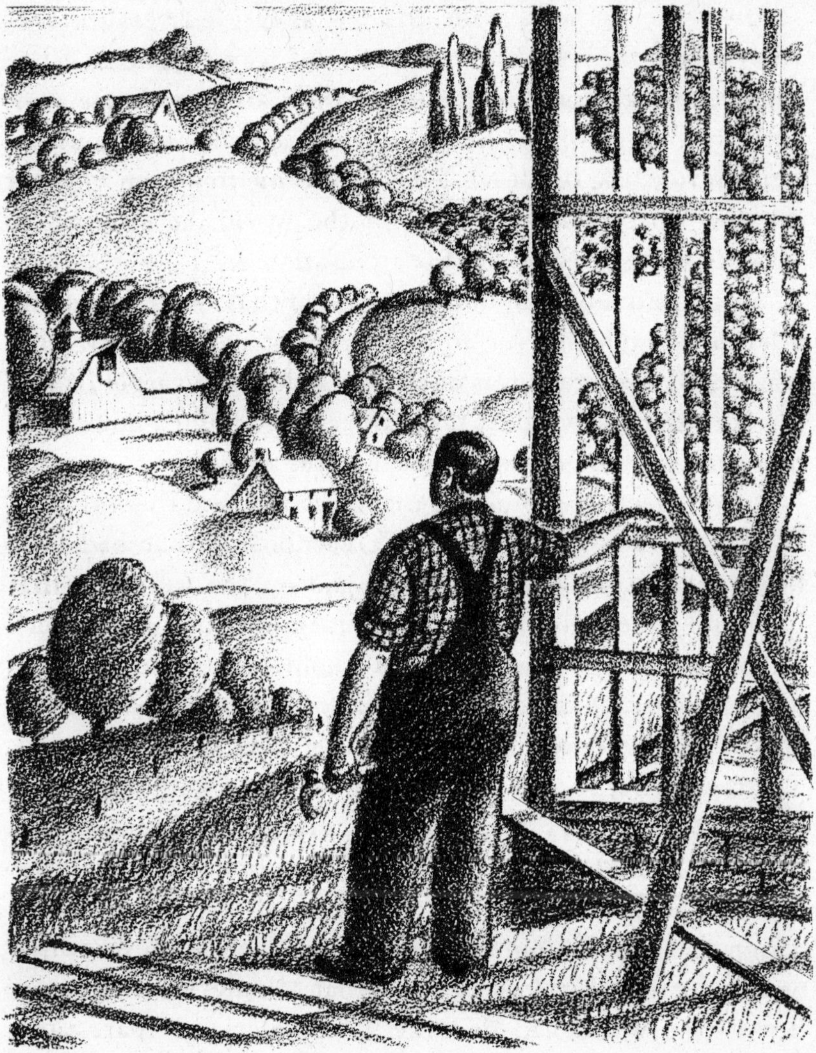

plentiful and the earth was as velvet soft as it had been back on the farm. As he raised the walls and laid on the roof, Grant saw hills closer, the rounded outlines of the trees, like green globes, toy-small houses set on the pattern of evenly spaced squares that the fields made. He saw as fertile rivers the furrows of the fields he had crossed on his way to school. When night came, the patter of rain on their lost farmhouse roof, the tangy scent of the buffalo robe when they had gone for a sleigh ride, the tinkle of sleigh bells came to him in pleasant dreams. There wasn't a thing in the world, he thought, so good as being alive in the Iowa countryside.

A pal, watching him build, suggested that Grant build him a house in exchange for an adjoining lot in Kenwood. That was a gift, for Grant was discovering that any carpenter can put up a bungalow but it takes an artist to build a home. The house he constructed on his new lot was a home.

Grant selected his building materials and used them as carefully as he had the cracker-box cardboards that had been his first canvases. He mixed and laid on the stucco so that it would take paint well. The dimensions of his mother's room, the deep window ledges to hold plants and the glass jars of the summer's jellies and jams, all the wood, plaster, and cement were combined to achieve their special purposes. The mellowing stucco made the house blend with the meadows. The windows were rightly placed for framing the sweep of the land. It was a small house but building it was important. Grant Wood's hands acquired the skill in strong design that grows from the ground up. There was everything needed for a new American art in that Middle-Western scene. But Grant Wood had no canvas, no colors, no spare time. And there was always his need of earning. He timed his hopes.

"Tomorrow." "When the building is done." "Next year." Then, "After the war." Next, "When this term's teaching is ended." For the popular new art instructor in a Cedar Rapids school, who taught in a faded Army uniform, was Grant Wood. But the stream of his longing flowed on.

At last he had saved enough money to go to Europe on his summer vacation. A year or so later he made a second trip to Europe and attended the Julien Academy in Paris.

Paris and Julien's Academy of Art were the goal of all art students at that time. Grant Wood never learned to speak French but he starved himself into a few terms at Julien's and quite a few trips through Europe between the Armistice of World War I and 1928. He never acquired a current fashion in painting, although it was a period of style. He still drew with as solid design as he built a house, arranged his compositions as neatly as he had plotted his vegetable garden. When he splashed many coats of paint on a canvas, achieving the brilliance of the impressionists but the colors of an Iowa landscape; when he took pains in painting bunches of flowers as he remembered the pattern of wall paper that had come from a Chicago, U.S.A., mail-order house, his fellow students ridiculed him. But he found what he had been looking for in Europe. He found that the greatest artists had been homespun. Their canvases were as honest as a hand-spun-and-loomed fabric. They had found their inspiration in their native countrysides.

Grant Wood in Paris painted many French doorways, those thresholds and lintels that opened upon gay gardens, river fronts, streets with book stalls, flower carts, and friendly neighbors. He painted cottages and farms.

In 1927 he was commissioned to design the stained glass World-War window for the Memorial Union in Cedar Rapids. This window took two years to design and Grant went to Munich to supervise the making of it.

There, in the great museums of Germany he discovered that the appeal of medieval Bible paintings came from the fact that the artists had drawn the saints and sages, the prophets and martyrs walking and living in the German countryside. Always in the back of Grant Wood's mind had been the idea of homespun American art; pictures that would say to whoever looked at them, "I remember that. I was there once upon a time and I want to go again."

When he went back to the countryside where he had grown up, he brought with him the inspiration of German primitives, and French peasant art, but mainly his conviction that all of that, and possibly something better, waited for his pencil and palette in Iowa.

He painted his mother's portrait first. Not with the elegance of Whistler's mother in silk and lace and folded hands, but the pioneer woman of the Iowa farmhouse. Because crops and hard work were necessary, the western settlers treasured their small luxuries, an old cameo pin, a rare plant however stiff that had come with them all the long way as a slip or root and had been nursed to growth on a kitchen window sill. Grant Wood's *Woman with Plant* was a portrait of his mother wearing her kitchen apron, holding a long-leafed plant, her hands as true as the toil-worn ones that Rembrandt painted, her eyes looking beyond homely tasks to the unknown boundaries that a line of light drew along the horizon. He chose his subjects as our pioneering people of Iowa had lived them. His pictures were as understandable as an Iowa cornfield. He painted each figure, tree, furrow, farmhouse, so as to make the whole canvas important, not alone from the picture-book of his boyhood memories but as today of our Middle West.

He remembered an old farmhouse not far from their farm that had an odd window, arched, like a church window. Perhaps the window frame had come from a church and the thrifty builder had used it to save buying a new one. The arched window was placed at the upper story and a curtain of figured stuff caught the light when the sun shone. That curtain and the poor glass that broke the sunlight into color resembled stained glass. Nobody except Grant Wood had seen anything unusual in putting a church window, a Gothic window at that, in an Iowa farmhouse, way up in the attic too; but he kept the idea in his mind for a long time.

In a field near the house with the Gothic window, he had noted a farmer, his pitchfork upright, resting a second. The three-pointed fork reaching toward the sky was shaped like an ancient church candle-holder. In the door of the house he had seen the farmer's wife, wearing a clean bright apron trimmed with rick-rack braid. The Gothic window was almost as old as the Iowa prairies in its design, and the woman and the man, keeper and builder of the pioneer home, belonged in a picture. He would like to paint the man just as he had seen him, holding the pitchfork high, the light tipping the three polished prongs like candle flames. The window would be a background, and the woman would have the far-seeing eyes of all pioneering women. Pioneer men looked down at the earth but women like his mother and his sisters kept their eyes on the hills.

He talked about that scene to his mother and sisters. Then he painted *American Gothic*. This painting surprised, shocked, then delighted us as it was exhibited in many galleries of the United States. The twentieth century of American art had discarded the simplicity of the old limners, the wall painters, and the craftsmen in iron, glass, and stone. Their efforts toward beauty had gathered cobwebs in attics for a century; they were forgotten legends. But here, in *American Gothic,* was a memory of covered-wagon days, brought into the present. Grant Wood dared to lay on the color thickly and with brilliance. Everything about *American Gothic* was American. The woman's dress, the man's overalls, the pitchfork might have been ordered from a mail-order catalogue. The shabby house with the Gothic window, the woman who made the home and the man who held his three-pronged fork like a candle-bearer told their story in the painting. When *American Gothic* was first shown in the All-American exhibit of the Chicago Art Institute in 1933, it had two results. It made people smile, then turn homesick for the kind of living it showed. Today the painting has another charm; it draws and colors the everyday living we are returning to and for which we are grateful.

Following *American Gothic* Grant Wood painted *Fall Plowing,* the plowman, a minute figure in the foreground, moving slowly against a panorama of ruddy earth broken into great furrows, mellow shocks of corn like Indian braves marching toward the hills and the landscape molded in squares of green, russet, and blue. It was a picture that attracted city people, one that country people were proud to recognize.

His *Arbor Day* might be a colored television of the thousands of country schools we pass when we follow dirt roads; a few children in bare feet and jeans, one overworked teacher for young and older pupils, together making sure that the woods shall not pass away.

Dinner for Threshers is an Iowa stage set. As Grant Wood knew the days of hot, bright harvest weather, so he painted the scenes. Big dinners cooked on a wood stove, a lot of hungry men in faded blue overalls and checked shirts seated around a long table, washing at the pump, the cackling of fowls, and the clatter of knives on thick crockery; these belonged together as surely as summer came. When that canvas was hung, we listened, smelled, as well as saw.

Each one of Grant Wood's paintings tells a good story. The hills are smooth enough to slide down. The trees toss their branches like pyramids of balloons. The fields are hot. The young corn is as straight and brave as a division of troops marching to victory. The patterns of prairies and horizon could be posters of cut bright paper in their clearness and truth. The modeling is like sculpture. The colors are startling; we never forget them.

The Midnight Ride of Paul Revere paints a tiny horseman disappearing around a curve in the road, but the white church steeple almost touches the top of the canvas and the little wooden houses, set primly on the Green, could have been built of blocks. *Quilts* reminds us of an ancient piece-bag crammed with the flowered and dotted cottons that Grant Wood's sisters drew from for dressing dolls; or laid themselves together and were handstitched into a patchwork of homely comfort and thrift. *Popcorn Feast* the artist drew on a sheet of wrapping paper. *Spring Corn* is a promise in purple, rose, and blue-greens. The portraits range from a group of gangling and plump fowls called *Adolescence* to childhood and wistful boyhood. *Midsummer* and *Autumn* are reminders of American abundance.

The most thrilling art is regional. That is to say, homespun art. Grant Wood once said, "I have a strong feeling for the ground itself." So did the artists who painted the early primitives of Germany, the farms and misty forests of France, the peasant-posed Madonnas of Italy. So shall we, in a new world, follow the examples of our own early-American limners, the designers in iron, silver, glass, clay, who created whatever they found at hand. American art from today is simple and kindly, it pictures our daily life and our hopes for tomorrow. It is, like the work of Grant Wood, an expression of something we have loved and always wanted to set down, painted exactly as we see it and with the courage and honesty of a free American.

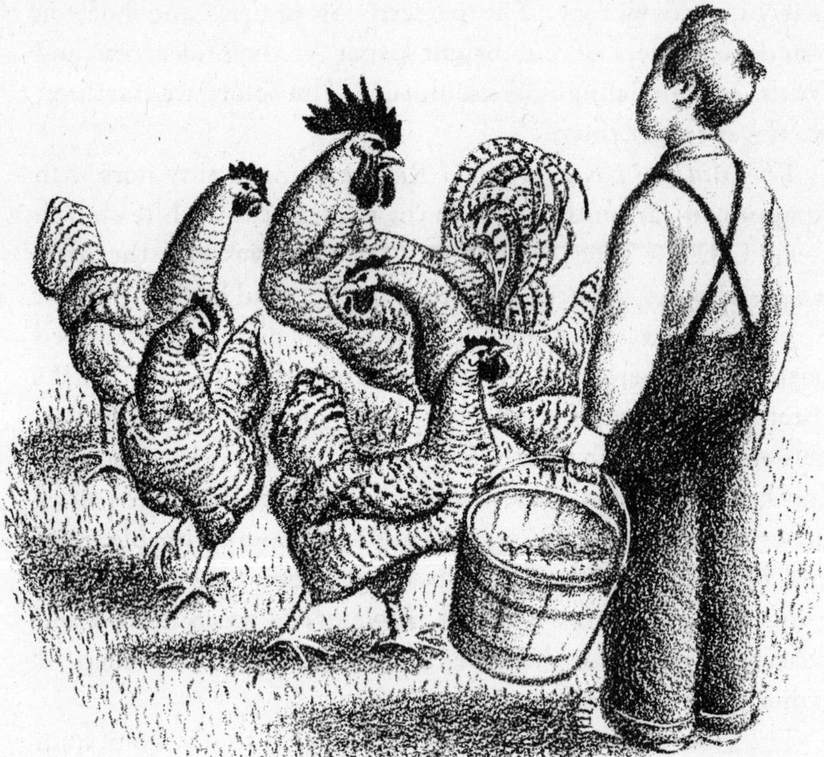

WHERE YOU MAY SEE GRANT WOOD'S PAINTINGS

American Gothic	The Collection of Friends of American Art, The Chicago Art Institute
Woman with Plant	The Collection of the Cedar Rapids Art Association, Cedar Rapids, Iowa
Fall Plowing	The Collection of Marshall Field, Chicago, Illinois
Arbor Day	The Collection of Edwin Hewitt, New York
Dinner for Threshers	The Collection of Stephen C. Clark, New York
Feeding the Chickens *The Blue Door* *The Cow Path* *The Old Sexton's Place*, and many others	The Collection of David Turner, Cedar Rapids, Iowa
Young Corn	The Collection of the Woodrow Wilson High School, Cedar Rapids, Iowa

Date D